The Little Black Book of
Pulmonary
Medicine

Series Editor: Daniel K. Onion

Edward Ringel, MD
MaineGeneral Medical Center
Waterville, ME
Adjunct Professor of Community
  and Family Medicine
Dartmouth Medical School

JONES AND BARTLETT PUBLISHERS
Sudbury, Massachusetts
BOSTON   TORONTO   LONDON   SINGAPORE

World Headquarters

Jones and Bartlett
  Publishers
40 Tall Pine Drive
Sudbury, MA 01776
978-443-5000
info@jbpub.com
www.jbpub.com

Jones and Bartlett
  Publishers Canada
6339 Ormindale Way
Mississauga,
Ontario L5V 1J2
CANADA

Jones and Bartlett
  Publishers
  International
Barb House, Barb Mews
London W6 7PA
United Kingdom

Jones and Bartlett's books and products are available through most bookstores
and online booksellers. To contact Jones and Bartlett Publishers directly, call
800-832-0034, fax 978-443-8000, or visit our website, www.jbpub.com.

Substantial discounts on bulk quantities of Jones and Bartlett's publications are available to corporations, professional associations, and other qualified organizations. For
details and specific discount information, contact the special sales department at
Jones and Bartlett via the above contact information, or send an email to
specialsales@jbpub.com.

Library of Congress Cataloging-in-Publication Data
Ringel, Edward.
    Little black book of pulmonary medicine / Edward Ringel.
        p. ; cm.
    Includes bibliographical references and index.
    ISBN-13: 978-0-7637-5244-6
    ISBN-10: 0-7637-5244-4
    1. Lungs—Diseases—Handbooks, manuals, etc.   I. Title.
    [DNLM: 1. Lung Diseases—Handbooks.   WF 39 R5811 2009]
      RC756.R56 2009
    616.2'4—dc22

                                                          2008029360

6048

Production Credits
Executive Publisher: Christopher Davis
Senior Acquisitions Editor:
  Nancy Anastasi Duffy
Associate Editor: Kathy Richardson
Editorial Assistant: Jessica Acox
Production Director: Amy Rose
Production Editor: Daniel Stone
Associate Marketing Manager: Ilana Goddess

Manufacturing and Inventory
  Coordinator: Therese Connell
Composition: ATLIS Graphics
Cover Design: Kristen E. Ohlin
Printing and Binding: Malloy, Inc.
Cover Printing: Malloy, Inc.

Printed in the United States of America
12   11   10   09   08   10   9   8   7   6   5   4   3   2   1

Dedication

This book is dedicated to the people of Central Maine, whom I have had the privilege to serve for these last 22 years. Thank you for all you taught me and your patience with me while I learned.

Contents

Preface

If you give a man a fish, you feed him for a day; if you teach a man to fish, you feed him for a lifetime.

—Author unknown

This book is intended for physicians and other clinicians in training and for the practicing primary care clinician. This target audience can benefit from a succinct guide and companion to the practice of pulmonary medicine. I avoid the use of the term *reference volume*; the *Little Black Book of Pulmonary Medicine* is not a reference. Rather, I have tried to write the book truly as a companion and guide. How does one approach the patient with cough? When should one refer a patient for bronchoscopy? How can one confirm a tentative diagnosis? It is my hope to help the reader learn to think out problems rather than matching patterns to descriptions of diseases. This volume is meant to teach the reader to fish.

The day-to-day practice of pulmonary subspecialty medicine is a mix of respiratory physiology, radiology, infectious disease, pulmonary medicine, and a dose of psychiatry thrown in on the side. A small number of diseases constitute a large component of daily practice and a thorough knowledge of the diagnosis and treatment of these problems and their common variants is the foundation of pulmonary primary care. At the same time, we must recognize when the peg is not fitting in the hole; to diagnose the less common condition, and to treat and/or refer as appropriate. To equip the reader to achieve these goals, the book is divided into three sections.

The first part of this book will help the reader understand the assessment process and provide practical guidance and algorithms for the evaluation of the cardinal signs of respiratory disease.

The second part of this book might be entitled "Tools of the Trade." Bronchoscopy, pulmonary function testing, and polysomnograms are often treated by the nonpulmonologist like a black box: If one puts the requisition or consult request in one end of the box, one gets a test result or therapeutic intervention out of the other. This often leads to suboptimal use of tests, results that are meaningless in the context of a particular patient, or a frightened, unprepared patient about to enter a procedure suite. This section will provide information on the tests and procedures that are unique to pulmonary medicine: how to use the test or procedure, how to understand the results, and how the more invasive procedures are conducted. Hopefully this will help the reader decide when a test or procedure is appropriate, understand the limitations of the procedure, interpret the results correctly, and counsel the patient wisely.

The last section is the largest, and is a discussion of the common and not so common diseases of respiratory medicine. It mostly adheres to the *Little Black Book* format of presentation and its signature feature of embedded references. The one area where the reader may take issue with my choice of subject matter is critical care. Although critical care is sometimes thought to be a subset of pulmonary medicine, it is not. I will limit my discussion of critical care other than respiratory failure to a very brief detour into sepsis. These two topics are so intertwined that it is impossible to address one without the other.

Two final thoughts. First, the author of a textbook tries to maintain some degree of neutrality in the presentation of the material, particularly controversial material. I have tried to sustain this neutrality of tone. However, this is a single author text. Inevitably, my approach to life and medicine will surface. For the record: I am therapeutically conservative, believe strongly in evidence-based medicine, and am a great fan of common sense. Second, I believe that thinking out problems is better than memorization and pattern recognition. This is the key to lifelong learning and allows one not to panic when facing the unexpected or the new. Throughout the book, I will try to emphasize that aspect of analysis. I also hope that emphasis on the thinking process will give the primary care clinician some insight into how a consultant approaches a problem. This will improve communication and patient care, our collective goal.

Edward Ringel, MD

Acknowledgments

My thanks to:

Dan Onion, for asking me to write this book.

Chris Davis, Kathy Richardson, Nancy Duffy, Dan Stone, Mark Goodin, and all the good folks at Jones and Bartlett for their encouragement and assistance.

Dave Hay, an already published co-author in the series, for his unflagging encouragement and sympathetic ear while I grumbled and sputtered.

Cora Damon, our Waterville librarian at MaineGeneral Medical Center, who was amazingly helpful in getting references. This book could not have happened without her help. Also, Barbara Harness, our Augusta librarian at MaineGeneral, who did an equally wonderful job when Cora was not around. Thank you both!!

Drs. Kristin Holm, Rick Hobbs, and Jenny Pisculli for wading through sentence fragments and half-baked concepts and making sure I didn't say anything too outrageous. I thank you all for spending the time reading my drafts when you could have done something else far more interesting.

I reserve my greatest thanks for my wife, Eileen Ringel, MD, and my daughters Julia and Meredith. Their love, support, and patience as I ground through all things pulmonary was a gift.

How to Use This Book

First, some caveats:

1. I am not perfect. My editor is not perfect. My sources are not perfect. My reviewers are not perfect. Although every effort has been made to assure the accuracy of the statements and observations made, this book is not warranted as 100% accurate and should not be treated as the final arbiter of all things pulmonary. In particular, drug doses and interventional recommendations must be tempered with *your* knowledge of *your* patient. Many of the drugs mentioned are technically used off-label. That's not necessarily a bad thing, and it is done commonly by almost all physicians. However, it requires greater vigilance on the part of the prescriber.

2. This book is not, by any means, complete. It is a guide and introduction, and by necessity information has been left out. There is a rich and vibrant intellectual life in pulmonary medicine; we just scratch the surface here. Just because the condition isn't covered in this book doesn't mean it doesn't exist or is heretofore unreported. Please check original sources, and use the excellent search tools available to round out your understanding and education.

3. Use common sense. If the article doesn't make sense, perhaps there is a reason. Are you assessing your patient using methodology developed for a different target group? Have you overlooked some critical piece of information in the history? Do you need to consider an additional diagnosis? Inconsistencies can be more of an inspiration than an obstacle.

4. The use of brand names for equipment, drugs, or similar is for informational purposes only. With the exception of the Bibliography section, no explicit or implicit endorsement of any product is implied by any article.

5. Although I may incur the criticism of readers for this decision, I have elected to provide only general recommendations regarding medication dosages. Many patients have multisystem disease and may be taking multiple medications. Drug interactions, age, allergies and sensitivities, and chronic renal and/or hepatic insufficiency demand careful, individualized drug selection and dosing decisions. There are numerous tools and resources available electronically and in print to assist the reader in this regard. Use them.

This book is divided conceptually into three parts. The first part (Chapter 1) presents a methodology for approaching the most common presenting complaints in pulmonary disease. "Approach to the Patient with . . ." sections in most medical texts have addressed traditional signs and symptoms: dyspnea, chest pain, diarrhea, and so on. The cardinal signs and symptoms of pulmonary disease are, of course, included. I have added sections on the evaluation of other indicators of pulmonary disease: unexpected hypoxia from pulse oximetry, pulmonary hypertension identified on echocardiography, and unanticipated X-ray findings. In my interactions over the years with primary clinicians, I have been impressed at the frequency of referrals that stem from these unexpected test results.

The second section addresses the practical aspects of diagnosing and treating pulmonary disease. Pulmonary medicine uses tests and interventions that are widely prescribed and sometimes poorly understood. Interpretation of pulmonary function studies, the appropriate prescription of oxygen, inhaled medications, and the limitations of bronchoscopy are some of the items that are reviewed. These topics are not well covered in other introductory texts, and can be vexing to the house officer or frontline practitioner. These subjects are covered in Chapters 2 and 3.

The third section is a guide to many of the common diseases that affect the lungs. This encompasses the rest of the book, from Chapter 4 on. The list is not all-inclusive. Conditions covered, however, constitute over 95% of my specialist practice. Many texts take the approach of grouping airways diseases, parenchymal diseases, pleural diseases, and vascular diseases as separate sections. This approach is arbitrary and misleading. Sarcoid, commonly considered a parenchymal disease, has significant airway manifestations. Likewise, scleroderma can affect the vasculature and the interstitium. Classification, therefore is pretty much mix and match. The major exception is pulmonary infectious disease; divisions among pathogens are self-evident. Some diseases are quite uncommon but have historical interest, have unique pathology, or are instructive as to disease mechanisms, and I have included them to provide perspective and intellectual stimulation. For example, new cases of many of the inorganic dust diseases, such as silicosis and asbestosis, are today almost never seen because the older patients, exposed before occupational safety rules were implemented, have died.

When appropriate, I have tried to provide a brief overview in each article that explains how I integrate and assess the subject in the aggregate. When possible, pathophysiologic mechanisms are provided to help develop the reader's ability to extrapolate knowledge and data. Pathophysiology is worth the extra minute or two of reading. I have also made a decision to provide a large number of review and textbook references. These references have been chosen for their readability, conciseness, and interest as well as their information content. For most readers, the references will be an enjoyable and appropriate next step in expanding their knowledge base, and I urge you to read beyond this book. Where data is new, controversial, or seminal, primary sources will be provided. This book aims to teach solid, middle-of-theroad, high-quality 2008 pulmonary care and to ride neither the cutting nor bleeding edge of medicine.

Medical Abbreviations

ABPA	allergic bronchopulmonary aspergillosis	BOOP	bronchiolitis obliterans with organizing pneumonia
ACB	active cycle breathing	BX	biopsy
ACCP	American College of Chest Physicians	CAP	community acquired pneumonia
ACE	angiotensin-converting enzyme	CD4	cluster of differentiation 4 (marker on T lymphocyte cell surface)
ADL	activity of daily living		
AECB	acute exacerbation of chronic bronchitis		
AECOPD	acute exacerbation of chronic obstructive pulmonary disease	CDB	coughing and deep breathing
		CDC	Centers for Disease Control
AEP	acute eosinophilic pneumonia	CEP	chronic eosinophilic pneumonia
AHI	apnea hypopnea index	CF	cystic fibrosis
AICD	automatic implantable cardiac defibrillator	CFC	chlorofluorocarbon
		CFU	colony forming units
AIP	acute interstitial pneumonitis	CHF	congestive heart failure
		CMI	cell-mediated immunity
ANA	antinuclear antibody	CMS	Center for Medicare and Medicaid Services
ANCA	anti-neutrophilic cytoplasmic antibody		
ARF	acute respiratory failure	CoHB	carboxyhemoglobin
ATS	American Thoracic Society	COP	cryptogenic organizing pneumonia
		COPD	chronic obstructive pulmonary disease
BAL	bronchoalveolar lavage		
BHL	bilateral hilar lymphadenopathy	CPET	cardiopulmonary exercise testing
BNP	brain natriuretic peptide	CRP	C-reactive protein
		CSA	central sleep apnea

CSS	Churg-Strauss syndrome	HELLP	hemolytic anemia, elevated liver enzymes, low platelet count (variant of eclampsia/pre-eclampsia)
CT	computed tomography		
CWP	coal workers pneumoconiosis		
CXR	chest X-ray	HFA	hydrofluoroalkane
		HHT	hereditary hemorrhagic telangectasia
DFA	direct fluorescent antibody		
DIP	desquamative interstitial pneumonitis	HIT	heparin-induced thrombocytopenia
DLCO	diffusing capacity of the lung for carbon monoxide	HIV+	human immunodeficiency virus antigen positive
DM	diabetes mellitus	HP	hypersensitivity pneumonitis
DPI	dry powder inhaler		
DPLD	diffuse parenchymal lung disease	HRCP	health care related pneumonia
DRSP	drug resistant S. pneumoniae	HRCT	high-resolution computed tomography
		HRT	hormone replacement therapy
EG	eosinophilic granuloma		
EIA	exercise-induced asthma		
ENT	ear, nose, and throat	IBW	ideal body weight
ERS	European Respiratory Society	ICS	inhaled corticosteroids
		IDSA	Infectious Disease Society of America
ESR	erythrocyte sedimentation rate	IPAH	idiopathic pulmonary artery hypertension
ET	endotracheal		
FOB	fiberoptic bronchoscopy	IVDU	intravenous drug user
FRC	functional residual capacity	KS	kyphoscoliosis
GB	Guillain-Barre	LAM	lymphangioleiomyomatosis
GU	genitourinary		
		LBB	Little Black Book
H&E	hematoxylin and eosin	LED	light-emitting diode
H2	histamin-2 receptor	LFE	lesson from experience
HAART	highly active anti-retroviral therapy	LMWH	low molecular weight heparin

LOX	liquid oxygen	OSHA	Occupational Safety and
LTRA	leukotriene receptor		Health Administration
	antagonist		
LVRS	lung volume reduction	PAH	pulmonary artery
	surgery		hypertension
		PAP	pulmonary alveolar
M. Tb	*Mycobacterium tuberculosis*		proteinosis
MAC	Mycobacterium avium	PCJ	*Pneumocystis jerovicii*
	complex	PCP	primary care practitioner
MALT	mucosa associated	PCR	polymerase chain reaction
	lymphoid tumor	PCV	pressure controlled
MDI	metered dose inhaler		ventilation
MDRTB	multidrug- resistant	PE	pulmonary embolism
	tuberculosis	PEEP	positive end expiratory
MI	myocardial infarction		pressure
MPA	microscopic polyangiitis	PFT	pulmonary function test
MRC	Medical Research Council	PH	pulmonary hypertension
	(U.K.)	PLM	periodic limb
MRSA	methicillin-resistant		movement(s)
	staphylococcus aureus	PMF	progressive massive fibrosis
MSDS	material safety data	PMN	polymorphonuclear
	sheet	PND	paroxysmal nocturnal
			dyspnea
NIPPV	noninvasive positive	PPD	packs per day
	pressure ventilation	PPI	proton pump inhibitor
NOTT	Nocturnal Oxygen	pred.	predicted
	Therapy Trial	PSG	polysomnogram
NPMV	negative pressure	PSS	progressive systemic
	mechanical ventilation		sclerosis
NSAID	nonsteroidal anti-	PTX	pneumothorax
	inflammatory drug		
NTG	nitroglycerin	RAST	radioallergosorbent test
NTM	non tuberculous	RB	respiratory bronchiolitis
	mycobacteria	RBILD	respiratory bronchiolitis
			interstitial lung disease
OLB	open lung biopsy	RCP	respiratory care
OSA	obstructive sleep apnea		practitioner

RCT	randomized controlled trial	TMP	trimethoprim
RDI	respiratory distress index	TMP/ SMX	trimethoprim/ sulfamethoxasole
RF	radio frequency	TTNB	transthoracic needle biopsy
RILI	radiation-induced lung injury		
		UIP	usual interstitial pneumonitis
SDB	sleep-disordered breathing		
SIADH	syndrome of inappropriate antidiuretic hormone secretion	V/Q	ventilation/perfusion
		VATS	video-assisted thoracic surgery
SIRS	systemic inflammatory response syndrome	VCD	vocal cord dysfunction
SLE	systemic lupus erythematosus	VILI	ventilator-induced lung injury
SPN	solitary pulmonary nodule		
		WBC	white blood cell
TBLB	transbronchial lung biopsy	WG	Wegener's granulomatosis
TLC	total lung capacity		

Journal Abbreviations

Acad Radiol	Academic Radiology
Acta Cytol	Acta Cytologica
Am J Emerg Med	American Journal of Emergency Medicine
Am Fam Physician	American Family Physician
Am Heart J	American Heart Journal
Am Rev Respir Dis	American Review of Respiratory Disease
Am J Med	American Journal of Medicine
Am J Med Sci	American Journal of Medical Science
Am J Hematol	American Journal of Hematology
Am J Kidney Dis	American Journal of Kidney Diseases
Am J Respir Crit Care Med	American Journal of Respiratory and Critical Care Medicine
Am J Physiol Lung Cell Mol Physiol	American Journal of Physiology: Lung Cellular and Molecular Physiology
Am J Roentgenol	American Journal of Roentgenology
Anaesthesia	Anaesthesia
Anesthesiology	Anesthesiology
Anesthesiol Clin North America	Anesthesiology of North America
Ann Oncol	Annals of Oncology
Ann Pharmacother	Annals of Pharmacotherapy
Ann Intern Med	Annals of Internal Medicine
Ann Rheum Dis	Annals of the Rheumatic Diseases
Ann Thorac Surg	Annals of Thoracic Surgery
Annu Rev Med	Annual Review of Medicine

Antimicrob Agents Chemother	Antimicrobial Agents and Chemotherapy
Arch Dis Child	Archives of Disease in Childhood
Arch Neurol	Archives of Neurology
Arthritis Rheum	Arthritis and Rheumatism
Aust Crit Care	Australian Critical Care
Br Med Bull	British Medical Bulletin
Br Med J (BMJ)	British Medical Journal
Br J Dis Chest	British Journal of Diseases of the Chest
CJEM	Canadian Journal of Emergency Medicine
CMAJ	Canadian Medical Association Journal
Cancer Control	Cancer Control (Journal of the Moffitt Cancer Center)
Cardiol Clin	Clinical Cardiology
Chest	Chest
Chest Surg Clin N Am	Chest Surgery Clinics of North America
Cleveland Clin J Med	Cleveland Clinic Journal of Medicine
Clin Chest Med	Clinics in Chest Medicine
Clin Infect Dis	Clinical Infectious Diseases
Clin Immunol Immunopathol	Clinical Immunology and Immunopathology
Clin Microbiol Rev	Clinical Microbiology Reviews
Crit Care Clin	Critical Care Clinics
Crit Care Med	Critical Care Medicine
Curr Opin Infect Dis	Current Opinions in Infectious Diseases
Curr Infect Dis Rep	Current Infectious Disease Reports
Curr Opin Pulm Med	Current Opinion in Pulmonary Medicine

Curr Opin Rheumatol	Current Opinion in Rheumatology
Drugs Today	Drugs of Today
Dis Chest	Diseases of the Chest
Emerg Infect Dis	Emerging Infectious Diseases
Emerg Med Clin North Am	Emergency Medical Clinics of North America
Emerg Med J	Emergency Medical Journal
Environ Health Perspective	Environmental Health Perspectives
Eur J Clin Microbiol Infect Dis	European Journal of Clinical Microbiology and Infectious Diseases
Eur Radiol	European Radiology
Eur Respir J	European Respiratory Journal
Expert Opin Investig Drugs	Expert Opinion on Investigational Drugs
Expert Opin Pharmacother	Expert Opinion on Pharmacotherapy
Geriatrics	Geriatrics
Hazard Review	Hazard Review
Infect Dis Clin N Am	Infectious Disease Clinics of North America
Indian J Chest Dis Allied Sci	Indian Journal of Chest Diseases and Allied Sciences
Int J Tuberc Lung Dis	International Journal of Tuberculosis and Lung Disease
Int J Clin Pract	International Journal of Clinical Practice
JAMA	Journal of the American Medical Association
J Am Coll Cardiol	Journal of the American College of Cardiology

J Am Paraplegia Soc	Journal of the American Paraplegia Society
J Clin Invest	Journal of Clinical Investigation
J Clin Oncol	Journal of Clinical Oncology
J Clin Microbiol	Journal of Clinical Microbiology
J Clin Virol	Journal of Clinical Virology
J Emerg Med	Journal of Emergency Medicine
J Gen Intern Med	Journal of General Internal Medicine
J Heart Lung Transplant	Journal of Heart and Lung Transplantation
J Intensive Care Med	Journal of Intensive Care Medicine
J Med Invest	Journal of Medical Investigation
J Neurol	Journal of Neurology
J Pain Symptom Manage	Journal of Pain and Symptom Management
J Rheumatol	Journal of Rheumatology
J Thorac Cardiovasc	Journal of Thoracic and Cardiovascular Surgery
J Thorac Imaging	Journal of Thoracic Imaging
Kidney Int	Kidney International
Lancet	Lancet
Lancet Infect Dis	Lancet Infectious Diseases
Mayo Clin Proc	Mayo Clinic Proceedings
Mastery of Surgery	Master of Surgery
Med Clin North Am	Medical Clinics of North America
Medicine [Baltimore]	Medicine (Baltimore)
Nat Clin Pract Oncol	National Clinical Practice Oncology
N Engl J Med	New England Journal of Medicine

Occup Environ Med	Occupational and Environmental Medicine
Postgrad Med J	Postgraduate Medicine Journal
Prim Care	Primary Care
Radiographics	Radiographics: A Review Publication of the Radiological Society of North America
Radiology	Radiology
Respiration	Respiration: International Review of Thoracic Diseases
Respir Care	Respiratory Care
Respir Care Clin N Am	Respiratory Care Clinics of North America
Respir Med	Respiratory Medicine
Respir Physiol	Respiration Physiology
Rheum Dis Clin North Am	Rheumatic Disease Clinics of North America
Scand J Infect Dis	Scandinavian Journal of Infectious Disease
Semin Arthritis Rheum	Seminars in Arthritis and Rheumatism
Semin Neurol	Seminars in Neurology
Semin Respir Crit Care Med	Seminars in Respiratory and Critical Care Medicine
Semin Respir Infect	Seminars in Respiratory Infections
Semin Thorac Cardiovasc Surg	Seminars in Thoracic and Cardivascular Surgery
Sleep	Sleep
Thorax	Thorax
Thorac Surg Clin	Thoracic Surgery Clinics
Thromb Res	Thrombosis Research
Treat Respir Med	Treatments in Respiratory Medicine
West J Med	Western Journal of Medicine

Notice

We have made every attempt to summarize accurately and concisely a multitude of references. However, the reader is reminded that times and medical knowledge change, transcription or understanding error is always possible, and crucial details are omitted whenever such a comprehensive distillation as this is attempted in limited space. And the primary purpose of this compilation is to cite literature on various sides of controversial issues; knowing where "truth" lies is usually difficult. We cannot, therefore, guarantee that every bit of information is absolutely accurate or complete. The reader should affirm that cited recommendations are reasonable still, by reading the original articles and checking other sources, including local consultants as well as recent literature, before applying them.

Drugs and medical devices are discussed that may have limited availability controlled by the Food and Drug Administration (FDA) for use only in research study or clinical trial. The drug information presented has been derived from reference sources, recently published data, and pharmaceutical tests. Research, clinical practice, and government regulations often change the accepted standard in this field. When consideration is being given to use of any drug in the clinical setting, the clinician or reader is responsible for determining FDA status of the drug, reading the package insert, and prescribing information for the most up-to-date recommendations on dose, precautions, and contraindications and determining the appropriate usage for the product. This is especially important in the case of drugs that are new or seldom used.

Chapter 1

Approach to the Patient with Pulmonary Disease

1.1   Introduction

Pulmonary diagnosis depends on history, imaging, and pulmonary function testing. Physical examination plays a lesser role. Initial evaluation often consists of a history, exam, chest X-ray, pulmonary function testing if indicated, and some basic blood testing. If a diagnosis is not clear, further testing and sometimes further interviews are indicated. Because the respiratory system interfaces so intimately with our physical surroundings, environmental history, in the broadest sense, is much more important than in many other areas of medicine. Additionally, because the lungs are the target of so many infectious agents and environmental insults, a clear picture of the patient's immune status, nutrition, habits, work and home environment, travel, and comorbid conditions is critical. I refer to this gestalt view of the patient as *host ecology*.

The majority of patients with respiratory illness will present with a limited number of complaints. Cough, wheeze, sputum, and dyspnea are the most common. Chest pain can be associated with respiratory disease, but the clinician should be mindful of the many nonpulmonary conditions that cause chest pain; the lungs may not be at the top of the list. Hemoptysis is a less common but serious complaint. The sections on taking the pulmonary history and initial analysis of presenting complaints are complementary and should be used together.

Increasingly, because of the wide net of tests cast when evaluating a medical problem, the practitioner may find him- or herself responding to an abnormal test result as the sole presenting symptom of pulmonary disease. Hypoxia identified by finger oximetry (the 5th vital sign in many emergency rooms), pulmonary hypertension on echocardiography, and the incidental pulmonary nodule found on a shoulder X-ray are sufficiently common that they warrant review. Some sense of how to handle these problems will be reviewed. A basic introduction to chest radiology, particularly with an eye to initial diagnostic decision making, will also be presented.

Finally, the practitioner is faced with complaints of snoring and sleep disruption. These are increasingly identified by the public as legitimate issues to bring to their practitioner, and the obesity epidemic is making sleep-disordered breathing more common. A short introduction to assessing the patient with sleep complaints is presented.

1.2 The Pulmonary History

Zackon 2000;885

General: It is important to get a sense of the general "ecology" of the patient. Age is decisive. Major chronic illnesses such as congestive heart failure, diabetes, and alcohol abuse markedly increase morbidity of respiratory infections. Alcohol abuse and drug use predispose to aspiration and some specific infections. Recent or concurrent contact with the medical care system alters empiric therapy of pneumonia. Some medications are associated with specific hypersensitivity and lung injury syndromes. Neurologic conditions are associated with restrictive thoracic disorders, hypoventilation, and aspiration. Prior radiation therapy (for malignancy of breast, lymphoma, thymus, lung, thyroid) can cause radiologic abnormalities and pneumonitis. Concurrent collagen vascular diseases have specific pulmonary syndromes (see **Rheu-**

matologic **Lung Disease**). Malnutrition alters immunity. Underlying cardiovascular disease confounds evaluation of dyspnea and can produce chest X-ray changes.

Immunocompetency: HIV predisposes to certain infectious and noninfectious conditions. Transplant recipients and patients with chronic use of prednisone have different infections than neutropenic patients undergoing chemotherapy. Congenital immune deficiency syndromes, although rare, have specific associated infections. Asplenic patients control *S. pneumoniae* infection poorly and are more likely to have septicemia. Gastrectomy, HIV infection, and diabetes predispose to TB infection.

Tobacco Use: Quantification in pack-years (1 PPD × 10 years = 10 pack-years; 2 PPD × 5 years = 10 pack-years, etc.). Time interval since quitting should be sought as risk of various complications recedes as time passes.

Dyspnea: Dyspnea evaluation assists both diagnosis and monitoring of therapy. It is a nonspecific symptom, and the clinician may need to help the patient differentiate true air hunger from fatigue ("Are you tired or out of breath?"). Course of dyspnea may be chronic or acute; onset may be abrupt or insidious. Character may be steady, progressive, or intermittent. Positional characteristics (orthopnea, platypnea) are often associated with cardiac disease. Precipitating factors should be elicited (exercise, cold air, smoke, medications, specific activities such as arm work vs. leg work). Ameliorating factors (stopping activity, inhaler, NTG) should be identified. Respiratory dyspnea, like cardiac dyspnea, can be associated with a bandlike feeling around the chest. Do not assume dyspnea is pulmonary in origin. Quantification of dyspnea may be difficult. It is appealing to use tools such as the Borg scale or other metrics, but there are drawbacks as well (see **Dyspnea**). Many clinicians find it more useful to put the question in context of personal activity. From the standpoint of therapeutic monitoring, it is much easier to ask "Since we started that inhaler, can you now walk up to your bedroom?" Useful metrics include: stairs, inclines, flat ground, with or without packages, up and down stairs to do laundry, vacuuming (uses both arms and legs), outside chores; in a rural area the walk out to the mailbox. In a vigorous, healthy person scaling of dyspnea may be different ("I can only run 1 mile instead of 2; this is a problem.") Be careful to avoid the gotchas: "Sure, I can mow the lawn," but the patient uses a riding mower; "I play 18 holes of golf," but she uses a cart, etc. *Do not* ask "Can you do everything you want to?" Many chronically ill patients unconsciously circumscribe their activity and believe they are doing everything they want to. Use specific tests of activity.

Cough: This is a nonspecific symptom. It may be generated by lower or upper respiratory tract, and distinguishing between the two is the first task. The characterization of cough with respect to duration, abrupt or insidious onset, progressive, intermittent, or stable all characterize the problem. Exacerbating and ameliorating factors should be elicited. Determine if the cough is productive, nonproductive, and/or associated with hemoptysis. Medication history may be important (e.g., ACE cough). Associated gagging and cough syncope are nonspecific ancillary findings that mean the patient can achieve high intrathoracic and intra-abdominal pressures. Initial evaluation should include appropriate ENT and GI questions (postnasal drip, hoarseness, reflux). Morning cough is a common respiratory complaint and is nonspecific.

Sputum Production: This is a nonspecific symptom. Sputum may be generated by the upper or lower respiratory tract. Association with fever should be considered pneumonia until proven otherwise and mandates vigorous, immediate workup. Green/yellow color is due more to presence of neutrophils than bacteria and is not a reliable indicator of bacterial infection. Foul smell can be associated with anaerobic infection. Sputum can have descriptors including thick, thin, watery, color, amount per day, and if the amount is increasing or decreasing over time.

Hemoptysis: New onset hemoptysis is frightening to the patient and should be to the clinician. The first step is to differentiate from oral, ENT, and GI bleeding. "Coughing up blood" is *not* reliable. Both ENT and dental bleeding are often coughed out of the upper airway. The bleeding should be characterized as to how long, new or old blood, increasing or decreasing in amount and severity. Amount (as with bleeding symptoms from all organ systems) is routinely misreported. Association with sputum, dyspnea, and chest pain can provide direction. Association with constitutional symptoms (weight loss, fever, malaise, lack of energy) suggests malignancy or chronic infection. The use of anticoagulants will not cause spontaneous bleeding from normal tissue at normal levels of anticoagulation; the tissue is abnormal and/or there has been injury such as cough. Chronic low-grade hemoptysis of limited clinical significance is common with bronchiectasis and bronchitis, but this must be an established, long-standing diagnosis before the clinician elects no further workup.

Chest Pain: Pain from the lower respiratory tract implies irritation of the chest wall and/or pleura. The presence of pain receptors within the airways or lung parenchyma is controversial (see **Chest Pain**). Chest pain can be characterized using the usual pain template: where, how long, how bad, character, what makes it better, what makes it worse. Pleuritic chest pain is typically associated with respiration. Chronic unremitting chest pain is often musculoskeletal but can represent invasion of pleura/chest wall by malignancy, infection, or rib fracture. Acute chest pain in the adult, unless "classically" musculoskeletal or pleuritic, is cardiac until proven otherwise. A complete discussion of cardiac chest pain is beyond the scope of this book, but should be thoroughly reviewed (see **Chest Pain**).

Wheezing: This symptom is specific for obstruction of the airway in either the lower or upper respiratory tract. The symptom may be characterized as abrupt or insidious in onset, constant or intermittent. Ameliorating and exacerbating factors and triggers should be explored. Circadian and seasonal variation may be present. Wheezing may occur on inspiration, expiration, or both, and may be a sign of possible aspiration. Association with voice change or hoarseness suggests upper airway location. If wheezing disappears when the patient is distracted, consider psychogenic causes or vocal cord dysfunction. A monophonic wheeze (single note of one pitch) suggests single airway obstruction such as with malignancy or foreign body. Polyphonic wheeze (lots of notes, many pitches) suggests diffuse airway obstruction such as that seen in asthma.

Snoring/Disturbances of Sleep: It is useful to have bed partner (if there is one) available at the interview. Major issues here are to see if: (1) is there more than snoring present (snoring is prevalent in the population almost to the point of being unusable as a symptom), (2) if daytime somnolence has a respiratory or nonrespiratory etiology, and (3) what the best diagnostic strategy is. Ask about snoring, movement, leg jerking. Is there a sleep position that worsens snoring? Determine if sleep talking or sleep walking are present. Violent, repetitive dreams with physical activity during the dream suggests REM behavior disorder. Sleep paralysis or hypnogogic hallucinations may be present. Daytime sleepiness is sometimes difficult to quantify. Many patients with significant disease on polysomnography can drive, work, etc. but crash when they come home. Differentiate sleepiness ("I want to lie down and take a nap") from physical fatigue ("I've worked hard for 3 hours; I'm tired and going to put my feet up"). A convincing history of cataplexy, a symptom associated with narcolepsy, can be elusive. The classic description is that of the patient losing tone in postural muscles in the context of strong emotional experience (anger, laughter, surprise). However, patients may not have classic symptoms; ask about strange feelings, "electric shocks," momentarily can't speak, anything out of the ordinary in the context of an experience with a strong emotional content (good or bad.). Stimulants, sedatives (Rx or not, caffeine, alcohol), and relation to bedtime should be explored. Determine bedtime and bed activities: exercise prior to bedtime, bedtime activities (reading, TV/radio on/off, etc.), actual bedtime, and rise time. Characterize awakenings if present: activities during awakenings, how does patient try and get back to sleep? Bedroom conditions: comfortable temperature, comfortable bed, dark, quiet, pets (not mentioned in texts, but pets are a common source of sleep disruption). In addition to daytime sleepiness, presence of headaches, cognitive impairment, sexual dysfunction, emotional lability/depression, and cardiovascular disease are associated with sleep-disordered breathing.

Environmental History: Home type: manufactured, carpenter built on site, apartment. Concrete or dirt basement. Carpets, animals. Heating fuel (wood, oil, gas, coal) and system (forced hot air, baseboard hot water, radiator). Wet or dry basement, kitchen, bathroom. Use of humidifiers, dehumidifiers. Hobbies. Vermin: mice in the basement, bats in the attic, birds in the eaves, pigeons on the air conditioners, cockroaches in the walls. Clinician should be aware of local environmental factors such as types of polluting industry, local heating practices (e.g., lots of wood stoves in Maine), endemic illnesses (histoplasmosis, coccidioidomycosis), local types of pollen.

Occupational History: (1) Find out *every* job the patient ever held (many patients do not count their military experience or summer jobs in college as jobs; often need to ask specifically). (2) Understand exactly what the patient did in that job, what materials they used, where they did their work, and what other people were doing around them (example: electrician putting cabling in the hold of a warship in 1940s handled no asbestos but had a massive exposure because coworker was insulating steam pipes 3 feet away in an enclosed space). Taking an occupational history is fun. Patients love to talk about their work even if they hate their job (Turkel, Working 1970), and your questioning gives you time to learn about your patient and to establish rapport. Clinician should have some knowledge of local industry and local occupations that present a respiratory exposure hazard. Individual worksite issues include presence or absence of respiratory protection, ventilation, and OSHA citations. Review MSDS if appropriate. If litigation or workmen's compensation case, meticulous documentation is mandatory. Many exposures have a significant latency to disease; the clinician may need to be a detective.

Other Relevant Organ Systems: Useful to inquire about ankle edema, paroxysmal nocturnal dyspnea, angina, and anginal equivalents (see **Chest Pain**). Recent loss of consciousness or dental work, or intoxications may be associated with aspiration. Reflux symptoms, allergic symptoms, and postnasal drip symptoms are relevant to asthma history.

1.3   Chest Pain

Introduction: Chest pain is a cardinal presentation of disease and is often an indication of serious illness. Misdiagnosis of chest pain is potentially lethal, and research has been applied to the development of accurate, cost-effective algorithms for this problem. Multiple disease etiologies can cause chest pain: cardiac, pulmonary, gastrointestinal, musculoskeletal, and vascular. Many etiologies have overlapping presentations, and diagnosis frequently requires additional testing. Pulmonary etiologies of chest pain often cannot be dissected out of a patient's complaint at presentation. *Almost all authorities agree that in the absence of trauma, acute chest pain should be considered cardiac in etiology until actively* *proven to be otherwise*. Chronic chest pain does not have this stipulation, but still should be approached with caution.

Pathophysiology: Chief sources of acute chest pain include the heart, the esophagus, the pulmonary vasculature, and the pleura. In most practitioners' experience, musculoskeletal chest pain is far and away the most common. Visceral organs have a dual innervation with visceral and somatic fibers. Visceral innervation for organs in the chest is the vagus nerve. Somatic fibers are spinal afferents. This dual innervation interaction is probably responsible for perception of visceral pain on the skin surface, difficulty localizing pain, and referred pain. The chest wall has somatic innervation alone. Although long thought that the respiratory tract did not have pain receptors, this is probably incorrect, and the tracheobronchial tree can respond to irritation with a sensation of pain.

Characterization: Location: substernal, back, diffuse, lateral, shoulder, arm, unilateral, bilateral. Character: crushing, burning, pleuritic (associated with breathing), ripping, fullness, band of constriction are common terms. Associated symptoms: nausea, dyspnea, diaphoresis, eructation, cardiovascular collapse, hemoptysis. Exacerbates: activity, food, position. Ameliorates: rest, nitrates, antacids, position.

Differential Diagnosis: There are a limited number of acute syndromes of chest pain that the clinician will encounter commonly. Unfortunately, this comes down to pattern recognition. See Table 1.1 for the patterns.

Further Testing: Most patients presenting with acute chest pain at an emergency care center will have an electrocardiogram, chest X-ray, and cardiac enzymes including troponin. Biochemical indicators of cardiac injury such as troponin have limitations in terms of both sensitivity and specificity (J Emerg Med 2002;23:57). Further testing may include hospitalization with observation for serial enzymes and ECG, acute stress testing, and acute imaging

Table 1.1   Prototypical Chest Pain Syndromes

Acute Coronary Syndrome	Substernal, crushing or squeezing with radiation into neck or jaw, associated with nausea, diaphoresis, relieved by rest, nitrates, or opiates. Sustained pain suggests infarction rather than ischemia. Variability is very wide.
Pulmonary Embolism	Sudden, pleuritic, associated with dyspnea, occasionally with hemoptysis. Also highly variable presentation.
Pneumonia	Onset often over hours. Pain is pleuritic, usually unilateral. Fever, sputum, and hemoptysis commonly accompany the pain.
Pneumothorax	Sudden, unilateral, pleuritic or sharp, associated with dyspnea.
Pericarditis	Gradual onset, pleuritic, often relieved by change in position. May not lateralize, or may lateralize to either side of the chest.
Aortic Dissection	Severe, sudden ripping or tearing pain, sense of impending doom, often radiates to back. May be associated with cardiovascular collapse.
Esophageal Disease	Burning, may also mimic angina. Can be partially or completely resolved with antacids.
Costochondritis	Dull, achy, worse with cough or movement. May reproduce with palpation of the chest wall.
Zoster	Burning, dysesthesia, unilateral. Symptoms may precede typical vesicular lesions
Tracheobronchitis	Central, described as raw or pleuritic.
Chronic Chest Pain	Occurs from chronic conditions: malignancy, chronic infections, pleural effusion, pericardial effusion, arthritic conditions of chest wall. Post-herpetic pain is common, described as burning. Post-traumatic and post-surgical pain may persist for months, especially with involvement of costal nerves.

with CT, cardiac catheterization. A full discussion of the cardiac evaluation is beyond the scope of this book. Suspected pumonary embolism may be further evaluated with D-dimer assays, ventilation perfusion scanning, and spiral CT scanning. Diagnosis of pulmonary embolism is complex (see **Pulmonary Embolism**).

Pneumonia or other infection is usually evident on chest X-ray. For further testing and treatment appropriate to presentation see **Approach to the Patient with Suspected Pneumonia.** Pneumothorax, pleural effusion, and malignancy are usually evident on chest X-ray. Zoster is usually evident on exam but can occasionally be confusing when pain precedes rash. Aortic dissection is suggested by mediastinal widening, proven by CT scan or echocardiogram. Esophageal disease may be diagnosed by response to therapy, upper GI, endoscopy (Ann Emerg Med 2006;47:1, Am Fam Physician 2005;72:2012).

Specific Therapy: Opiates, nitrates for cardiac pain; opiates for pleuritic pain of pulmonary embolism. NSAIDs for pleuritic, costochondritic pain if appropriate. Esophageal pain often responds to nitrates, antacids; PPIs and H2 blockers may be helpful acutely and chronically. Pain of malignant or infectious invasion of bones, pleura may require high-dose opiates and specialized techniques such as nerve block. Neuropathic and postherpetic neuralgia respond to gabapentin (Cochrane Database Syst Rev 2005;CD005452) and capsaicin (J Neurol 1991;238:452), although the latter works only in a limited number of patients.

1.4 Cough

N Engl J Med 1979;300:633, a classic; Am J Respir Crit Care Med 2002;165:1469, interesting and provocative

Introduction: Cough is a common symptom of respiratory disease, upper respiratory tract disease, and gastrointestinal disease. In evaluating a cough, the main questions are: (1) Is this coming from the respiratory tract? (2) Is it a nuisance, or is it a manifestation of a serious problem? (3) What are the appropriate steps to achieve a diagnosis? As with many other pulmonary symptoms, the company it keeps provides the answer. Cough is a nonspecific symptom that gives little direction to the clinician. When cough is a presenting symptom, its course can also be monitored as an indicator of therapeutic success/failure as the patient is treated.

Pathophysiology: The respiratory tract has few means of expressing its displeasure or its irritation. The airways and pulmonary parenchyma have some receptors, but cough is the primary pulmonary response to noxious stimuli. Irritant receptors throughout the respiratory tract can trigger cough in an effort to clear injurious materials. Only irritation of structures with vagal innervation can precipitate involuntary cough. These structures include the larynx, tracheobronchial tree, posterior oropharynx, and middle ear. Any process that irritates these structures can precipitate cough. ACE cough is produced by sensitization of irritant receptors by accumulating prostaglandins and bradykinins. Interstitial lung disease provokes cough by irritation of the smallest airways rather than the alveoli. Voluntary cough (clearing throat or a deeper cough) is also possible. The mechanism of cough is forced expiration against a closed glottis which suddenly opens and permits a very high velocity stream of air through the airway, presumably taking noxious material with it (Murray and Nadel 2005;1:831).

Characterization: Main distinction is between chronic and acute. Chronic cough variously defined as 3–8 weeks in duration (Thorax 2003;58:901). Acute cough is often associated with infection, inhalation or aspiration, or activation/exacerbation of latent/chronic lung disease (asthma, COPD). Chronic cough has a very broad differential diagnosis. It is helpful to associate it with activities such as exercise (EIA), eating (aspiration, neurologic disease), season (asthma), environment (workplace, home, friend's house with cats), heartburn (reflux-associated cough). Clearing throat type of cough is more often associated with upper airway irritation. Presence of sputum suggests infection, airway inflammation. Nocturnal cough can be associated with postnasal drip, reflux, and asthma. In an established asthmatic, persistent nocturnal cough is a reliable indicator of incomplete control of disease. Acute or chronic hemoptysis is a red flag and raises possibility of malignancy or process that is destructive of lung tissue (such as lung abscess or TB). Smoking changes ecology of illness and raises probability of COPD and malignancy.

Differential Diagnosis: Differential for acute cough is limited: bronchitis, pneumonia, asthma exacerbation, COPD exacerbation. Rarely foreign body. Cough is common in CHF, PE, but rarely is the sole presenting complaint. Differential in common practice for chronic cough will be reflux, postnasal drip, medication (ACE), airway disease, ENT disease, parenchymal disease, and malignancy (N Engl J Med 2000;343:1715). Initial differentiation will depend upon the history (ENT problems, reflux, associated dyspnea, sputum, wheeze, medications), exam (wheezing, rales, mucoid material on posterior oropharynx, nasal congestion), and chest X-ray.

Further Evaluation: Cough with abnormal chest X-ray will be driven mostly by the chest X-ray findings. See Figure 1.1 for a possible algorithm. Note the absence of bronchoscopy in the evaluation of cough in the presence of a normal X-ray; the yield of bronchoscopy in this setting is quite low (Chest 2006;129:147S).

Direct Treatment: Identify and treat underlying problem first. A cough should not be suppressed without a diagnosis. That said, control of symptoms can be very helpful short term while definitive therapy is under way or for palliation when the underlying problem is untreatable. In rare circumstances there may be need to use as adjunct long term. Dextromethorphan is effective and nonnarcotic. Narcotics generally are effective, but there is risk of addiction (Thorax 2004;59:438, Murray and Nadel 2005;1:831). Older patients may become unsteady from the sedative effect and injure themselves. In rare circumstances, narcotics for cough can precipitate respiratory failure in patients with CO_2 retention or untreated sleep apnea.

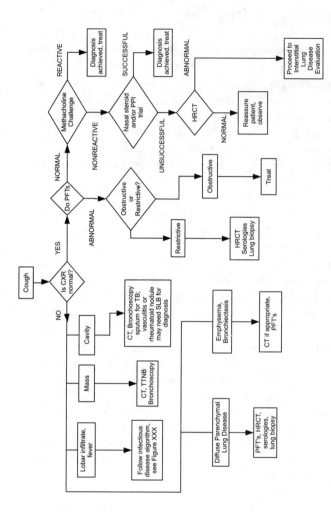

Figure 1.1 Algorithm for the evaluation of cough based on initial chest X-ray findings. Proposed further testing would depend upon the clinical situation and the individual needs of the patient. All tests mentioned would not be applicable to all patients.

1.5 Dyspnea

Excellent further reading: Am J Respir Crit Care Med 1999;159:321, Am Fam Physician 2005;71:9

Introduction: Dyspnea is an elemental manifestation of disease. It is variously described as air hunger, shortness of breath, inability to take a deep breath, and many other complaints. Dyspnea is a manifestation of the disruption of the brain's interpretation of the balance among multiple afferents and efferents that control oxygen delivery to the tissues. The main diagnostic task is to differentiate pulmonary dyspnea from nonpulmonary dyspnea. Once determined as pulmonary, further characterization of the symptom can be of value. Dyspnea in one form or another accompanies most respiratory disease. Monitoring and quantifying dyspnea is valuable in disease management. Occasionally there is a need to treat the symptom of dyspnea rather than the root cause.

Pathophysiology: The brain expects certain relationships among blood oxygen tension, blood carbon dioxide tension, chest wall stretch receptors, pulmonary interstitium stretch receptors, oxygen demand of the tissues, oxygen delivery, and work of breathing. Disruption of the balance causes dyspnea. In practice, four major conditions cause dyspnea: pulmonary disease, cardiac disease, anemia, and deconditioning. Patient perception of noxious sensation varies widely complicating patient-to-patient comparisons.

Characterization: Can categorize as chronic/acute, episodic/constant, progressive/stable. Orthopnea is recumbent dyspnea. Platypnea is dyspnea produced by sitting up or standing. There have been multiple efforts at developing objective measures such as the Borg scale, but psychological and perceptual issues can confound inter- (as opposed to intra-) patient comparisons. I have found it useful to quantify in terms of ADLs: stairs, flat ground (how many, how far), indoor and outdoor chores, work, (LFE: vacuuming uses arm and leg work; often the first to go for patients responsible for the housework). Patients often modify activities to fit their exercise capacity; don't take at face value statement "I can do anything I want to." Get patient to quantify their exercise capacity. Improvement in dyspnea with treatment is a reliable sign of success. The New York Heart Association uses a Grade I through IV gradation of dyspnea (Cleveland Clin J Med 2003; 70:S9), which can be useful in classifying severity of disease (I no impairment; II dyspnea with ordinary physical activity; III dyspnea with less than ordinary physical activity; IV dyspnea at rest).

Differential Diagnosis: Pulmonary dyspnea is usually associated with other pulmonary symptoms. Cardiac dyspnea is usually associated with other cardiac symptoms. Deconditioning and anemia can mimic either but more often seem cardiac. PND and orthopnea strongly suggest a cardiac etiology. Complaints of arm work perceived as harder than leg work is associated with pulmonary disease (N Engl J Med 1986;314:1485). Some authorities state that precise characterization of complaints can help differentiate, but in practice this may be hard to do. Chronic, constant, progressive dyspnea suggests COPD, DPLD, and CHF. Episodic, chronic dyspnea that does not worsen suggests asthma, or ischemic heart disease. Acute dyspnea raises concerns for PE, MI, acute respiratory failure, or pneumonia of any etiology. Like other pulmonary symptoms, dyspnea is evaluated by the company that it keeps. In practice, it is often difficult to differentiate cardiac from pulmonary dyspnea, and the two frequently coexist often along with deconditioning.

Further Evaluation: Chronic: See Figure 1.2 for a proposed algorithm. Acute: At minimum, a thorough history and examination, chest X-ray, arterial blood gases, electrocardiogram, and CBC are required. The diagnosis will often be apparent with these first steps. Pulmonary edema, MI, asthma, AECOPD, pneumonia,

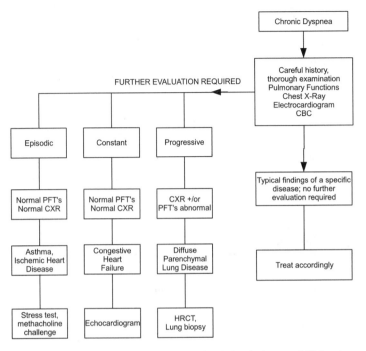

Figure 1.2 Proposed algorithm for the evaluation of chronic dyspnea. Initial evaluation will lead to a prompt diagnosis or further evaluation will be required. Depending upon the character of the dyspnea (episodic, constant, progressive) and key initial findings, common diagnoses are suggested. Initial diagnostic interventions are proposed in the lowest set of boxes. Not every patient requires every test, and this list may not be appropriate for all patients. It's a start.

sepsis, and PE will be most common ER presentations of acute dyspnea, *but be alert for less common etiologies.* In particular, if the CXR is normal, P_{O_2} low, and cardiac, obstructive lung disease, and infections are excluded, consider pulmonary embolism and do a V/Q scan or spiral CT. There has been considerable interest in the BNP and D-dimer as means to screen for heart failure and PE respectively. These tests can be helpful but also very misleading. BNP is increased in pulmonary disease, renal disease, and the aged as well as CHF (Am Heart J 2004;147:1078); D-dimer is elevated in *many* inflammatory states (Thromb Res 1993;69:125). See **Pulmonary Embolism** for a more complete discussion of the role of the D-dimer. In all cases CXR will play a major role in determining direction of evaluation. Consider CPET (see **Cardiopulmonary Exercise Testing**) for refractory diagnostic cases of chronic dyspnea.

Direct Treatment: Opiates excellent for control of dyspnea of advanced lung disease, also benzodiazepines. Oxygen also recognized as helpful.

1.6 Wheezing

Eur Respir J 1995;8:1942, interesting short review of the mechanisms of wheezing as well as differential diagnosis

Introduction: Wheezing is an adventitious lung sound that is produced exclusively by the respiratory tract. It is defined as a continuous (sustained) musical note produced by the airways, including the large airways and larynx. Sounds with a dominant frequency of 400 Hz and higher are defined as wheezes; those with a dominant frequency of 200 Hz and below are defined as rhonchi. Wheezes and rhonchi have an identical pathophysiology, and have the same differential diagnosis. In evaluating the patient with wheezing, avoid the temptation to assume that wheezing (1) emanates from the lower respiratory tract and (2) represents either asthma or COPD. In this text, wheezes refer to both wheezes and rhonchi.

Pathophysiology: Researchers have hypothesized that wheezing is produced in a manner similar to a musical instrument: either generating a vibrating air jet (flute), or by a vibrating reed (clarinet). The mechanism is complex and probably has a component of both means, but more along the line of the vibrating reed. All models require a critical narrowing of the airway so that the walls almost touch. The sound depends on the velocity of air in the airway, and the mass and elasticity of the airway wall at the site of critical obstruction. Under the right conditions, the airway walls and the enclosed column of air vibrates, and sound is created. The character of the sound does not reliably indicate large or small airway obstruction.

Characterization: Given the pathophysiology described above, the question is whether or not wheezes are present. Although inspiratory wheezes are reported as associated with upper airway obstruction, inspiratory wheezing can be heard in severe lower airway obstruction. Wheezes can be described as monophonic and polyphonic. Monophonic implies one site of obstruction; polyphonic implies multiple. A true persistent monophonic wheeze should prompt a search for a single anatomic obstruction.

Differential Diagnosis: From a practical standpoint, asthma and COPD are the most common sources of wheezing. Other sources: tracheobronchitis, laryngitis, tracheal or bronchial stenosis, large airway tumors, foreign bodies, and extrinsic airway compression. States with high mucus production such as bronchiectasis and cystic fibrosis also produce wheezing. The clinician should be aware of VCD, the misdiagnosis of which can cause months or even years of unnecessary medications. Severe degrees of fibrosis can cause a "squeaking" that can mimic wheezing. Pulmonary edema can precipitate wheezing as well.

Further Testing: Careful history directs further evaluation. Most obstructive lung diseases have a distinctive pattern of presentation (see **Asthma, COPD, Bronchiectasis**). Once obstructive lung disease is a consideration, formal PFTs are recommended: determine severity, determine reversibility, and confirm diagnosis. Methacholine challenge testing may help determine reversibility. Chest X-rays and CT scans may help diagnose bronchiectasis, emphysematious changes, or lung masses. Bronchoscopy may be useful if there is a consideration of large airway anatomic abnormality. When a patient does not fit into a category with assurance, psychogenic issues should be considered.

Symptomatic Treatment: Treatment of the underlying condition is the only feasible approach.

1.7 Sputum

Zackon 2000;885

Introduction: Sputum production is a nonspecific symptom associated with many pulmonary diseases. In general, sputum will be a product of airway inflammation or infection, but can have an alveolar source as well. Major goal of evaluating sputum production is to characterize the produced material and then try and determine an etiology. Additional testing holds varying degrees of favor with different authors; much of this depends upon anticipated etiology. Occasionally "sputum" will be from the upper airway; it's worth a quick question to make sure that the patient really is coughing up material from the lower airway.

Pathophysiology: Mucus is a normal component of the airways, forming a protective layer over the respiratory endothelium. This layer prevents dehydration of surface cells, traps foreign materials, and is the medium in which cilial transport functions. Mucus hypersecretion is pathologic, with excessive stimulation of both goblet cell and submucosal gland sources of mucus. A large number of mediators of hypersecretion have been identified and are closely linked to various components of the inflammatory cascade: neurotransmitters and neuropeptides; inflammatory mediators such as leukotrienes, prostaglandins, and histamine; bacterial enzymes; and proteases, especially those from neutrophils. Precise mechanism varies from disease state to disease state. Consequences of mucus hypersecretion include cough, airway plugging, and airway obstruction (Murray and Nadel 2005;1:330).

Characterization: Color: Clear/white usually implies very few inflammatory cells. Yellow/green is associated with pus cells, less reliably with bacteria (can have purulent sputum with viral pneumonia, viral bronchitis). Bright green is associated with pseudomonas. Brown, red sputum is associated with blood and tissue destruction. Consistency: thick, tenacious sputum can be associated with CF, but many conditions can cause this. Thin copious secretions are characterized as bronchorrhea and associated with bronchoalveolar cell carcinoma. Pulmonary alveolar proteinosis can be associated with "gelatinous" sputum. Quantity: Unreliable helper. Classically bronchoalveolar cell carcinoma and bronchiectasis are associated with massive (cups) amounts of sputum per day. In practice this is encountered uncommonly, even in specialty practice. Odor: Deliberately smelling sputum is inappropriate and contrary to principles of universal precautions. However, a foul, stoollike odor suggests anaerobic, tissue-destructive infections. Grapelike, fruity odor is associated with pseudomonas. Macroscopic, visible abnormalities are also possible: Visible parasites (e.g., ascaris), and the classic copious "layering" sputum of bronchiectasis are two examples. Obvious food, foreign material is prima facie evidence of aspiration.

Differential Diagnosis: Patients are unlikely to confuse sputum with secretions from other organ systems. Rarely, the clinician will need to distinguish from nasal discharge, gastric contents. Primary differentiation will be based on accompanying symptoms. *In general, sputum, especially acute appearance of sputum, should be considered to be infectious until proven otherwise.*

Further Testing: Primary testing is primarily based on microscopic examination of the sputum, culture of the sputum, and occasional other tests such as PCR. Before testing, the laboratory must make certain that the material is representative of the lower respiratory tract. Presence of bronchial columnar cells, alveolar macrophages, and neutrophils suggest a lower tract specimen. Squamous cells, saliva-like consistency of expectorated material, and high concentration of a broad range of bacteria with occasional fungi suggest oral-nasal etiology. Authors vary widely in their level of confidence in the results of sputum testing. Presuming a representative lower tract specimen in a patient with an intact upper airway (no tracheostomy or endotracheal tube) a single pathogen associated with neutrophils is likely a true positive finding; likewise positive sputum cytology is likely a true positive. A negative finding for pathogens or a benign cytology does not conclusively exclude the disease in question; pretest probability and associated findings drive the need for further testing. Finally, certain diseases are notorious for their difficulty in isolating from the sputum; atypical pneumonia agents such as *Legionella, Chlamydia,* and *Mycoplasma* are extremely difficult to identify in sputum, and other means should be used for diagnosis. When a patient has chronic airway disease, a tracheotomy, or an endotracheal tube, presence of bacteria in sputum may be infection or colonization. Presence of infiltrates on chest X-ray, fever, and other signs of infection may be important ancillary pieces of information. Specific diseases: community acquired pneumonia: an etiologic agent can be identified in approximately 60–80% of cases in research studies (Eur J Clin Microbiol Infect Dis 2005; 24:241). The experience of most practicing clinicians is 20–30%. Tuberculosis: 60–80% with multiple induced sputa and culture results (Int J Tuberc Lung Dis 2004;8:945, Int J Tuberc Lung Dis 2001;5:855). PCJ in HIV patients: as high as 90% with three induced sputa (Eur Respir J 2003;21:204, Chest 1998;113: 1555). Sputum cytology for malignancy: as high as 80% in some series (Acta Cytol 2003;47:1023). This test is dependent on the skills of the pathologist. Some authors feel that sputum cytology collection should be skipped, and the evaluation should proceed to bronchoscopy directly (investigate airway, evaluate suitability for operation, etc.). Some authors feel that sputum eosinophilia is helpful in diagnosis of asthma, chronic eosinophilic bronchitis (Chest 2006;129:1344). The reliable recovery of fungal agents and parasites is uncertain.

Symptomatic Treatment: Mucolytics such as guiafenesin 600 mg po bid, humidification, bronchodilators (beta agonists and anticholinergics), iodine preparations (SSKI), acetylcysteine inhaled, dornase alfa inhaled (CF patients only). Clearance enhanced by mechanical means as well: flutter valve, vibratory chest physiotherapy.

1.8 Hemoptysis

Introduction: This is a significant symptom that can be associated with serious and life-threatening illness. The clinician is faced with determining if the blood truly comes from the lower respiratory tract, if it is immediately life threatening, and the precise diagnosis. When hemoptysis is chronic, most pulmonary physicians will take the position that the etiology is lung cancer until proven otherwise. This may seem contradictory to the statistical material presented below, but forces a systematic, careful evaluation.

Pathophysiology: The lung has a dual blood supply: a systemic-pressure supply in the bronchi, and a low-pressure pulmonary artery supply presented to the alveoli for gas exchange. Bronchial arterial bleeding can be quite brisk and may be life threatening. Bronchial venous bleeding and parenchymal bleeding can also be massive, although it is less common. Respiratory tract bleeding is life threatening not only from blood loss, but from the ability of the clot to block the major airways and cause asphyxia. Massive bleeding can drown the alveoli. Disruption of vessels can be caused by infection, inflammation, primary vascular disorders, tissue necrosis, and tumor. Traumatic hemorrhage is self-evident and will not be addressed. Bleeding can be worsened by anticoagulants and antiplatelet drugs, but these agents will not cause a spontaneous bleed from normal tissue; they act as more of a "stress test."

Characterization: Quantify amount but patients often overestimate the severity of a bleed; admixture with sputum suggests infection; stomach contents suggests GI source. Frothy pink sputum suggests heart failure. Bright red, clotted blood suggests respiratory tract source. Coffee grounds or black material suggests hematemesis, but patients with hemoptysis often swallow some blood and may regurgitate the stomach contents

Differential Diagnosis: The clinician must first confirm that it is respiratory tract blood. ENT and oral exam are helpful. Patients with true hemoptysis will not have epistaxis. Oral blood with true hemoptysis is common, and clinician may want to have patient rinse out mouth for the exam. GI etiology of blood suggested by history, abdominal complaints, preexisting liver disease. Patients with massive hemoptysis (variously defined as 100–600 ml/24 h) require careful monitoring, stabilization, and early pulmonary/ thoracic surgery consultation. Localization of site of bleeding is as important as an etiologic diagnosis so that intervention can be planned.

In primary care practice, most bleeding will be infectious: bronchitis, pneumonia, TB. Fever, sputum, precise history, and imaging data are cornerstones of evaluation. Less common infections include parasites and fungi. Pneumonia will often have parenchymal infiltrates. Some patients with chronic airway diseases such as CF, bronchiectasis, and severe chronic bronchitis may have a combination of infection and structural abnormality leading to relatively frequent bleeding events. Some events can be massive and require therapeutic intervention. Necrotizing infections (TB, pulmonary abscess) can also cause hemoptysis. Malignancy is also common; the diagnosis is suggested by imaging results, weight loss, malaise, and smoking history; look for extrathoracic manifestations as well. Consider Kaposi's sarcoma in HIV+ patients, and remember that less common pathogens may be present (see **HIV and the Lung**). Vascular etiologies include PE, septic embolism, mitral valve disease, pulmonary hypertension, and CHF. History and exam, BNP and D-dimer when appropriate, imaging, and cardiac studies such as echocardiogram help make diagnosis. Pulmonary AVMs, such as those seen in HHT are suggested by imaging, evidence of telangectasia elsewhere, especially mouth (see **Pulmonary Arteriovenous Malformations**); or therapeutic misadventure with Swan Ganz catheter. Inflammatory/necrotizing diseases are interesting and difficult to diagnose: Wegener's granulomatosis, pulmonary hemorrhage associated with lupus, anti-GBM disease (Goodpasture's syndrome), and pulmonary hemosiderosis (see chapter on **Diffuse Parenchymal Lung Disease**). There are also syndromes of pulmonary hemorrhage that are poorly characterized.

Further Evaluation: Fiber-optic bronchoscopy and CT scan are complementary tests and are the primary means of evaluation. Aggressiveness of evaluation is dictated by imaging data, age, smoking history, and associated symptoms. Patients with an obvious pneumonia, PE, or trauma do not need diagnostic bronchoscopy for hemoptysis (although it may be necessary from a therapeutic standpoint). Patients with masslike lesions are usually bronchoscoped (see **Diagnostic Fiber-Optic Bronchoscopy**) if the lesion is technically accessible. CT scan will usually be performed as well to plan bronchoscopy and determine extent of disease. Patients with infiltrative lesions undergo bronchoscopy depending upon appearance of lesion: lobar or segmental infiltrates have a higher likelihood of association with an endobronchial lesion. Diffuse infiltrates will have a lower yield on bronchoscopy. Workup of diffuse infiltrates for immunologic or inflammatory disease is appropriate, possibly including surgical lung biopsy. HRCT is appropriate to characterize infiltrate and plan biopsy. A difficult and common problem is hemoptysis with normal chest X-ray. Young (<40), nonsmoking patients with a single episode of hemoptysis have a very low incidence of serious pathology and may be observed safely. This is especially true if HRCT is negative as well. If the CT is abnormal, further evaluation will depend on character of abnormality. Older smokers with persistent low-grade hemoptysis need both bronchoscopy and HRCT. A patient in the middle ground (older nonsmoker, 30-year-old smoker with 10 pack-year history) presents a difficult decision, and there are no explicit algorithms (Am Fam Physician 2005;72:1253, Chest 1989;95:1043, Arch Intern Med 1991; 151:171).

Direct Treatment: Treat the underlying condition. Stop anticoagulants and/or antiplatelet drugs if possible. Low-grade hemoptysis can be treated with narcotic antitussives to reduce excessive cough and to prevent dislodgement of clot; this problem usually can be treated as an outpatient. Massive hemoptysis requires admission; position the patient in bed with "bad lung down." Use antitussives, enough to reduce excessive cough but not so much that patient cannot protect airway. If the patient cannot maintain their airway and bleeding is profuse, endotracheal intubation is appropriate. An anesthesiologist or chest surgeon may try to intubate the good lung (uninvolved lung) only or use a double lumen ET tube. Pulmonary and thoracic surgery consults are mandatory. Bronchoscopy with a fiber-optic scope will localize bleeding in case of need for surgery, and hopefully identify the offending lesion as well. Rigid bronchoscopy is indicated for removal of clot, instrumentation, cautery, and/or laser. Bronchial artery bleeding associated with CF or bronchiectasis may be addressed with arterial embolization (though tricky and can injure spinal cord in small fraction of cases) (Clin Chest Med 1994;15:147).

1.9 Hypoxemia

Respiratory Physiology, The Essentials 2005;186; Pulmonary Pathophysiology, The Essentials 2003;205

Introduction: Inadequate tissue oxygenation is termed hypoxia. Inadequate oxygenation of the blood is hypoxemia; these terms are often mistakenly used interchangeably. A complete discussion of the mechanisms, diagnosis, and treatment of inadequate tissue oxygenation lies more within the realm of critical care and is beyond the scope of this book; we will limit ourselves to mechanisms of and defects of oxygenation of the blood.

Pathophysiology: Oxygen has limited solubility in plasma. Oxygen in sufficient quantity to meet tissue needs is carried by the hemoglobin molecule. Oxygen binding to the hemoglobin molecule is dependent upon the partial pressure of oxygen in the plasma, with increasing saturation of hemoglobin binding sites as the partial pressure of oxygen increases. Saturation vs. oxygen partial pressure follows a sigmoid curve, with an asymptotic approach to 100% occupancy of binding sites. See Figure 1.3.

At the level of gas exchange in the alveolus and at the alveolar-capillary membrane, oxygen is constantly taken up by the blood and carbon dioxide is excreted into the alveolus. A 70 kg man on a typical American diet will transfer approximately 250 ml of oxygen from the alveolus into the blood, and 200 ml of carbon dioxide into the alveolus per minute. The numerical relationship between oxygen uptake and CO_2 off-loading is termed the respiratory quotient, or R. (Diet is relevant because CO_2 production is influenced heavily by which fuel is oxidized.) Because the gases within the alveoli must obey the gas laws of chemistry and thermodynamics, it is possible to predict the composition of the gas within the alveolus, consisting of nitrogen and other inert gases, the partial pressure of water vapor, oxygen, and carbon dioxide. This relationship is expressed as the alveolar air

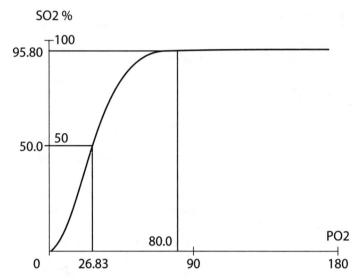

Figure 1.3 Oxyhemoglobin dissociation curve. The X axis represents pO_2, and the Y axis denotes hemoglobin saturation with oxygen. Fifty percent and 100% saturation-pO_2 relationships are noted, 90% saturation occurs at ~pO_2 55–60. Courtesy of www. ventworld.com

equation, and is: $PaO_2 = (PB − 47) * FIO_2 − PaCO_2/R$. PB is barometric pressure, 47 is the partial pressure of water vapor at body temperature, FIO_2 is the fraction of oxygen in the inspired gas, $PaCO_2$ is the partial pressure of carbon dioxide in the alveolus, and R is the respiratory quotient. PB and FIO_2 are both known, as is R. $PaCO_2$ is the same as the $PaCO_2$, the arterial partial pressure of carbon dioxide. In a normal person, the arterial oxygen tension, PaO_2 is 5–10 torr below PaO_2. This difference is termed the A-a gradient. The normal PaO_2 is approximately 95–100, and the normal $PaCO_2$ is 40. The normal hemoglobin saturation is approximately 98%.

With this information, it is possible to address the physiologic causes of hypoxemia.

1. Low oxygen tension secondary to low barometric pressure. This is the most common etiology of hypoxemia, and is seen in people who live at high altitude.
2. Low fraction of oxygen in inspired air. This is relatively uncommon and is seen in individuals enclosed in airtight structures where there is no replenishment of oxygen as it is consumed. Much research, for example, was done on this problem in conjunction with early and mid 20th-century submarine warfare.
3. Diffusion block—As the red blood cell traverses the capillary surrounding the alveolus, gas is diffused across the alveolar-capillary membrane. It is appealing to envision a pathologic state of diffusion block, where there is physical impediment to the transfer of gas across the membrane. Although this does occur, it is of limited physiologic significance. There is great redundant capacity in the gas transfer capability of each alveolar-capillary unit, and abnormal membrane function can be accommodated. Most alveolar-capillary units tend either to work or not, with relatively few units "impaired but functioning" because of a diffusion abnormality.
4. Hypercarbia—The alveolar air equation predicts that hypercarbia can cause hypoxemia. This phenomenon is of particular value clinically in determining if a patient has intrinsic pulmonary pathology or is simply hypoventilating, such as a healthy young person with a drug overdose. Solve the alveolar air equation and then calculate the A-a gradient. If the A-a gradient is normal (5–10), hypoxemia noted on blood gases is due solely to carbon dioxide accumulation, and one does not need to search for other causes (the etiology of the hypercarbia still remains to be determined).

5. Shunt—The clinical definition of *shunt* is hypoxemia that does not respond to supplemental oxygen. When an alveolar unit is not in communication with the rest of the airway, unsaturated blood with a low partial pressure of oxygen passes through the alveolar-capillary complex without raising the PaO_2 or increasing the saturation of the hemoglobin. This blood mixes with blood that has been reoxygenated. It is critical to recognize that this mixing takes place in the pulmonary veins, with the blood not exposed to the gases in the alveoli. Under these circumstances, hemoglobin saturation determines the PaO_2, rather than vice versa. Since the blood will always be less than 100% saturated, (because of the admixture of oxygen-depleted hemoglobin coming from the unventilated alveolus), the PaO_2 will always be low as well. Attempts to improve PaO_2 and hemoglobin saturation by increasing FIO_2 will fail. The blood in communication with a functioning alveolus cannot be supersaturated, and the oxygen-depleted blood will always pull down the saturation of the mixed blood.

6. Ventilation-perfusion mismatch—If the shunt situation is changed to permit poor (as opposed to zero) communication between the alveolus and the rest of the airway, it is easy to envision that some exchange of gas between the alveolus and airway will occur; oxygen in the alveolus will be replenished, albeit slowly; the higher the concentration of oxygen in inspired air, the higher concentration of oxygen in the alveolus; and oxygen concentration in the alveolus will also depend on how much oxygen is delivered from the inspired air and how much is taken away by the blood. This is ventilation-perfusion (V/Q) mismatch. In practice, in the vast bulk of clinical situations where hypoxia is encountered—pneumonia, COPD, heart failure, pulmonary embolism, etc.—the hypoxemia seen is secondary to V/Q mismatch.

Finally, it should be noted that the blood may lose its ability to carry oxygen as a consequence of poisoning of the hemoglobin molecule. The most common agent is carbon monoxide. Toxic levels of carboxyhemoglobin cannot be identified from either pulse oximetry or blood gases, and diagnosis is made from a combination of high index of suspicion, examination, and direct determination of carboxyhemoglobin levels. A discussion of CO poisoning is beyond the scope of this book, but warrants review. (Emerg Med Clin North Am 2004;22:985 is an excellent article on the subject.)

Characterization: A patient's oxygenation status is determined by pulse oximetry or arterial blood gases. Both methods have advantages and disadvantages, and these are covered in their respective sections (see **Pulse Oximetry** and **Arterial Blood Gases**). Normal PaO_2 is greater than 85–90 torr, and normal oxygen saturation is >95%. Signs such as cyanosis and dyspnea as indicators of hypoxia are too nonspecific to be reliable.

Differential Diagnosis: Hypoxemia is a consequence of almost any disruption of pulmonary physiology and many cardiac conditions as well. It is rare to have hypoxemia as the sole presenting finding, and a history will invariably turn up other signs or symptoms.

Further Evaluation: Hypoxemia should prompt history, vital signs, and physical exam. If hypoxemia is found to be part of a serious systemic illness, physiologic support including fluid resuscitation, supplemental oxygen, and ventilatory support is appropriate simultaneous with diagnostic evaluation and treatment of the precipitating problem. In a less critical setting, chest X-ray, pulmonary functions, and/or echocardiography often will provide an answer. HRCT and polysomnography may be helpful.

Treatment: A variety of methods for providing supplemental oxygen and positive pressure ventilation are available. See **Oxygen Therapy, Noninvasive Positive Pressure Ventilation,** and **Positive Pressure Mechanical Ventilation.**

A discussion of hypercarbia may be found in the section on COPD.

1.10 Pulmonary Hypertension

Introduction: Widespread use of echocardiography sometimes identifies pulmonary hypertension when it is unexpected. Although most of these patients will have some readily identifiable process that can account for the abnormality, occasionally the clinician will need to evaluate this finding as a primary presenting complaint. Until recently, pulmonary hypertension was classified as primary, a disease intrinsic to the pulmonary arteries, or secondary, where the pulmonary vasculature is affected by another process, and pulmonary hypertension is one of the consequences. In 2003 the WHO sponsored a consensus conference and the classification system was changed (J Am Coll Cardiol 2004; 43:5S). This new system of classification makes more sense and is more informative. See **Pulmonary Arterial Hypertension and Pulmonary Hypertension.**

Pathophysiology: Part of the echocardiographic evaluation is determination of pulmonary artery pressures (Cardiol Clin 1990;8:277). The reliability of this measurement has been proven in patients undergoing right heart catheterization immediately after echocardiogram (J Am Coll Cardiol 1997;30:1765, J Heart Lung Transplant 2005;24:745). These patients all had severe disease requiring heart catheterization, so the accuracy of the technique in milder PAH is less well defined. An elevated pulmonary artery pressure is considered to be greater than 25 mmHg at rest or 30 mmHg during exercise. Diseases of the arteries per se are now termed *pulmonary artery hypertension*, and conditions previously referred to as secondary are now termed *pulmonary hypertension*.

Differential Diagnosis: An outline of the differential diagnosis is developed in Table 1.2 (this table is identical to the classification table in the Pulmonary Hypertension section.) Idiopathic pulmonary artery hypertension (IPAH) is an uncommon disease

Table 1.2   WHO Classification of Pulmonary Artery Hypertension and Pulmonary Hypertension. The two rightmost columns describe recognized subgroups, examples, and/or further comments.

Type 1 Pulmonary Artery Hypertension (add'l diagnostic requirements of mean pulmonary artery pressure >25 mmHg at rest or >30 mmHg with exercise, AND pulmonary capillary wedge pressure <15 mmHg, AND pulmonary vascular resistance (PVR) >120 dynes/sec/cm5, AND transpulmonary gradient >10 mmHg, defined as the difference between the mean pulmonary arterial pressure and the pulmonary capillary wedge pressure)	Idiopathic Familial Collagen vascular Intracardiac shunt Anorexigens Stimulants HIV disease Portal hypertension	Preponderance in young women Similar molecular defect to idiopathic Scleroderma, lupus, RA VSD, ASD Fenfluramine, dexfenfluramine, diethylpropion Cocaine, amphetamines HAART appears to help hemodynamics [Eur Resp J 2004;24:861]
Type 2 Pulmonary hypertension with left heart disease	Left atrial or ventricular disease Left-sided valvular disease	Left heart failure, left heart diastolic dysfunction, pericardial disease Mitral stenosis, regurgitation
Type 3 Pulmonary hypertension associated with lung diseases and/or hypoxemia	COPD Interstitial lung disease Sleep-disordered breathing Alveolar hypoventilation	PH correlates with hypoxia PH correlates with hypoxia OSA Obesity hypoventilation, chronic musculoskeletal disease
Type 4 Pulmonary hypertension due to chronic thrombotic and/or embolic disease	Developmental abnormalities Prox. thrombotic occlusion Distal thrombotic occl. Occl. w/foreign material	Eisenmenger syndrome Acute PE, chronic PE Chronic embolization Schistosomiasis
Type 5 Pulmonary veno-occlusive disease	Obstruction of large pulmonary veins by fibrosing diseases such as fibrosing mediastinitis, tumor, sarcoidosis, Langerhans histiocytosis	

tending to occur in young women. Specific genetic abnormalities have been identified that render the pulmonary vasculature susceptible to further injury from a variety of sources and cause reduction in arterial caliber and a proliferative response of the vessel to the injury. Certain drugs, infections, and diseases may cause a process indistinguishable from IPAH (anorectics, HIV, scleroderma) and are therefore placed in group 1. Secondary pulmonary hypertension is produced by reduction in the total cross-sectional area of the pulmonary arterial bed or increase in downstream vascular resistance. Generally, this is caused by (1) hypoxic pulmonary vasoconstriction with diffuse arteriolar spasm, (2) obliteration of the alveolar-capillary bed by destruction of pulmonary parenchyma (COPD, DPLD), (3) obliteration of the arteriolar and capillary bed by luminal filling (PE, micro PE, sickle cell disease), (4) pulmonary vein occlusion, and (5) cardiac disease (mitral valve disease, left atrial hypertension, intracardiac shunts). Often, more than one mechanism is operant.

Further Evaluation: If idiopathic PAH is suspected, early consultation and referral is appropriate as these patients have a poor prognosis and require aggressive therapy. In general, an evaluation for causes of hypoxia (OSA), parenchymal and airway disease (PFTs, HRCT), rheumatologic disease (appropriate exam and serologic testing), and cardiac disease (echocardiography, which often has already been done). More recently, diastolic dysfunction has been identified as one of the important etiologies of pulmonary hypertension (through a mechanism of left atrial hypertension), and the echocardiogram should be reviewed for signs of this condition (N Engl J Med 2001;344:56, N Engl J Med 2001;344:17). Further evaluation is based on these first rounds of tests. If no etiology can be determined, the patient should be considered to have idiopathic PAH until proven otherwise (Cleve Clin J Med 2003; 70 Suppl 1:S9).

Direct Treatment: Treatment relies on addressing the underlying illness. Reversal of hypoxia with supplemental oxygen is required, irrespective of etiology. Anticoagulation, particularly for cardiac and thromboembolic disease, may be appropriate. If diastolic dysfunction is present, it should be treated. There are a number of specific pulmonary antihypertensive agents (calcium channel blockers, iloprost, nitric oxide, sildenafil, bosentan) that require careful evaluation of the patient and individually tailored therapy. There are no set guidelines for initiation or maintenance of treatment, and some of these agents are cumbersome and expensive. Consultation is recommended.

1.11 Radiologic Findings

General Introduction to Chest Radiology

Imaging is the most important test done in pulmonary medicine. Chest imaging has been available since the inception of roentgenography. The radiodensity differences among bone, tissue, fluid, and air make every chest X-ray a contrast study, so the lungs are suited to X-ray evaluation. The primary modes of imaging used are plain chest radiographs, CT scans, and ultrasound. Less commonly used modes include MRI and angiography.

X-ray technique and X-ray interpretation are beyond the scope of this book. The latter is a skill that is acquired over a number of years of experience and from deliberate efforts at education. Gaining this skill is recommended. It will always be to your advantage to review the films of your patients with your radiologist. This improves patient care and is interesting. This section assumes that you have correctly identified the pattern of abnormality on the X-ray and are ready to incorporate that information into your clinical decision making.

Imaging information alone is misleading and should be put in the context of the patient's clinical condition; that is your job, not the radiologist's. X-ray findings are best interpreted in the context of the patient's ecology and acuity of presentation. Each subsection addresses a basic abnormality. The final section deals with a common but difficult problem, the presumably acute pneumonia that fails to resolve in an appropriate period of time.

Cavity

Introduction: Pulmonary cavities are caused by destruction of lung tissue. To differentiate from other air-containing structures such as bullae, blebs, etc., cavities are arbitrarily said to have a wall thickness of >1 mm. Cavitation results from absence of blood flow with infarction and necrosis, necrotizing bacteria, or host defense response that is lethal to surrounding tissue. New cavities, irrespective of presumed age, require evaluation. Older texts differentiate between thin-walled and thick-walled cavities. Incremental benefit of this is probably limited as there is considerable overlap in diagnostic categories. Practically speaking, differentiation between single and multiple cavities may also be of limited benefit because of the differential diagnosis overlap.

Differential Diagnosis: Table 1.3 reviews common causes of cavities. Old cavities and cysts can become colonized and/or superinfected and may appear more alarming than warranted. Mycetoma, infected bullae are examples of this.

Further Evaluation: The primary concern is infection as this requires prompt treatment. Acute presentation should raise the question of anaerobic aspiration, staphylococcal, or *Klebsiella* infections. A chronic presentation should raise the question of nocardia/actinomycosis, TB, and atypical mycobacteria. Evaluation of pulmonary infection should be ecology/context driven. Empiric treatment per ATS/IDSA guidelines for treatment of aspiration pneumonia (Clin Infect Dis 2007;44 Suppl 2:S27) will address the majority of presenting organisms that cavitate. Sputum samples and blood cultures should be obtained (see **Approach to the Patient with Suspected Pneumonia**). Consider TB if the cavity is chronic. There may be sizeable overlap among illnesses, and

Table 1.3   Common Causes of Pulmonary Cavities

Mechanism of Tissue Injury	Etiologies	
Absence of Blood Flow	Pulmonary infarction Malignancy (growth outstrips blood flow)	
Necrotizing Infection	Bacterial	*Staphylococcus,* Aspiration pneumonia Other anaerobic infections *Klebsiella* Post-obstructive Rarely pneumococcus
	Mycobacterial and related	*M. tuberculosis* Atypical mycobacteria *Nocardia,* actinomycosis, rhodococcus Persistent cavity may be result of successfully treated TB
	Fungal	*Aspergillus* Histoplasmosis Coccidioidomycosis Mucormycosis Sporotrichosis
	Parasitic	Amebiasis Echinococcus Paragonimiasis
Inflammation and Tissue Destruction	Wegener Churg-Strauss Rheumatoid nodule(s) Coal workers' pneumoconiosis Sarcoid (rare in my experience)	

Data from Zackon, 2000.

invasive workup may be needed, especially if malignancy is a consideration. CT scan may provide accessory data such as mediastinal lymph nodes and additional unsuspected lesions. A patient with positive blood cultures and multiple cavitary pulmonary lesions does not need a pulmonary biopsy but does need a search for source of emboli. Similarly, some authorities feel that a patient with a positive ANCA, cavitary pulmonary lesions, and renal failure does not need a lung biopsy (this is somewhat controversial).

Emphysema and Bullae

Introduction: Although emphysema and bullous lung disease is usually (and correctly) associated with smoking, there are several other etiologies worth mentioning. These include congenital malformations, alpha 1 anti-trypsin deficiency, and several rare disorders. Additionally, true bullae and blebs must be differentiated from other airspace conditions of similar appearance. Bullae are thin-walled (<1 mm wall) airspace cavities. Blebs are subpleural bullae. Emphysema consists of destruction of alveolar walls and terminal/respiratory bronchioles to create air-containing spaces.

Differential Diagnosis: Bullous emphysema is associated with smoking (COPD) and congenital bullous lung disease (sometimes occurring in otherwise normal individuals). Subpleural bullae (blebs) are associated with smoking or may be spontaneous. Blebs are associated with Marfan syndrome, homocystinuria, and ankylosing spondylitis. Alpha-1-antitrypsin deficiency is associated with emphysema and bullous lung disease. Pneumatoceles are bullae that are a consequence of infection, typically staphylococcal infection. Bronchogenic cysts can appear to be bullae, as can cystic bronchiectasis. Honeycombing (extensive fibrosis with loss of alveoli and extensive scar tissue and large, nonfunctional air spaces) can be confused initially with emphysema but can be distinguished with CT scan.

Further Evaluation: It is uncommon that emphysema or bullae will be identified as isolated findings on CXR; the CXR evaluation is usually in the context of a suspected underlying illness. Physiologic consequences of hyperinflation, loss of radial traction with elevated expiratory airflow obstruction, and compression of functional lung tissue can cause significant dyspnea; pulmonary function testing is indicated. HRCT can be helpful in differentiating emphysema from other conditions, identifying location of disease, and disease unapparent on CXR. Intervention will be based on underlying disease and degree of impairment.

Interstitial Lung Disease/Diffuse Parenchymal Lung Disease

Zackon 2000;885, Fraser and Pare 1999;3:3076

Introduction: The term *interstitial lung disease* is a misleading term that is used by clinicians to refer to diffuse parenchymal lung disease. Diffuse parenchymal lung disease (DPLD) can affect the interstitium, terminal airways, and alveolar spaces. The list both of diseases and etiologies is long, and although it is possible to make some predictions as to final diagnosis from the plain film and clinical history, an invasive diagnostic procedure will often be required. Characterization of DPLD has been altered by the availability of high-resolution CT scanning of the chest and video-assisted thoracoscopic lung biopsy. The former permits biopsy planning and occasionally will even provide a definitive diagnosis when the "signature" appearance of a lesion is evident on HRCT. The latter has reduced the risk and recovery time involved in obtaining sufficient tissue for histological and cytological analysis.

Differential Diagnosis: A list of common diseases causing DPLD is in Table 1.4. Practically, the frontline clinician will see a limited number of illnesses. Acute DPLD will usually be CHF, ARDS, viral pneumonia, or mycoplasmal pneumonia. Chronic conditions causing DPLD will often turn out to be sarcoidosis, UIP, or malignancy.

Further Evaluation: Successful diagnosis and treatment requires close collaboration among primary clinician, pulmonary specialist, and radiologist. A complete algorithm for the diagnosis of these illnesses is beyond the scope of this book. However, the approach

Table 1.4 Common Causes of Diffuse Parenchymal Lung Disease Pattern on Chest X-Ray

Infectious	Hemodynamic	Inhalational	Drugs	Idiopathic	Collagen Vascular	Malignant
Miliary TB Pneumocystis Viral *Mycoplasma* Rickettsiae *Nocardia*	Congestive heart failure Mitral stenosis	Pneumo- conioses Extrinsic allergic alveolitis	Amiodarone Nitrofurantoin Chemotherapeutic agents	Interstitial pneumonias UIP, DIP, AIP, LIP Sarcoidosis Lymphangioleio- myomatosis BOOP (COP) Eosinophilic pneumonia Eosinophilic granuloma Langerhans histiocytosis	Rheumatoid Scleroderma Dermato- myositis Polymyositis	Bronchoalveolar carcinoma Lymphangitic carcinomatosis Pulmonary lymphoma

described below has served me and many of my colleagues well for patients with a chronic or subacute presentation. First, very careful history regarding exposures (remote exposures, hobbies, home environment, occupation, travel, drugs, concomitant/ remote diagnosis of malignancy, smoking) as well as general evaluation regarding patient ecology. Second, evaluation for identifiable systemic disease (lupus, Goodpasture's, Wegener's, scleroderma, dermatomyositis/polymyositis) including examination and serologies. Third, pulmonary function testing. Even if this does not contribute to diagnosis, it will be required for further treatment and management. Fourth, HRCT. Direct consultation with the radiologist including providing him/her with a detailed clinical history helps. There are numerous excellent atlases of HRCT appearance of pulmonary parenchymal illness (we favor Webb, Muller, and Naiditch, see **Bibliography**) and some degree of pattern matching between patient image and textbook image is necessary. Referral to a pulmonary physician is proper. If sarcoid, eosinophilic pneumonia, Langerhans histiocytosis, PCJ, or lymphangitic carcinomatosis are likely, TBLB and/or BAL are useful. All other patients should be subjected to surgical lung biopsy. The reason for this more invasive approach is that the histology of many of these diseases is inhomogeneous with large parts of the lung either normal or having nonspecific inflammation/fibrosis. Biopsy of a skip area is more likely with a transbronchial biopsy and a larger piece of tissue is required to assure diagnosis. The primary exceptions to biopsy are the patient with severe multisystem disease who may not withstand even VATS and the patient with obvious end-stage lung disease (extensive honeycombing, severe symptoms) where a specific diagnosis and prognosis may be academic. From a practical standpoint, the threshold to biopsy should be low, and the specimen should be referred to a pulmonary pathologist if there are any doubts or reservations about the diagnosis. Prognosis and therapy depend heavily on diagnosis (and varies widely among diseases) so precision is vital. My bias toward invasive biopsy notwithstanding, there are situations where it is perfectly appropriate not to do so. This would include situations such as obvious CHF, a HRCT picture compatible with carcinomatosis in a patient with known active malignancy, coexisting active immunologic disease known to affect the lung, etc.

Patients presenting acutely with DPLD are potentially at risk for their life and should be treated as such. Early consultation, rapid evaluation, early biopsy, and possible hospitalization are proper. The clinician should assume the patient is salvageable and treatable until proven otherwise. ARDS, CHF, viral pneumonia, mycoplasma, PCJ, and acute lung injury syndrome will be seen most commonly; pulmonary hemorrhage syndrome should be considered because of its lethality.

Lobar and Segmental Infiltrates and Atelectasis

Introduction: X-ray abnormalities in a lobar/segmental distribution imply an abnormality in bronchial or pulmonary circulation distribution. Atelectasis is a result of obstruction to airflow or loss of surfactant, the latter often the result of reduced blood flow or parenchymal injury. Focal consolidation can also occur without complete opacification of a segment or lobe. Peribronchial infiltrates may also be included in this group. The patient should be approached remembering that common things happen commonly. The most common problem with this acute presentation is infection, with airway obstruction and pulmonary embolism a distant second and third. Chronic presentation of this pattern suggests obstruction and/or a noninfectious etiology. Older texts spend time defining subtle differences among X-ray appearances of various infections, e.g., staphylococcal vs. pneumococcal vs. *Klebsiella*. This exercise offers little incremental benefit and is not consistent with current approach to pneumonia. ATS and IDSA have developed comprehensive patient ecology/context-based guidelines (see **Approach to the Patient with Suspected Pneumonia** and **Community-Acquired Pneumonia**) and are recommended as the basis for treatment. *Use the protocols. The clinicians who created them are far wiser than you and I.*

Differential Diagnosis: The spectrum of disease includes pneumonia, malignancy with obstruction, pulmonary embolism with or without infarction, BOOP, bronchiectasis, mucus plugging, impaction, aspiration, bronchial stenosis (there are many benign etiologies for this including sarcoid, previous pneumonia or TB, lymph nodes [right middle lobe syndrome]), or a foreign body. Loculated fluid may have the appearance of infiltrate. Often, it is difficult to differentiate between mass, infiltrate, and combination of the two on plain X-ray and CT scanning; invasive evaluation or serial observation may be required. Differentiation among pleural fluid, infiltrate, or both can be difficult. In the ICU setting, a misplaced ET tube can cause whole lung or lobe atelectasis. Generally, patients without indicators of infection (fever, sepsis, etc.) have greater likelihood of noninfectious etiology.

Further Evaluation: If the suspicion for acute pneumonia is high, follow empiric therapy guidelines and obtain sputum and blood cultures, sputum gram stain, and initiate antibiotics. Do *not* waste time with extensive imaging. Survival of community-acquired pneumonia is highest with antibiotics started within 4 hours of presentation (Arch Intern Med 2004;164:637). CT scan may help if a noninfectious etiology is considered and is the test of choice for bronchiectasis. The presence of an air bronchogram within the infiltrate argues against complete obstruction of the airway. Absence of any air within abnormality suggests that endobronchial obstruction is present. Evaluation for PE (see **Pulmonary Embolism**) usually relies on spiral CT or V/Q scan. D-dimer will be unhelpful if the differential diagnosis includes pneumonia or other inflammatory infiltrate unless the D-dimer level is normal (common pitfall [Thromb Res 1993;69:125]). If there is a strong suspicion for endobronchial obstruction, bronchoscopy may be diagnostic. Refractory, nonresolving infiltrate may be approached using the nonresolving pneumonia algorithm (see **Nonresolving Pneumonia**).

Mass

Introduction: Mass is defined as a very dense opacity without airspace visible or bronchi visible (air bronchogram). The primary concern is that this is pulmonary malignancy. Appearance of a previous CXR, smoking history, symptoms of infection, and known extrathoracic malignancy help define patient's ecology. Lesions <3 cm are addressed in the **Nodule** section.

Differential Diagnosis: Malignancy is favored by size (>3 cm), age (>45), smoking history, and presence of mediastinal adenopathy on imaging. Commonly associated symptoms of malignancy include cough, hemoptysis, dyspnea (sometimes), and constitutional symptoms. Many patients with advanced lung cancer have few or no symptoms. Clubbing is unreliably associated with malignancy and has little predictive value. Infections are suggested by fever and purulent sputum. Infections may include atypical presentation of common pathogens (*S. pneumoniae*, etc.) or typical presentation of uncommon pathogens (nocardiosis). Pleural disease can appear to be a mass, as can fluid trapped in a fissure. Inflammatory diseases can include BOOP/COP and Wegener's. Developmental abnormalities include bronchogenic cyst and pulmonary sequestration (Semin Thorac Cardiovasc Surg 2004;16:209). Previous X-rays can be useful in this setting. Multiple masses favor inflammatory/infectious process. Cavitation of a mass (see **Cavity**) can occur with multiple etiologies and is an unreliable marker of anything. Other etiologies include aspiration, progressive massive fibrosis (Radiographics 2006;

26:59), pseudolymphoma, rounded atelectasis (Respir Med 2005;99:615), and vascular abnormalities (AV malformation).

Further Evaluation: CT scan can help define the presence of calcification, mediastinal lymph nodes, or other lesions, and help plan biopsy approach. Unless there is a good explanation for the lesion (signature appearance such as progressive massive fibrosis, obviously infected patient, appearance of AVM), the lesion should be considered for biopsy. If likely malignant, bronchoscopy or TTNB is appropriate. Proximity to airways/pleura will determine from a technical standpoint the best approach. If likely inflammatory, a surgical lung biopsy is favored because histology as well as cytology will be available from the specimen. MRI may help define vascular abnormalities (Eur Radiol 2006;16:1374). PET scanning is used less for mass and more for nodule diagnosis, but PET may be helpful in defining extent of disease (see **Bronchogenic Carcinoma**).

Nodule

Zackon 2000;885, Fraser and Pare 1999;3:3076, N Engl J Med 2003; 348:2535

Introduction: Pulmonary nodules are defined as <3 cm and fully surrounded by pulmonary parenchyma on imaging. Multiple nodules have a different meaning and diagnostic algorithm from solitary nodules. There is a wide differential diagnosis that depends upon imaging characteristics, patient ecology, and acuity. Particularly for solitary nodules, history and previous images play an important role. Because the approach to multiple and solitary nodules is so different, they will be addressed separately.

Solitary Nodules (SPN)

The lesion is often asymptomatic and an incidental finding on CXR for cough, rib fracture, or shoulder pain. As with other masslike lesions, the primary concern is malignancy. Risk of malignancy rises sharply with age and smoking history, with over

60% of new lesions malignant at age 50 or greater (Chest 1974; 66:236). Early, small lung cancers have the best prognosis, and excision offers the best hope for cure. However, enthusiasm for biopsy must be balanced against unnecessary procedures when at all possible. There are established criteria for determining if a lesion is benign or malignant.

The most reassuring characteristic of an SPN is presence on an X-ray taken greater than 2 years previously. If old films are not present (or old films do not show lesion), the patient should have a CT scan. Smooth borders of a lesion are also suggestive of benign status. Uniform calcification, concentric laminar calcification, "popcorn" calcification (hamartoma), and central calcification suggest a benign lesion. Fat density also suggests a benign lesion. Smaller lesions tend to be benign (<2 cm) but many of the malignancies identified are <2 cm.

Malignancy is suggested by a spiculated edge, eccentric calcification, and/or doubling in size over 20–400 days. Cavitation may not be malignant, but indicates a metabolically active lesion that deserves further workup irrespective of etiology. Metastatic malignancy should be a consideration, and the clinician should assure him/herself that an extrapulmonary primary has been excluded.

Differential Diagnosis: Primary pulmonary malignancy, metastatic malignancy, granuloma (TB, fungal, atypical mycobacteria; old or active), and hamartoma (especially with fat, popcorn calcification) are most common. Bacterial abscess, solitary lesion of Wegener's granulomatosis, parasite infestation, rheumatoid nodule, carcinoid, vascular malformation, rounded atelectasis, loculated fluid, intrapulmonary lymph node, and PCJ in patients with AIDS are less common but reported. Despite the wide differential diagnosis, lung cancer is the primary diagnosis of concern in routine clinical practice. An algorithm addressing the evaluation of the SPN based on malignant potential is in the article on **Bronchogenic Carcinoma.**

Further Evaluation: If lesion is not assuredly benign (present on previous films, obvious benign pattern of calcification, fat density), PET scan with FDG (radioactive glucose) has become next test of choice. PET uses the differential (greater) uptake of glucose by metabolically active tissues. PET-CT combines the anatomic data of CT scanning with the nuclide data of the PET component to provide greater anatomic delineation. PET scanning, even with CT data, has significant limitations in terms of a high false-positive rate (Ann Thorac Surg 2000;70:1154), limited spatial resolution (problems with lesions <1 cm) (J Clin Oncol 1998;16: 1075), inaccuracy in the presence of hyperglycemia, and tumors with a low metabolic rate (Respiration 2006;73:267). Nonetheless, PET scanning is the test of choice for SPN after initial characterization, with sensitivity and specificity for malignancy in the 85–90% range.

At least two formal decision-making algorithms have been unable to differentiate fully between benign and malignant lesions (Am Rev Respir Dis 1986;134:449, Radiology 1993; 186:415, Mayo Clin Proc 1999;74:319). A predictive formula has been derived that can offer a reasonable pretest probability of malignancy (Chest 2005;128:2490). See Figure 1.4. (Don't panic; this is easily adapted to an Excel or Excel-compatible spreadsheet.) This probability calculation can be helpful in driving further testing, but is not definitive. For this reason, the primary care clinician should obtain early consultation with a pulmonary physician. Most pulmonary physicians and thoracic surgeons recommend excisional biopsy for a positive PET nodule (assuming this is the only PET-positive area on scan) with completion lobectomy if the frozen section indicates cancer; safety of this procedure has been improved considerably by VATS (see **VATS, Open Lung Biopsy, and Mediastinoscopy**). TTNB is reserved for the high-risk patient who will not undergo surgery. Although negative PET is reassuring, I (and most other pulmonary physicians) will continue to follow these patients for 1–2 years to assure stability of the nodule.

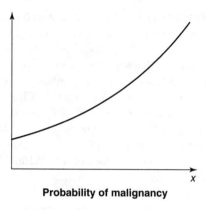

Probability of malignancy

Figure 1.4 Pre-test probability of a solitary pulmonary nodule being malignant. Data from Herder, 2005.

Multiple Nodules

Differential Diagnosis: The likelihood of primary lung cancer drops significantly, but is still present. Metastatic malignancy is more likely, with colon, renal, breast, testes, ovary, melanoma, and sarcoma common culprits. Metastatic disease is often peripheral. Consider Kaposi's sarcoma in HIV+ patients. Infections include multiple abscesses, septic emboli, fungi (*Aspergillus*, histoplasmosis, coccidioidomycosis, *Cryptococcus* in HIV+ patient), and parasite (paragonimus, echinococcus). Multiple nodules are an uncommon presentation of mycobacterial disease. Other noninfectious conditions include AVM, Wegener's granulomatosis, BOOP/COP, lymphoma, sarcoid, pneumoconiosis (CWP), and rheumatoid lung nodules. The patient's ecology is an important consideration.

Further Evaluation: Driven primarily by context. Evaluation should depend on the most likely diagnosis. CT scanning is recommended by most authorities. There should be a careful evaluation for solid organ malignancy. As with SPN, cavitation is an unreliable sign, although it will suggest infection especially if the patient is febrile or septic. PET scanning may be less helpful. If solid organ malignancy likely, TTNB of one of the lesions may be helpful. Often, a search for the primary is more valuable. A patient with positive ANCA and renal failure should have a renal, rather than pulmonary, biopsy. A patient with positive blood cultures and cavitating nodules has septic emboli and usually does not need biopsy. Likewise, a patient with very active rheumatoid arthritis and asymptomatic nodules may not need a biopsy. When an inflammatory condition is the primary consideration, VATS rather than TTNB is probably the best sampling method so that histology and cytology may be evaluated.

Pleural Abnormalities

BMJ 2005;330:1493, Clin Chest Med 2006;27:193

Introduction: Pleural abnormalities include inappropriate presence of air, liquid, or solid tissue in the pleural space. Normal pleural space contains ~5 cc of fluid acting as a lubricant. A balance between hydrostatic pressures, oncotic pressures, and the capillary membrane barrier allows continuous circulation of fluid maintaining this small residual quantity in the pleural space. When hydrostatic pressures increase, oncotic pressure is lost, or capillary membrane integrity is violated, fluid will accumulate. The character of the fluid will suggest an etiology. The presence of air in the pleural space is a consequence of violation of either the chest wall or the visceral pleura. Solid tissue usually is a consequence of scarring or malignancy.

Air: Air in the pleural space is termed *pneumothorax*. This may be air alone, or with fluid in which case it is called a hydropneumothorax.

Differential Diagnosis: Common causes of pneumothorax are outlined in Table 1.5.

Fluid: Fluid in the pleural space is termed *pleural effusion*. Fluids are broadly classified as exudates and transudates. Criteria for differ-

Table 1.5 Common Causes of Pneumothorax

Penetrating chest trauma
   Low-velocity penetrating injury (stab wound)
   High-velocity penetrating injury (gunshot wound)
Iatrogenic
   Thoracentesis
   Biopsy needles
   Central venous catheter placement
Bleb rupture (in otherwise healthy person)
Ruptured bulla in patient with bullous lung disease
Barotrauma from positive pressure ventilation
Asthma exacerbation
Rupture of cavity
Rupture of honeycomb lung in advanced pulmonary fibrosis
Rib fracture with resultant lung laceration
Cystic fibrosis and related bronchiectasis
Catamenial (pleural endometriosis)
Diffuse parenchymal lung disease
   Lymphangioleiomyomatosis
   Langerhans histiocytosis
   Radiation pneumonitis

entiation are presented in **Pleural Disease.** Transudates occur when fluid enters pleural space because of hydrostatic pressure or low plasma oncotic pressure. Exudates are result of bleeding, loss of capillary membrane integrity (usually a consequence of infection, malignancy, or inflammation), or rarely lymph (chylothorax).

Differential Diagnosis: When fluid is a transudate, congestive heart failure, liver disease, and iatrogenic fluid overload are overwhelmingly the most frequent etiologies. Meig's syndrome (ovarian benign tumor associated with a transudate) is also described, although some authorities describe this as an exudate. Exudates have a much broader differential and include bleeding (trauma, embolism/infarct), infection, malignancy, inflammatory lung disease, and systemic immunologic disease (rheumatoid arthritis, lupus). Chylothorax can be spontaneous, associated with yellow nail syndrome (Postgrad Med J 1997;73:466) or with malignancy or trauma.

Solid Tissue: Solid tissue in the pleural space is due to scarring or malignancy. Rare benign tumors are described (Cancer Control 2006;13:264).

Differential Diagnosis: Calcified thin fibrous scars are plaques, usually associated with asbestos exposure. Scarring as a consequence of infection or hemothorax usually leaves nonspecific pleural thickening. Occasionally the pleura may be calcified, especially with TB. Mesothelioma and metastatic malignancy have a variety of morphologies: multiple implants on pleural surface, smooth "rind," or a "lumpy-bumpy" mass covering the pleural space.

Further Evaluation: If sufficient fluid is present to be easily visible on plain film and there is a question about diagnosis (patient does not have obvious CHF, fluid overload, resolving pneumonia) thoracentesis is appropriate (see **Thoracentesis**). CT scanning may also be appropriate for any pleural abnormality. If possible, CT scanning should be delayed until lung is reexpanded (fluid drained, pneumothorax relieved) to maximize diagnostic value. Subsequent evaluation will depend upon the results of the thoracentesis and CT scan. Ultrasound evaluation of the pleural space is available at the bedside, is quick, accurate, and inexpensive. It is capable of identifying small effusions and pneumothoraces. (Radiology 1993;186: 297). This is a good general reference to pleural imaging as well.

Widened Mediastinum

Fraser and Pare 1999;3:3076, strongly recommended for this topic for a more advanced and authoritative introduction

Introduction: Widening of the mediastinal contour results from enlargement of structures within the mediastinum, migration of normal structures into an abnormal place, infiltration by abnormal tissues, and by bleeding, air, and infection. Although many problems in the mediastinum are unrelated to the lungs, assessment of these abnormalities often falls to the pulmonologist.

Differential Diagnosis: Mediastinum is bounded by the thoracic inlet, the diaphragm, left and right medial lung borders, vertebral column and surrounding structures, and anterior chest wall. Most discussions of mediastinal pathology are based on anatomy. The mediastinum is conceptually divided into the anterior, middle and posterior compartments. Differential diagnosis of masses or enlargement of the various compartments is outlined in Table 1.6. Lesions infiltrating from the lung or bronchus (usually tumor) may be difficult to distinguish from primary mediastinal disease, even with advanced imaging techniques. Purulent material can track into the mediastinum from a cervical infection or abdominal infection. Mediastinal air may be secondary to alveolar rupture and tracking "inward" of air into mediastinal planes rather than "outward" to the pleura. Air in the mediastinum in association with a history of trauma, severe vomiting, and/or unstable vital signs is a red flag requiring evaluation and prompt consultation with pulmonary and/or GI and thoracic surgery because it raises concern for bacterial contamination of the mediastinum (mediastinitis). Acute mediastinitis is a catastrophe that needs immediate attention. The mediastinum may also be widened for several weeks after cardiac surgery (Am J Roentgenol 1983;140:475). Mediastinal calcification has a broad differential, not necessarily benign, and is beyond the scope of this section.

Further Evaluation: The clinical presentation will drive the evaluation. Examples (all in conjunction with a visible X-ray abnormality): severe chest pain and hypotension implies ruptured aortic aneurysm; severe pain, hypotension, and fever after vomiting implies ruptured esophagus with mediastinitis; fevers, malaise, and weight loss over 6 months suggests lymphoma or

Table 1.6 Causes of Mediastinal Widening Categorized by Compartment. Multiple implies that multiple compartments may be involved, or that any of the compartments may be affected.

Anterior	Middle	Posterior	Multiple
Thymus tumors or enlargement Lymph nodes Germ cell tumors (teratoma) Substernal thyroid/parathyroid (and assoc tumors)	Lymphoma Vascular lesions (e.g., aortic aneurysm) Lymphadenopathy from metastatic disease Bronchogenic cysts Pleuropericardial cysts Pericardial effusion Cardiac aneurysm	Lymphoma Vascular lesions Neurogenic tumors (neurofibroma) Extramedullary hematopoeisis GI hernias (hiatus, paraesophageal) Neurenteric cysts Thoracic duct cysts	Neoplasm Aneurysms Esophageal enlargement (e.g., achalasia) Diffuse adenopathy Fibrosing, granulomatous mediastinits Acute mediastinitis Hemorrhage Fatty infiltration (more common with increasing incidence of severe obesity)

other malignancy. Thymoma may be associated with symptoms of myasthenia gravis. A patient with thalassemia may have extramedullary hematopoiesis and a posterior compartment mass. History of TB raises the question of granulomatous mediastinitis. CT scan will almost always be the next test, and results will drive the next round of testing. MRI may be helpful especially for thyroid or neurofibroma imaging. MRI is quite good for vascular lesions, but many vascular lesions in mediastinum will be emergent, and MRI is often a difficult procedure in the critically ill.

Nonresolving Pneumonia

Med Clin North Am 2001;85:1511, Semin Respir Infect 1993;8:59, Clin Chest Med 2005;26:143. Rome (Med Clin North Am reference) recommends a more aggressive approach than other authors and is probably in a minority.

Introduction: Most patients who develop a typical bacteria pneumonia resolve their clinical and radiographic findings promptly. When a patient's clinical symptoms linger and their CXR remains abnormal, the original diagnosis must be reconsidered and the patient reevaluated. Much of the confusion in the management of this situation revolves around the definition of nonresolution and the expected time course of events. A nonresolving pneumonia should be considered a malignancy, treatment failure, or other serious condition until proven otherwise.

Pathophysiology and Definitions: Pathogens commonly associated with CAP usually have resolution of clinical symptoms within 4–7 days. Radiographic resolution often takes longer. Studies have reviewed the resolution of multiple agents; N Engl J Med 1975;293:798 is the seminal article, identifying a cadre of patients whose *S. pneumoniae* took as long as 6 to 8 weeks to resolve. Clin Chest Med 1999;20:623 reviewed this in greater detail. They and other authors cite the impact of pathogen, comorbidities, and underlying immune status of the patient, the presence or absence of structural lung disease, and age on the

Table 1.7 Causes of Non-Resolving Pneumonia

Correct Diagnosis, Incorrect Treatment	Correct Diagnosis, Correct Treatment, Complications	Incorrect Diagnosis, Infectious Etiology	Incorrect Diagnosis, Malignant Etiology	Incorrect Diagnosis, Inflammatory Etiology	Incorrect Diagnosis, Vascular Etiology
• Penicillin resistant *S. pneumoniae* • Resistant gram negative rod • MRSA	• Empyema • Cavitation • Mucus plugging with atelectasis • Airway malignancy or adenoma causing obstruction and preventing drainage • Recurrent aspiration	• Atypical pneumonias such as *Legionella*, *Chlamydia*, *Mycoplasma* • Tuberculosis, esp. primary TB • Fungal infection, *Nocardia* • HIV + patients: fungal, PCJ, mycobacterial	• Bronchoalveolar cell carcinoma ("classic") • Kaposi sarcoma (in HIV + patients)	• BOOP/COP • Amiodarone toxicity • Wegener granulomatosis or other vasculitis • Rheumatoid lung disease • Sarcoid • Pulmonary alveolar proteinosis	• Pulmonary embolism or infarction

expected rate of recovery. Consensus puts clinical response first. As long as the patient is improving clinically, invasive evaluation is not indicated until somewhere in the range of 6–8 weeks. At that time point, if there is no resolution of radiographic abnormalities, evaluation is warranted even if the patient is clinically well. If the patient is worsening under treatment, earlier reevaluation is indicated. Some pneumonias produce permanent scarring and will not resolve to normal lung. In these infections, resolution to a stable, "chronic" appearance (stranding, linear streaking, enhanced lung markings in a circumscribed area) is an acceptable endpoint.

Differential Diagnosis: The differential diagnosis of nonresolving pneumonia encompasses most respiratory diseases that present with an infiltrate and a subacute time course. Table 1.7 presents common diagnoses that may be seen in this setting. Two points deserve further mention. In HIV+ individuals, the differential diagnosis is very broad and care must be taken not to miss an infectious diagnosis. Second, the possible diagnosis of greatest concern in most normal hosts is malignancy, and the fear is justified. A nonresolving infiltrate must be correctly diagnosed, or it may come back to haunt both patient and practitioner. The "classic" malignancy in this setting is bronchoalveolar carcinoma (Chest 2007;132:306S). This is a form of adenocarcinoma that tracks along the alveolar walls and bronchioles and has the appearance on chest X-ray more of an infection than a mass. However, any form of lung cancer may be responsible for a nonresolving pneumonia.

Further Evaluation: History and exam should offer clues in which direction to start evaluation. However, most pulmonary clinicians will have a low threshold for invasive evaluation, usually starting with bronchoscopy. This procedure permits inspection of the airways, biopsy of endobronchial lesions, transbronchial lung biopsy and BAL, and retrieval of microbiological specimens. CT scan is also appropriate. VATS for lung biopsy may be necessary in a refractory situation.

Chapter 2

Pulmonary Diagnostic Testing

2.1   Introduction

This section deals with the tests and procedures used in diagnosing and managing pulmonary diseases. Many of these tests are ordered and interpreted by both pulmonary specialists and primary care clinicians. To the frustration of both parties, there are often different expectations as to how to order these tests and interpret their results. The pulmonary physician is frustrated when a patient is referred for bronchoscopy when the procedure is technically inappropriate; the primary care clinician is discouraged when presented with dense tables of numbers purporting to be the results of pulmonary function testing.

Many of the tests and procedures have entire books devoted to the subject, and it is impossible to provide that kind of detail in this work. This section will review how each test is performed, the physiology on which the test is based, general interpretation of results, and how and when to order the test. This should help the clinician order tests, interpret their results, and refer for consultation appropriately and confidently.

2.2   Arterial Blood Gases

Respiratory Physiology, The Essentials 2005;186, Weinberger,
     Principles of Pulmonary Medicine 2004;403

Introduction: Arterial blood gases reflect both oxygenation and ventilation. Ventilation in turn interacts with renal homeostatic mechanisms to maintain the body's acid-base balance.

Physiology: Blood from the systemic circulation returns to the right atrium and ventricle where it mixes; different levels of metabolic activity cause differences in venous oxygenation and acid load. Venous blood samples from the leg veins during running will be different from arm vein samples taken from the same patient under the same conditions. Mixed venous blood is transported to the alveolar capillary membrane where gas exchange takes place. Oxygenation depends upon a carrier molecule (hemoglobin) for adequate oxygen delivery to the periphery and uptake is non-linear. Although saturation measurements express the percentage of oxygen binding sites on hemoglobin that are occupied, PaO_2 reflects the actual partial pressure of oxygen in the plasma. This difference is the basis of understanding shunt, A-a gradients, and similar issues of pathophysiology (see **Hypoxia**). Carbon dioxide elimination (or retention) is inversely proportional to alveolar ventilation. Alveolar ventilation in large part is governed by the body's maintenance of acid-base homeostasis, using a carbon dioxide bicarbonate buffering system. The body defends pH, not CO_2 or $[HCO_3^-]$. Carbon dioxide dissolved in the blood forms carbonic acid with acceleration of the reaction by red blood cell carbonic anhydrase, and is in equilibrium with hydrogen ions and bicarbonate. The Henderson-Hasselbach equation $pH = 6.1 + \log([HCO_3^-]/.03 * PCO_2)$ governs this relationship and implies that reduction in PCO_2 creates a more alkalotic environment, and an increase in PCO_2 causes a more acidotic environment. In the same line of reasoning, retention of bicarbonate by the kidney causes alkalosis, and reduction in bicarbonate levels causes acidosis. Increased excretion of CO_2 can compensate for reductions in bicarbonate concentration, and increases in bicarbonate can compensate for increases in CO_2 (Respiratory Physiology, The

Essentials 2005;186). When an acid-base perturbation occurs, compensation by the other organ (kidney for lung, and vice versa) will return the blood pH to close to (but not exactly) normal. If the initial perturbation is in P_{CO_2}, the disturbance is considered a respiratory acidosis ($\uparrow CO_2$) or respiratory alkalosis ($\downarrow CO_2$). If the initial perturbation is in $[HCO_3^-]$, the disturbance is considered a metabolic acidosis ($\downarrow$) or metabolic alkalosis ($\uparrow$). Efforts by the body to return pH to normal is termed *compensation*, and acidosis and alkalosis are termed *acute* (*uncompensated*) or *compensated*. It is also possible to have complex disturbances where there are multiple pathological processes occurring simultaneously with multiple primary disturbances.

Indications for Testing: Arterial blood gases are indicated any time the clinician requires precise knowledge of the patient's oxygenation, P_{CO_2}, and acid-base status. Common situations include diagnosis and treatment of respiratory distress and respiratory failure, sepsis, hypotension, obstructive lung disease, acute asthma, and weaning from mechanical ventilation. Blood gases are valuable for the diagnosis and treatment of a multitude of metabolic derangements such as diabetic ketoacidosis and renal failure. Although not reviewed in this section, blood gas analysis of mixed venous blood is used in the treatment of shock states, particularly severe septic shock. With the advent of noninvasive pulse oximetry, there has been a tendency to do fewer blood gases. Oximetry can give a false sense of security by providing an incomplete picture of the patient's status. Arguably, if you even think about getting a blood gas, do so.

Testing Procedure: Analyzing arterial blood gases requires obtaining an arterial blood sample. This is done most commonly by radial artery puncture. The blood must be collected anaerobically and immediately heparinized. Special preheparinized syringes that permit filling from blood pressure alone (don't need aspiration, and differentiate arterial from venous flow) are commonly used for this test. Allen's test for evaluation of collateral circulation is recommended by some but not universally. 0.1 or 0.2 cc 1% lidocaine infiltrated into the site of the proposed puncture can reduce pain; digital massage of the wheal returns landmarks. Radial artery catheterization is used in critical care units where repeated ABG determinations are anticipated, and there is the added benefit of continuous arterial pressure monitoring. Both of these procedures have a learning curve and require training for safe and efficient specimen collection. Analysis of the arterial blood is by electrode or optode (an optical-chemical transducer used in many point-of-care portable systems) with computer or microprocessor control. There are defined protocols for analysis proficiency and quality control that are required for laboratory certification and reimbursement. Complications of puncture and catheterization include bleeding, hematoma, thrombosis, distal ischemia, and arterial laceration. These are all uncommon in the hands of trained operators.

Interpretation of Test Results: Evaluation of oxygenation status requires knowledge of the FIO_2. This permits a calculation, at least roughly, of the A-a gradient using the alveolar air equation ($PAO_2 = (PB - 47) * FIO_2 - PACO_2/R$; see **Hypoxemia**). While PaO_2 of 100 at room air is respectable, the same PaO_2 at 100% FIO_2 indicates severe shunt or V/Q mismatch. Most blood gas analyzer reports also include saturation information. The saturation curve can be shifted by pH, PCO_2, temperature, and 2,3 DPG levels, and the analyzer will take this into account. Once a defect in oxygenation is identified, it is the responsibility of the clinician to track down the etiology. Analysis of acid-base abnormalities can be daunting at first, but can be approached systematically. First, determine if the patient has a normal, acidotic, or alkalotic pH. Above 7.45 is considered alkalotic, and below 7.35 is considered acidotic. Next, determine the primary disturbance. If the patient is alkalotic, for example, and the PCO_2 is low, the patient has a respiratory alkalosis. The degree of counterbalancing change in $[HCO_3^-]$ determines the degree of compensation present. Similarly, a low bicarbonate with an acid pH would indicate a metabolic acidosis, and the compensation would manifest as a reduction in the PCO_2. Here, however, the low PCO_2 is *not* associated with a high pH, and so the primary disturbance is a metabolic acidosis. The clinician should be alert to the possibility of a complex disturbance when both the PCO_2 and $[HCO_3^-]$ are outside of normal values, a primary disturbance cannot be identified, or the pH is normal. Analysis of simple acid-base disturbances is aided by full knowledge of the patient's electrolyte and volume status, and this knowledge is mandatory for the analysis of a complex disturbance. Many clinicians find the use of an acid-base map to be helpful, and this is my favored tool for rapid bedside ABG analysis. See Figure 2.1. Plotting the patient's pH, PCO_2, and bicarbonate places the patient's values as a point on a grid of pH, PCO_2, and $[HCO_3^-]$ and gives a quick answer. If the point is within one of the map areas indicating a simple disturbance (with or without compensation), analysis is complete. If the plot point falls outside one of the simple disturbance bands, a complex disturbance is likely. If the PCO_2, pH, and blood gas bicarbonate level cannot be made to converge on a single point on the map (i.e., the math doesn't work), testing error is likely. The etiology of metabolic disturbances is beyond the scope of this book; the reader is referred to the companion volume **LBB of Nephrology.** Respiratory alkalosis stems from excessive ventilation. Common etiologies include hypoxia (including high altitude), pulmonary embolism, sepsis, aspirin intoxication, pregnancy, liver disease, and alcohol withdrawal. Respiratory acidosis arises from inadequate ventilation. This can arise from an intrinsic pulmonary defect (COPD, advanced interstitial lung disease, pulmonary edema), respiratory muscle dysfunction or bellows dysfunction (kyphoscoliosis, myasthenia, ALS, diaphragmatic paralysis,

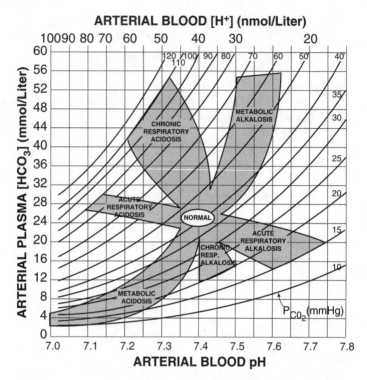

Figure 2.1 Acid-base nomogram. Shown are the 95% confidence limits of the normal respiratory and metabolic compensations for primary acid-base disturbances. This figure was published in Brenner and Rectors' The Kidney, Volume 1, Barry Brenner, Acid Base Nomogram, p. 942, Copyright Elsevier, 2000.

muscle metabolism syndromes, high quadriplegia), or control dysfunction (obesity hypoventilation syndrome, narcotic overdose, neurological injury).

Limitations of Testing: Blood gas analysis does not provide a specific etiology or mechanism for the acid-base and oxygenation status.

Metabolism in the sample must be stopped if there will be a delay in analysis, even just transportation to a lab; icing the sample is recommended. Additionally, samples must be obtained and maintained anaerobically until analyzed. Blood gas analysis proficiency testing and quality assurance procedures must be maintained for reliable results, accreditation, and reimbursement. Although only a small aliquot of blood is necessary for actual sample analysis, it is possible to waste a considerable amount of blood when the sample is obtained through a radial artery catheter in the ICU; blood conserving pressure monitoring/flush/access systems are recommended.

2.3   Cardiopulmonary Exercise Testing (CPET)

Eur Respir J 2007;29:185, Prim Care 2001;28:159, Prim Care 2001;28:5

Introduction: CPET is a noninvasive or minimally invasive means of assessing the work capacity of a patient. If work capacity is judged to be abnormally low, CPET offers an opportunity to determine the physiologic factor(s) limiting work capacity. CPET is also used as a means of assessing a patient's response to therapy, prescribing an exercise program, and determining suitability for surgery and/or other invasive procedures. CPET requires both professional and ancillary staff expertise and an investment in equipment and space. For this reason, the test is not available universally. Additionally, much of the information provided by CPET can be derived from other simpler tests. Nonetheless, CPET can be a useful tool in the appropriate clinical circumstance.

Physiologic Basis for Testing: CPET evaluates the work capacity of a large-mass muscle group, usually the legs and less frequently the arms. Effective function of these muscles depends on multiple factors: ability of the lungs to provide gas exchange, ability of the heart to pump blood, oxygen-carrying capacity of the hemoglobin molecule, and function of the muscle oxidative mechanism (pathologic states and deconditioning.) Abnormalities present at any point in the oxygen delivery and utilization chain can produce reduced work capacity. By measuring oxygen utilization, CO_2 production, electrocardiogram, pulse oximetry, and minute ventilation, it is possible to calculate a series of parameters that define the patient's work capacity and the limiting factors. Oxygen consumption (VO_2 max) is the best overall indicator of exercise capacity. This is the amount of oxygen extracted from inspired gas per minute and is a reflection of integrated function: uptake, transport, and utilization. This variable is usually expressed as an absolute value and percent predicted. When the muscle mass function outstrips its oxygen supply, lactate is produced, in turn creating a metabolic acidosis. This crossover point is termed the anaerobic threshold. Like oxygen uptake, it is a reflection of integrated function. Heart rate serves as a good proxy for cardiac output, because at higher levels of exercise an incremental increase of cardiac output is a function of an incremental increase in heart rate. Normal values for age have been established. Ventilatory reserve refers to the relationship between minute ventilation used to achieve a certain oxygen uptake and the maximal voluntary ventilation of the patient. As actual minute ventilation increases as a fraction of maximum voluntary ventilation, oxygen uptake is then limited by ventilation. The efficiency of ventilation (the formal physiologic definition of ventilation is carbon dioxide excretion) is measured by the ratio of minute ventilation to minute CO_2 elimination. Arterial blood gas determinations can be used here also so that assessment of oxygen transfer can be evaluated as well. Pulse oximetry is used to monitor oxygen saturation in real time, and the patient's perception of effort is also an important parameter (Clin Chest Med 2001;22:679).

Testing Procedure: CPET often uses a stationary bicycle for loading the muscle groups being tested, because work can be precisely measured, and it is somewhat easier to do exhaled gas analysis on someone who is sitting. Heart rate, blood pressure, ECG, pulse oximetry, and exhaled gas composition are measured. Prior to testing, it is common to perform spirometry and maximal voluntary ventilation maneuvers. Various protocols are used for testing (Am J Respir Crit Care Med 2003;167:211). The parameters described above are collected by the operator and by computer monitoring and are usually presented in both graphic and tabular form for interpretation.

Interpretation of Results: CPET is inexact and is dependent upon the cooperation of the patient and the skills of the testing facility. Nevertheless, it is possible to obtain useful information from the protocol. The test provides physiological information, and does not point to an etiologic diagnosis. Inability to reach a target work output (maximum oxygen uptake below predicted for age) can be caused by pulmonary limitation (inability to sustain adequate gas transfer in the lungs), cardiac limitation (inability to meet peripheral demand for oxygenated blood), or peripheral limitation (muscles inefficient, muscles deconditioned, lack of effort). Each abnormal condition will have its own pattern of abnormal measurements, but there is some overlap. Competent interpretation of results takes experience, practice, and a knowledge base beyond that provided by this text. Clin Chest Med 2001;22 page 693 has a good overview of the interpretation strategy, and is a good place to start for further reading. Figure 2.2 Am J Respir Crit Care Med 2003;167:211 provides a basic algorithm of interpretation.

Indications for Testing: Diagnostically, CPET is useful for evaluating dyspnea when less complex, less expensive tests have yielded inconclusive or contradictory results. Several algorithms are

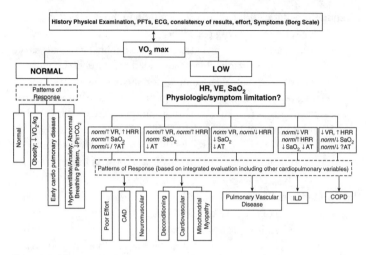

Figure 2.2 Strategy for the interpretation of peak CPET results. Weisman I, et al. 2003 ATS/ACCP Statement of Cardiopulmonary Exercise Testing. *American Journal of Respiratory and Critical Care Medicine* 167: 211–277. *Official Journal of the American Thoracic Society* © *American Thoracic Society*.

available for determining who will benefit from CPET in specific clinical contexts, but usually CPET is invoked when simpler evaluations such as echocardiography, cardiac stress testing, and pulmonary function testing fail to provide a clinically usable answer. See **Bronchogenic Carcinoma** for a specific example. When CPET is completed, the patient will be judged to have a normal study or abnormal work capacity. If abnormal, the pattern of limitation will indicate a pulmonary, cardiac, or peripheral defect. Testing can be particularly valuable where there is a disassociation between patient complaints and initial objective testing results. Although we would prefer not to consider our patients dishonest, malingering can also be identified with CPET. When disease management requires an objective assessment of work capacity, CPET can be useful. CPET is used frequently for generating exercise prescriptions for rehabilitation, evaluation of suitability for pulmonary resection, assessing suitability for heart and/or lung transplants, and exercise oxygen prescriptions. Newer indications include identifying high-risk patients for bariatric surgery (Chest 2006;130:517). CPET can also be used to determine functional impairment in the context of legal issues (disability, work-related injury, other litigation).

2.4 Diagnostic Fiber-Optic Bronchoscopy

Chest 2004;125:712, Semin Respir Infect 2003;18:87, Chest Surg Clin N Am 1999;9:19, Eur Respir J 2002;19:356, Murray and Nadel 2005, 617–650, Clin Chest Med 2001;22:263.

Introduction: Ikeda, in 1964, transformed bronchoscopy with the introduction of the flexible fiber-optic bronchoscope (Keio J Med 1968;17:1). Since that time, the diagnosis of pulmonary disease, in particular cancer, pneumonia, and some forms of DPLD, has been revolutionized. Despite the value of the instrument, it has a number of limitations, and expectations of the capabilities of the device are sometimes not accurate. This section will review the diagnostic use of the fiber-optic bronchoscope.

Physiologic Basis of Testing: The tracheobronchial tree subdivides 18 times (generations) before terminating in the alveoli. The pertinent divisions are trachea → mainstem bronchi → lobar bronchi → segmental bronchi → subsegmental bronchi → sub-subsegmental bronchi. The qualified bronchoscopist, using a "standard" bronchoscope, encountering normal anatomy, absence of obstruction, and a cooperative patient should be able to inspect all segmental bronchi. The same assurance cannot be made about smaller airways, particularly when the bronchoscope must make multiple turns to arrive at the orifice in question. Despite the six-generation limitation, pathology is often encountered in the central airways retaining the investigation's value. It is possible to perform a number of maneuvers beyond direct vision that enhance the reach of the instrument. The healthy airway is a yellow-pink color covered with a thin mucus layer. Cartilage rings are anterior and U-shaped, providing rigidity to the airway. The posterior wall of the large airways is a flat membrane; this asymmetry helps provide an anterior-posterior orientation. Bronchial anatomy is not fixed (Respir Physiol 1985; 59:289). Most bronchoscopists consider "normal" anatomy as a statistical rather than absolute statement, and exploration includes looking for accessory bronchi, etc. Because of this variability, bronchoscopists identify locations within the tracheobronchial tree by keeping track of the landmarks and generations already traversed and the appearance of the airway at the current point of inspection. Bronchi do not have pain fibers, and airway punctures and biopsies will produce cough rather than pain. The bronchial tree has a separate circulation with bronchial arteries at systemic pressure; extensive bleeding is possible with a biopsy. The bronchi are in close proximity to the pulmonary circulation, and it is possible (and common) to puncture the pulmonary artery or vein with a transbronchial needle aspiration. The upper airway—posterior oropharynx, base of tongue, epiglottis, and true and false vocal cords—can be inspected with the bronchoscope as well; many bronchoscopists (myself included) have found at least one unanticipated laryngeal cancer.

Description of Procedure: Conscious sedation with local, topical anesthesia is used for the majority of procedures. A discussion of the various sedation and anesthetic techniques is beyond the scope of this section. Once the patient is comfortable and sedated, the instrument is passed transnasally or transorally. Upper airway structures are inspected as possible. The larynx is evaluated for lesions and mobility with phonation. The trachea and airways are then inspected. Bronchoscopists make an effort to inspect the entire airway, not just the area of suggested pathology from X-ray or CT. Modern bronchoscopic equipment permits digital image documentation of abnormalities (or normal structures). Microbiologic and cytological samples are obtained using a variety of techniques. The choice of procedure(s) used depends on the anticipated diagnosis, the anatomic location of the abnormality, and whether or not the lesion can be directly visualized through the bronchoscope. Procedures used for visible lesions include saline washings, brushings, forceps biopsy, and needle aspiration. A visible, malignant lesion can be diagnosed ~90% of the time with combined brushings, washings, and forceps biopsy. Needle aspiration is generally used for submucosal lesions (a visible bump under the mucosal surface) and successfully makes a diagnosis ~80% of the time. Lymph nodes can be sampled for metastatic spread using transbronchial needle aspiration. Either cytology and histology needles can be used (21 vs. 19 gauge). Sampling can be performed using fluoroscopic or CT guidance, but many practitioners simply mentally correlate bronchial and CT anatomy. Success of this procedure varies widely from institution to institution. Good results appear to correlate with experience (both operator and pathologist), use of histology needles (vs. cytology needles), anatomic location of the sampled lymph nodes, and use of point-of-care cytology preps to confirm adequate sampling. The literature reports successful sampling in 50–80% of cases. Peripheral mass lesions (defined as visible pulmonary parenchyma between the lesion and the hilum on plain X-ray) can be sampled using needle aspiration, cytology brushings, and forceps biopsy. Some practitioners will also use bronchoalveolar lavage. Successful sampling correlates with proximity to the hilum and size of the lesion. A peripheral lesion <2 cm in diameter near the pleural surface has a 50% chance or less of adequate sampling. Evaluation of infection uses a different set of techniques. Isolation of the bronchoscopic specimen from oral/nasal contamination is required for bacterial specimens, and many practitioners will use a protected brush for sampling. In this system, a sealed catheter within a catheter is opened once the collecting end of the unit is in position, and a collection brush is then advanced. This system permits quantitative assessment of bacterial load and drives treatment decisions, particularly in nosocomial pneumonia and ventilator-associated pneumonia. Greater than 10^3 CFU/ml collected with a protected brush indicates significant infection. Bronchoalveolar lavage consists of wedging the bronchoscope into a bronchial orifice and injecting a sufficient amount of fluid to reach the alveoli, and then retrieving the liquid. In this setting, a CFU/ml of 10^4 is considered diagnostic of infection. Etiologic diagnosis of presumed infectious infiltrates in the immunocompromised patient uses a combination of bronchoscopic and less invasive techniques to achieve an etiologic diagnosis between 50% and 80% of the time; a substantial proportion of the final diagnoses are noninfectious, and no diagnosis is made in 20–30% of cases even with surgical lung biopsy and/or postmortem exam. Fungal and mycobacterial infections are amenable to diagnosis using bronchoscopic techniques. PCJ is diagnosed 90% of the time with bronchoalveolar lavage. The successful evaluation of DPLD using bronchoscopy varies depending upon the ultimate diagnosis. Bronchoalveolar lavage and transbronchial lung biopsy can provide a diagnosis when there is a high density of uniformly abnormal architecture: sarcoidosis, hypersensitivity pneumonitis, PAP, Langerhans histiocytosis, viral pneumonia, PCJ, and lymphangitic carcinomatosis have success rates of 70–80% and greater. Lesions with skip areas, complex architecture, and infections with a low organism burden are much harder to diagnose. Transbronchial lung biopsy uses fluoroscopy to guide biopsy forceps beyond direct vision to the periphery of the lung in order to take a biopsy of alveolar tissue. Other techniques used diagnostically include endobronchial ultrasound (Chest 2008;133:264) and endobronchial photofluorescence (J Med Invest 2007;54:261). Once the procedure is complete, the patient is recovered for 1–2 hours and discharged. Use of general anesthesia for diagnostic bronchoscopy in an adult is rare, but it can be used for patients who are agitated, fearful, or do not have the capacity to cooperate. Newer diagnostic tools include electromagnetic navigation. In this method, the patient has a large antenna placed under them and an RF emitting probe introduced through the bronchoscope. The probe is localized real time and the bronchoscope and an extended working channel can be directed to the abnormality (Thorac Surg Clin 2007;17:159).

Indications for the Procedure: Bronchoscopy is used in a wide variety of diagnostic clinical situations. Abnormal chest X-ray and CT suggesting an endobronchial lesion or obstruction are among the least controversial indications. Undiagnosed pneumonia, DPLD where the expected diagnosis is likely to be identified, suspicion for foreign body (aspiration pneumonia not responding to therapy), inspection in context of thermal or chemical injury are also widely accepted indications. Bronchoscopy can also be performed for the express purpose of sampling mediastinal lymph nodes or biopsy of a peripheral lesion. Cough, hemoptysis, wheeze, and stridor are not universal indications for bronchoscopy. For example, persistent cough with a normal CXR leads to a malignant diagnosis in 4% or less of patients. Hemoptysis in the context of a typical pneumonia with appropriate resolution of X-ray does not always need an invasive investigation. There are also a number of technical indications for bronchoscopy that are of lesser interest to the primary clinician: evaluation of a surgical anastomotic site, evaluation for TE fistula, and injury to the airway from an endotracheal tube. Although lists of indications for bronchoscopy will typically include pleural effusion, diaphragm paralysis, and persistent pneumothorax, bronchoscopy is clearly a secondary procedure and is not always indicated. Indications for therapeutic bronchoscopy are reviewed in that section.

Complications and Limitations: Complications of bronchoscopy relate to physical injury to the lungs and the upper and lower airway, uncontrolled bleeding, and precipitation of cardiovascular instability. Serious complications are well under 1% of procedures and include bleeding, pneumothorax, hypoventilation/refractory hypoxia, precipitation of bronchospasm, precipitation of arrhythmia, and myocardial infarction. Individuals at elevated risk of complication can often be identified prior to a procedure: recent MI, uncontrolled bronchospasm or hypoxia, and severe COPD. Risk of conscious sedation and topical anesthesia carry their own risks; local topical anesthetics that can induce methemoglobinemia, such as tetracaine, are avoided. Most bronchoscopists will stop anticoagulant and antiplatelet drugs for an appropriate interval prior to a procedure. Recent literature indicates that it is safe to do BAL with a platelet count of 20,000, and a biopsy should be performed at <50,000–75,000. Stopping aspirin is probably not necessary, but clopidogrel and other highly active antiplatelet drugs should be stopped 5–7 days before the procedure. Pneumothorax is rare outside the context of TBB, and occurs in ~1% of procedures with TBB under fluoroscopic guidance. Pneumonia is uncommon after bronchoscopy, although a low-grade temperature after the procedure is not. On a practical level, delayed complication (unlike colonoscopy or endoscopy) after bronchoscopy is unusual, and if a patient is stable at the time of discharge they will almost certainly do well. Most institutions have guidelines for conscious sedation, conduct of the bronchoscopy, and recovery that minimize risk. Limitations of the procedure relate primarily to sampling error (a TBB only retrieves a dozen or so alveoli, metastatic disease in a lymph node is not uniformly distributed, etc.), physical inability of the bronchoscope to pass beyond the sixth or seventh airway generation, and the radius of curvature of the bronchoscope (scope needs to make too tight a turn to get into a given airway.) The working channel in a bronchoscope is small (1–2 mm) and can be easily overwhelmed by blood and secretions. The lens is also small, and vision can be lost from a clot the size of a pinhead. Unlike GI scopes, there is only one channel, so an instrument needs to be withdrawn before suction to clear secretions can be applied. Additionally, experience predicts limited utility of bronchoscopy in certain clinical scenarios. Bronchoscopy is not the procedure of first choice for sampling a small peripheral lesion, for cough with a normal chest X-ray, for limited hemoptysis with a resolving pneumonia in a nonsmoker, and patients with DPLD (except for the previously described high-yield situations). Elderly patients, patients after a recent MI, patients who are experiencing massive hemoptysis, have unstable oxygenation, or have a bleeding diathesis may have greater risk than benefit from the procedure. In all but exceptional cases empiric treatment of pneumonia should not be delayed for bronchoscopy.

Further Interventions: Patients who are not suitable candidates for FOB may benefit from transthoracic needle biopsy, rigid bronchoscopy, CT scanning, or VATS biopsy or OLB. These are often technical decisions and close collaboration with your consultant is of great value.

2.5 Polysomnography

Kryger, Roth and Dement, Sleep 2005;28:499, Sleep 1997;20:406, Respir Care Clin N Am 2005;11:709, Sleep 1993;16:748, Sleep 1992;15:173.

Introduction: Sleep medicine is a rapidly evolving field that 20 years ago was outside the medical mainstream. The identification of noninvasive positive pressure ventilation as a treatment for obstructive sleep apnea has altered sleep medicine profoundly, providing an effective, safe treatment for the most common medical sleep problem. Sleep centers are found throughout the United States, and many labs permit the primary clinician to order testing without consultation by a sleep specialist (or neurologist or pulmonary physician). With that ordering privilege is the responsibility to use the test wisely and understand the results. This section will cover testing as it relates to sleep-disordered breathing.

Physiologic Basis for Testing: Human adult sleep consists of five stages: Stage I, a transition stage between wakefulness and deeper sleep; Stage II, a stage of deeper non-REM sleep; stages III and IV, sometimes lumped together as delta wave sleep, which are the deepest non-REM stages; and REM stage, a stage of consciousness where dreaming takes place. Non-REM sleep is characterized by preservation of muscle tone and an EEG demonstrating slowing (lower overall average frequency of the signal than awake), indicating a reduction in brain function. REM stage is characterized by an EEG similar to that of an awake person, rapid eye movements, penile tumescence in men, and a marked reduction in muscle tone with the exception of eye muscles and respiratory muscles. Humans descend in progressively deeper stages of non-REM sleep, return to stage II, and then have a period of REM sleep. This cycle repeats itself anywhere between three and five times per night. Because of the disruption in normal sleep in the sleep laboratory, the first REM period is sometimes absent. This is termed *first night effect*. Humans typically wake up for very short periods of time during the night and return to sleep easily. For a person to wake in the morning feeling refreshed, he or she must have enough time in bed, normal cycling through stages, uninterrupted, nonfragmented sleep, and normal EEG waveforms. During sleep, a variety of pathological entities can be encountered. Abnormalities can be architectural, where sleep is fragmented or stage sequence or fraction can be anomalous. Pathologic events can occur, such as parasomnias, sleep-disordered breathing, leg movements, desaturations, arrhythmias, or abnormal arousals. Pathological events often cause architectural abnormalities. Sleep is monitored by EEG (usually just a vertex and occipital lead bilaterally), electrooculogram, and submental electromyogram. Cardiorespiratory status is monitored by ECG, oral and nasal airflow, abdominal and thoracic respiratory efforts, and noninvasive pulse oximetry (see **Oximetry**). Limb movements are monitored using bilateral anterior tibial electromyograms. Low light or infrared video and sound recordings of the night are often collected. Although studies can be limited to cardiorespiratory parameters, and EEG monitoring can be more complex, the configuration described above is the most common for apnea-related polysomnography. It should be noted that presently (first half of 2008), most third-party payors still require EEG monitoring as part of the polysomnogram to qualify for reimbursement and equipment prescriptions. Medicare regulations have just changed to permit home sleep testing including testing without an EEG component. Local implementation of national policy and the response of other Medicaid and commercial insurers to this change are under development.

Testing Procedure: The patient reports to the sleep lab in the early evening and usually is interviewed by the technologist. A sleep history is obtained. Electrodes and sensors are applied, and the patient is put to sleep. The majority of modern laboratories use computerized data acquisition because of greater ease of use, more compact equipment, and greatly reduced storage space requirements for studies compared to paper-based recordings. Most laboratories have protocols that permit the application of oxygen and CPAP/BiPAP if abnormalities are identified. SDB-related studies can be performed as diagnostic tests, where no therapeutic intervention is provided, titration studies where the sole purpose of the test is treatment, and split night studies where diagnosis and treatment are performed in a single study. Titration refers to the fitting of NIPPV mask equipment, determining mode (CPAP, BiPAP, or BiPAP with backup rate), and determining the pressure appropriate to the patient. Titration is more of an art than a science, and the initial titration is sometimes only a starting point. Patients may require empiric adjustments in pressure and occasionally the patient will need to return to the laboratory for further modification of the prescription. The patient fills out a post-test questionnaire in the morning and is discharged. The testing procedure is completed by scoring and interpretation. The night is arbitrarily divided into epochs, usually 30 seconds in length. Each epoch is assigned a sleep stage and relevant events (desaturations, leg movements, apneas, hypopneas, arousals, etc.) are recorded. Sleep milestones (time to sleep onset, percentage of night asleep, percentage of the night in each stage, etc.) and events are tabulated. This process is usually computer assisted. Scoring is usually performed by a technologist, and the technologist may often offer a preliminary report and interpretation. The study is then given to the sleep professional (MD, DO, or PhD) for interpretation. It is expected that the sleep professional will review every epoch and briefly review the accuracy of the technologist's scoring. An evaluation of the patient's sleep and recommendations for treatment will be provided. Many labs issue a report that is difficult for the primary clinician to understand, and recommendations tend to be boilerplate. Although the pages of tabular data are necessary for the sleep physician, the durable medical equipment supplier, and the insurance company, individualized recommendations and a comprehensible summary should be expected.

Indications for Testing: Sleep testing is indicated in a variety of situations. Testing related to SDB is the most common. As a rule, diagnostic and split night polysomnography will have the highest yield of results that change therapy when performed for conditions that manifest excessive daytime somnolence. Formal, validated assessment tools, such as the Berlin questionnaire (Ann Intern Med 1999;131:485), can also be used to stratify patients into groups with high- and low-pretest probability of sleep apnea. Patients with abnormalities of overnight oximetry without obvious cardiovascular or pulmonary disease, patients with pulmonary hypertension and/or right heart failure of uncertain etiology, and patients with hypoxia-related erythrocytosis of uncertain etiology may also benefit from testing. Increasing recognition of the interplay of sleep apnea with cardiac disease lends urgency to testing patients with poorly controlled left heart failure and poorly controlled hypertension when other risk factors (obesity, snoring, abnormal airway) are present. Referral for testing to initiate NIPPV, to assess continued need for therapy after surgery or weight loss, or because of persistent symptoms despite therapy are also appropriate. It is unusual for SDB to present with insomnia, and PSG testing should be considered after other causes for the insomnia are excluded. Indications for testing are frequently circumscribed by third-party payors, and these general comments should be interpreted in the context of local insurance behaviors and misbehaviors.

Interpretation of Results: Polysomnogram reports contain much information, most of which is of little value to the primary clinician. Most reports contain a description of the testing environment and the observations of the technologist. Sleep is described using a series of milestones. Sleep latency, the time to persistent sleep, is usually under 30 minutes. Sleep efficiency, the amount of time spent asleep from lights out to lights on, is usually greater than 85–90%. Stage I sleep makes up about 5% or less of the night, Stage II about 50% of the night, Stages III and IV combined about 20–25%, and REM about 20–25%. Obviously, there is some room in these numbers to account for normal patient-to-patient variation. Stage II is distributed throughout the night, Stages III and IV predominate in the earlier part of the night, and Stage REM in the latter part of the night. Patients who have abnormalities of the fraction of time spent in a given stage, or who have abnormalities of stage delay or advancement (early REM, late III/IV) are said to have architectural abnormalities. Oxygen saturation and ECG parameters are reported. Rates of sleep fragmentation expressed as arousals per hour, leg movements as leg movements per hour, and respiratory events as apneas and hypopneas per hour (AHI, used interchangeably with RDI, or respiratory distress index) are provided, usually in tabular form. While there are generally accepted severity standards based on RDI for normal (<5), mild (5–15), moderate (15–30), and severe (>30) sleep apnea, a generally accepted severity score has not been defined for leg movements and arousals. Periodic leg movements and successions of leg movements meeting certain criteria have particular pathologic significance and an index of 5 or greater is considered pathologic. There is no such threshold for an arousal index. Some labs will report a snoring index. RERA's, respiratory-related arousals are events where a respiratory event triggers an arousal, but the event does not meet the definition of an apnea or hypopnea. When CPAP or BiPAP are applied and titrated to effect, the report will reflect the scorer's and interpreter's opinion as to best pressure, whether there was rebound sleep (intense, long runs of III/IV and REM sleep), suppression of snoring and apneas, suppression of desaturations, and if the REM stage while the patient was supine was seen. This last observation has to do with apnea being the most severe during supine REM. Sometimes omitted but of value is the hypnogram, a plot of time vs. various sleep parameters. This tool correlates parameters such as stage and body position with various events. Results of the polysomnogram will drive intervention, further testing, and consultation.

2.6   Pulmonary Function Testing

The West books (Respiratory Physiology, The Essentials 2005;186, Pulmonary Pathophysiology, The Essentials 2003;205) are the classics in the field and are the first step in any effort at serious further study. Extensive documentation regarding testing procedures and standards are available on the ATS Web site (www. thoracic.org/sections/publications/statements/index.html).

Introduction: Pulmonary function testing is the term commonly used for assessing the physiologic function of the lungs. A range of tests fall under this umbrella term, but in common practice it refers to spirometry, lung volume determinations, and carbon monoxide diffusing capacity determination. This group of tests evaluates physiologic function and does not (and cannot) by themselves provide a diagnosis or etiology for the presenting complaint. These tests are dependent upon the cooperation of the patient and the skill of the operator. Major professional associations (ATS, ERS) have written extensive guidelines to assure maximum reliability and reproducibility of results and to provide a framework for standardized interpretation.

Physiologic Basis for Testing: The physiology of respiration has been well understood for decades. The lungs always contain air, even at the end of forced exhalation. Normal lungs have elastic recoil that causes the lungs to tend to collapse. The chest wall and diaphragm form a bellows that increases and decreases the volume of the lungs. The chest wall and diaphragm have an inherent elasticity that causes them to expand. The lungs within the chest wall counterbalance each other and govern the volumetric excursion from forced exhalation to full inspiration. Inspiration and expiration occurs through the trachea and bronchi. The airways are not rigid (partially collapsible), and because of this there is an interaction between the pulmonary parenchyma, the chest wall, and the airways during respiration. In practice, this means that the higher the absolute lung volume, the higher the rate of airflow, and that there is an absolute maximum rate of airflow at any given point in the breathing cycle that is dependent upon lung volume and is independent of effort. This is termed *expiratory flow limitation*. Oxygen is transferred from the alveoli to the red blood cells, and carbon dioxide from the blood (both plasma and red cells) to the alveoli; this is termed *gas transfer*. Pathologic conditions can cause increases or decreases in lung volumes, reductions in flow rates of gas in the airways, and abnormalities of gas transfer. Common pulmonary function testing evaluates the absolute amount of gas in the lungs (lung volume determination), airflow rates and some relative lung volumes (spirometry), and gas transfer (diffusing capacity). Reduction in lung volume is termed *restriction*; reduction in airflow greater than would be expected for a given reduction in lung volume is called *obstruction*.

Although there are measurements made of lung volumes at many stages of inspiration and expiration, there are four important measurements: total lung capacity is the maximum gas capacity of the lung after maximum inhalation; residual volume is the minimum gas left in the lung after forceful exhalation; vital capacity is the difference between the two (volume of excursion between total lung capacity and residual volume; and functional residual capacity is the volume of gas in the lung at the conclusion of quiet breathing exhalation. The last value is of physiologic significance as it is the point of balance between the tendency of the lung to collapse and the tendency of the chest wall to expand. Lung volume determinations require more complex equipment than spirometry because the amount of gas in the lung is measured referenced to a theoretically completely collapsed, gasless lung. It is simple, however, to measure the vital capacity ("breath all the way in, and now blow out 'til there's nothing left") and spirometry is performed more frequently. Spirometry is valuable in assessing airway disease, the most common form of lung disease requiring PFT evaluation and monitoring.

Spirometry measures vital capacity (as described above) as well as dynamic lung performance. The most common and standardized measurement of airflow is termed the FEV1 (forced expiratory volume in one second). The patient must participate fully in this evaluation, as the purpose is to force expiratory flow limitation so that the test is reproducible. Another measurement calculated from the plot of volume exhaled vs. time (the spirogram) is the FEF 25-75. This measurement is particularly sensitive to obstruction in the smaller airways.

The most commonly used method to measure gas transfer in the clinical setting is called the carbon monoxide diffusing capacity. Tracer amounts of carbon monoxide, a gas avidly bound by hemoglobin, are introduced into the inhaled gas. Because all CO that comes into contact with hemoglobin will be bound tightly for the duration of the test, the amount of CO removed from the inspired gas is an approximation of the amount of hemoglobin in the lung at test time, and the efficiency of interaction between the alveoli and the capillaries. This is a sensitive but nonspecific test for any parenchymal pulmonary dysfunction. One interesting side issue is the presence of free blood in the alveoli after pulmonary hemorrhage or contusion. In this setting, the amount of CO uptake will be well above normal, with the noncirculating blood acting as a CO sink.

Lung volumes and flow rates vary in the population. These variations are due to differences in age, sex, height, and race. Multiple predictive equations are available for estimating normal function based on these parameters. Many pulmonary physicians do not think of pulmonary function test results in absolute numbers, but rather as a percentage of predicted value.

Test Procedure: A wide variety of testing equipment are available. Spirometry-only units are often fairly small and portable. Lung volume determination equipment is usually operated out of a fixed base. Spirometry correlates exhaled volume with time elapsed from the beginning of exhalation. Exhaled volume can either be measured in a collection system (reference units use a water seal bell jar) or inferred by electronically integrating flow rate vs. time. The latter is commonly used in hospital laboratories and clinician offices, and with current technology these units are very accurate. Lung volume determination is performed by a dilution technique or plethysmography. In the dilution technique, a tracer gas (usually helium or nitrogen) in a known volume of air is measured in the patient's breathing circuit, and the air in the patient at the time of the connection equilibrates with the air containing the tracer gas. By measuring the tracer gas before and after equilibration, the volume of air in the patient at the time of the connection can be determined. Plethysmography ("the box") encloses the patient in an airtight box and the patient is asked to perform breathing against a closed airway while airway pressure is being measured. It is possible to measure the pressure swings in the box (volume of box minus volume of person is precisely known) and infer the volume of compressible gas in the patient. The physics and physiology are quite elegant (J Clin Invest 1956; 35:322). Both systems have their advantages and disadvantages. Diffusing capacity measurement capacity is usually built into the lung volume machine. There are a number of different techniques, but many labs use the single-breath technique, where the patient inhales a single breath of gas containing CO, holds their breath for 10 seconds, and then exhales. The exhaled gas is sampled and the amount of CO removed is calculated. This figure, along with the amount of tracer gas inhaled, permits calculation of a transfer function.

The technician should be specifically trained and experienced. The patient should be able to follow directions. For diagnostic purposes, the patient is usually told to refrain from any respiratory medications for 24–48 hrs prior to testing (if possible). Spirometry is usually performed first, so that if the patient fatigues at least the spirometric data is available. Testing may also include response to inhaled bronchodilators. Occasionally, provocative testing to elicit airways hyperreactivity may be performed. The agent usually used in the United States is methacholine (sometimes exercise). The procedure is safe and discriminates well between patients with airway hyperreactivity and those without (Am J Respir Crit Care Med 2000;161:309).

Most patients have no difficulty with the testing procedures. Some patients, particularly those with significant degrees of underlying lung disease or those who are severely deconditioned, can find the testing quite tiring. Some patients complain of claustrophobia with the plethysmograph. If the patient exhales too forcefully during testing, it is possible to precipitate a syncopal episode.

At the conclusion of testing, the test is reviewed for reproducibility, technical error, and suitability for interpretation. It is then given to the interpreting physician. Some testing units provide a computerized preliminary interpretation.

Indications for Testing: Pulmonary function testing provides functional rather than diagnostic information and can describe the kind of functional impairment present. Diagnostically, pulmonary function testing can provide objective confirmation of a complaint of dyspnea. Testing can distinguish between obstructive functional impairment and restrictive functional impairment. Although not diagnostic in itself, this distinction has influence over how the remainder of the diagnostic evaluation is conducted. PFTs provide an objective measure of the severity of the functional abnormality. Within each category, obstruction can be shown to be reversible or fixed. Restrictive disease can be described as parenchymal or extrapulmonary. In both types of abnormality, the presence or absence of a gas transfer function abnormality can be ascertained. Once a diagnosis is established, PFTs can be used to monitor the course of the disease and to evaluate the efficacy of treatment intervention. PFTs are used as part of disability evaluations to provide objective confirmation and documentation of a patient's complaints of impairment. Pulmonary function testing can be used as a kind of "reality check" in patients with an established diagnosis of lung disease. If there is a significant difference between observed dyspnea and dyspnea expected from the pulmonary function test results, extrapulmonary or pulmonary vascular contributors to dyspnea should be sought.

In practice, this translates to ordering PFTs at an initial workup to confirm the presence of a functional defect; characterize the defect as restrictive, obstructive, or mixed; and grade the severity of the abnormality. The pattern of impairment drives the direction of the subsequent evaluation. Severity grading is increasingly important as guideline-based therapy of asthma and COPD becomes mainstream and helps stratify the patient into the correct treatment category. During treatment, periodic testing can indicate the need for changing therapy or altering prognosis.

Interpretation of Test Results: Pulmonary function testing reports usually provide a table of data outlining actual test values as well the relation of the results to the predicted values. There has been an evolution of thinking about the meaning of normal. Older texts approached the issue of normal as ±20% of predicted value. More recently, the lower limit of normal has been defined as a confidence limit. The report will indicate the prediction equations used and scheme of interpretation. There is usually a statement from the technician as to the technical adequacy of the test, and finally there is the physician interpretation. Spirometry, lung volumes, and diffusing capacity are often reported as separate line items. Obstruction is addressed in the spirometry results, restriction or hyperinflation in the volumes results, and abnormal gas transfer is described in the diffusing capacity results. Severity of the abnormality is usually graded as normal, mild, moderate, moderately severe, severe, and very severe, and specific ranges of percentages predicted correspond to these categories. The criteria in Table 2.1 and Table 2.2 and the algorithm in Figure 2.3

Table 2.1   Types of Ventilatory Defects and Their Diagnoses

Obstruction	• FEV_1/VC <5th percentile of predicted. • A decrease in flow at low lung volume is not specific for small airway disease in individual patients. • A concomitant decrease in FEV_1 and VC is most commonly caused by poor effort, but rarely may reflect airflow obstruction. Confirmation of airway obstruction requires measurement of lung volumes. • Measurement of absolute lung volumes may assist in the diagnosis of emphysema, bronchial asthma, and chronic bronchitis. It may also be useful in assessing lung hyperinflation. • Measurements of airflow resistance may be helpful in patients who are unable to perform spirometric maneuvers.
Restriction	• TLC <5th percentile of predicted. • A reduced VC does not prove a restrictive pulmonary defect. It may be suggestive of lung restriction when FEV_1/VC is normal or increased. • A low TLC from a single breath test should not be seen as evidence of restriction.
Mixed Defect	• FEV_1/VC and TLC <5th percentile of predicted. • FEV_1: forced expiratory volume in one second; VC: vital capacity; TLC: total lung capacity.

Pelligrino et al. Interpretative strategies for lung function tests. Eur. Respir. J., Nov 2005; 26:948–968. Copyright European Respiratory Society Journals Ltd. Used with permission.

Table 2.2   Severity of Any Spirometric Abnormality Based on the Forced Expiratory Volume in One Second (FEV₁)

Degree of severity	FEV₁ % pred
Mild	>70
Moderate	60–69
Moderately severe	50–59
Severe	35–49
Very severe	<35

% pred: % predicted

Pelligrino et al. Interpretative strategies for lung function tests. Eur. Respir. J., Nov 2005; 26:948–968. Copyright European Respiratory Society Journals Ltd. Used with permission.

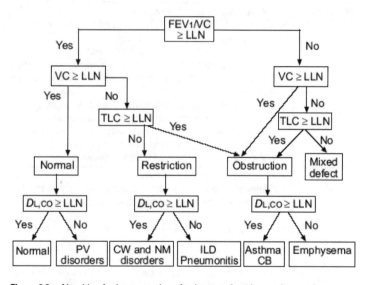

Figure 2.3   Algorithm for interpretation of pulmonary function testing results. Pelligrino et al. Interpretative strategies for lung function tests. Eur. Respir. J., Nov 2005; 26:948–968. Copyright European Respiratory Society Journals Ltd. Used with permission.

provide the analytic strategy used by most pulmonary physicians for PFT interpretation (Eur Respir J 2005;26:948).

Some Final (Editorial) Comments: A hurried clinician, cattle prodded by an MBA in an office for productivity, hears a smoker cough and complain of dyspnea. That patient is labeled as having COPD, told to stop smoking, given a handful of inhalers, and sent on their way. Consider the injustice afforded that patient. The diagnosis has not been confirmed; bronchodilator response is unknown; severity is undefined. The patient may have pulmonary fibrosis; she may be inundated with expensive medications that don't work; she has been denied an opportunity to have therapy directed by progressive guidelines; and she has been denied the opportunity to have an objective, serious discussion about prognosis and smoking cessation. Pulmonary function testing should be as integral to the evaluation of the pulmonary patient as echocardiography is to the evaluation of the cardiac patient.

2.7 Pulse Oximetry

Introduction: The ability to monitor a patient's oxygenation status is a critical component of modern medical care. With the advent of pulse oximetry in the early 1980s this can now be done noninvasively. However, there are practical and theoretical limitations on the information that can be provided by this instrument.

Physiologic Basis of Testing: Oxygen content of the blood can be calculated by multiplying the oxygen carrying capacity of hemoglobin by the percent of hemoglobin-binding oxygen molecules, the saturation. (Dissolved oxygen contribution is negligible.) Oxygen content is a function of oxygen transfer from the alveoli and oxygen off-loading at the tissue level. Venous oxygen content will reflect both oxygen transfer and oxygen uptake, also termed *oxygen extraction*. Arterial oxygen content will depend primarily on gas transfer in the lung (see **Hypoxia**). Venous oxygenation status becomes important in low perfusion states and shock, but is difficult to measure and does not play a role in all but the sickest patients. Arterial oxygen saturation is easily measured and has a variety of clinical uses. The oxygen hemoglobin saturation curve reflects the relationship between the partial pressure of oxygen in the blood and percent of hemoglobin receptor sites carrying oxygen. This sigmoid curve is 50% saturated at a PaO_2 of 25–30, 90% saturated at PaO_2 55, and essentially 100% saturated at PaO_2 of 90 or above. At sea level a normal individual breathing 100% oxygen can easily achieve a PaO_2 in excess of 600. This means there is a great range of PaO_2 over which saturation will not change even when there may be considerable interference with gas transfer. Oxygenated hemoglobin and deoxygenated hemoglobin have different absorption spectra. By measuring the relationship between absorption at 660 and 910 nm, the proportion of oxygenated and deoxygenated hemoglobin can be determined. Pulse oximetry uses two LEDs and two detectors to make these measurements. The LED light is passed through the skin; it is unaffected by skin pigmentation and tissue water content. This raw signal is processed to remove the venous contribution to saturation/desaturation by only examining pulsatile changes in saturation (http://www.oximetry.org/pulseox/principles.htm 2002;2007). Although there are clinical problems in using this data, there are a number of methodological and mechanical limitations as well. Common problems with conventional oximeters include sensitivity to motion, poor perfusion, and in some instances venous flow (forehead probes). They do not identify abnormal hemoglobins (carboxyhemoglobin, methemoglobin) (http://www. oximetry.org/pulseox/limitations.htm 2002;2007). Newer-generation oximeters have digital signal processing algorithms to reduce noise, improve reliability, and improve performance in low perfusion states (http://www . masimo.com/pdf/technology/LAB1035M.pdf 2005;2007).

Testing Procedure: Emitter/detector probes are applied to the finger, earlobe, forehead, or other easily accessible areas. Many oximetry units are freestanding, providing a pulse reading, indicator of signal quality, and saturation. Other oximeters are integrated into larger diagnostic or therapeutic units, such as ICU monitors, anesthesia machines, and CPET testing units.

Interpretation of Results: Saturations above 90% are generally considered to be safe saturations, indicating that there is adequate gas exchange under conditions of testing to oxygenate hemoglobin to 90% or better. Saturations below 90%, if accurate, indicate impaired gas exchange. A rising oxygen saturation in response to therapy is reassuring; a falling oxygen saturation suggests very significant cardiopulmonary impairment.

Indications for Testing: Use of pulse oximetry is ubiquitous in the developed world, and has almost become one of the vital signs. Its use is seen in operative areas, critical care areas, emergency rooms, delivery suites, procedure suites, and the like for promoting patient safety. Oximetry is integral to CPET, graded cardiac exercise testing, and polysomnography.

Limitations: Mechanical and technical limitations of the technique have been addressed above. From a clinical perspective, consider what oximetry *does not* do. Saturations must be interpreted in the clinical context. A patient may have an adequate saturation, yet this saturation is achieved at the cost of a high FIO_2, respiratory rate of 40, and all accessory muscles of respiration in use. The patient is still clinically in respiratory failure. Oximetry does not provide any information about the patient's acid-base status. Even if a patient is severely hypercarbic, the alveolar air equation allows saturations of close to 100% provided the FIO_2 is sufficiently high. Oximetry cannot distinguish between a saturation of 100% produced by a PaO_2 of 100 or 600; the PaO_2 in this setting will correctly reflect saturation, not gas exchange. A common personally observed error is to derive false reassurance that a patient is clinically stable from an adequate saturation because the clinician has not taken into account the conditions of testing (Aust Crit Care 2006;19:139).

2.8 Thoracentesis

Introduction: Thoracentesis is used to sample the contents of the pleural space. A variety of pulmonary and nonpulmonary diseases have manifestations as pleural effusions. Safe sampling of the pleural fluid is essential to the diagnosis of infection, malignancy, a variety of inflammatory conditions, cardiac disease, and hepatic disease. The combination of modern imaging techniques such as ultrasound with traditional physical examination of the pleural space permits smaller effusions to be tapped with greater safety.

Physiology: The visceral and parietal pleura form a potential space between the chest wall and the lung. In normal circumstances, there is 5 cc or less of fluid present in the pleural cavity, and the liquid acts as a lubricant between the two surfaces during respiration. Fluid flows into the pleural space from the systemic vessels in the parietal and visceral pleura, and fluid exits the pleural through the parietal lymphatics. There is a normal turnover of fluid in the pleural space, and for fluid to collect it must enter in sufficient quantity to overwhelm the drainage capacity of the lymphatics. Fluid can collect in the space because of increased hydrostatic pressure in the blood vessels increasing inflow, breakdown of the capillary barrier also increasing inflow, blockage of lymphatics impeding drainage, and entry of fluid from other sites (ascites entering through diaphragmatic defects, blood from injury, lymph [chyle] from thoracic duct injury or obstruction, esophageal contents). Effusions that arise from malignancy, inflammation, and infection have higher protein content than effusions arising from simple increased hydrostatic pressure or liver disease. High-protein effusions are termed *exudates;* low-protein effusions are termed *transudates*. Diagnosis of pleural disease usually begins with the identification of the fluid as an exudate or transudate.

Procedure: The presence of fluid is identified by imaging or examination. Assurance that the fluid is free flowing can be made using decubitus imaging. Once a decision is made to sample the fluid, a site for suitable sampling is found. Traditional physical exam is used to find an area of dullness consistent with the X-ray findings. More recently, ultrasound localization of pleural fluid permits the safe sampling of fluid pockets and smaller effusions (Chest 2006;129:1709). Some authors feel that the standard of care requires the use of ultrasound for localization and determining depth of penetration necessary. My personal experience is that the value of percussion has gone down as the average weight of the patient has gone up; everywhere is dull. Once a suitable site at a rib interspace is selected, it is marked. Standard sterile preparation with povidone iodine or chlorhexidine and appropriate draping is performed. Local anesthesia is injected intradermally and subcutaneously. The initial needle is exchanged for a longer thin needle to bring anesthesia down to the level of the rib and pleural surface. Recalling that the neurovascular costal bundle runs under the caudal edge of the rib, the needle is "walked" over the top of the lower rib of the interspace, injecting anesthesia as the needle is moved. Entrance into the pleural space is momentarily painful even with injection of anesthesia, and location of the end of the needle is confirmed by the ability to withdraw pleural contents. The needle is withdrawn, and a needle-catheter system is introduced along the anesthetized track. There are a number of different collection systems available and choice is a matter of economics and personal preference. Once the catheter is in place, fluid is withdrawn from the pleural space. Many pulmonologists will limit drainage to 2 liters at a time to avoid postexpansion pulmonary edema. Short of that limit, as much fluid as possible is collected to increase diagnostic yield when the fluid is tested. Removal of a substantial amount of fluid also can reduce dyspnea, and is another motivation to drain the pleural space when dyspnea is a significant symptom. Fluid is removed using either a vacuum bottle or a syringe-based pump mechanism. When flow of pleural fluid slows, the catheter is withdrawn slowly until flow returns. When this maneuver produces no more flow, the catheter is withdrawn. A chest X-ray is usually performed to evaluate for pneumothorax.

Indications for Procedure: Thoracentesis is performed primarily to diagnose the etiology of fluid in the pleural space. In some cases, such as obvious CHF, it is not necessary to sample the pleural space. In general, however, the clinician should have a low threshold for thoracentesis, particularly in the setting of pneumonia or possible malignancy. Thoracentesis is also performed to reduce dyspnea (Am J Med 1983;74:813). Thoracentesis may also be used to treat empyema if the collection is relatively small and free flowing.

Interpretation of Results: Pleural fluid is sent for cytology analysis, cell count and differential, and microbiologic analysis. The latter usually includes routine culture and sensitivity, anaerobic culture, gram stain, fungal culture, and AFB smear and culture. This may be modified for the particular patient, but generally it is better to order too many tests rather than too few when the consequence of inadequate testing may be another invasive procedure. Fluid pH is useful, but the fluid must be collected anaerobically and processed with an electrode/optode system (i.e., same as a blood gas). For chemistry analysis most practitioners will obtain at minimum glucose, protein, and LDH. Additional tests may include cholesterol, amylase, pro-BNP, triglycerides, and other disease-specific tests. The first diagnostic differentiation is between an exudative and transudative effusion. The most widely accepted method of differentiation is the application of Light's criteria (pleural fluid is an exudate if any one of the following criteria are met: pleural fluid protein/serum protein ratio >0.5; pleural LDH/serum LDH >0.6; pleural LDH >2/3 upper normal limit of serum LDH). Some authors advocate the use of cholesterol levels or other more complex analyses (Clin Chest Med 2006;27:241). Transudates have a circumscribed differential diagnosis: CHF, liver disease, Meig's syndrome (ovarian neoplasm), nephrotic syndrome, and peritoneal dialysis are most common. Once a transudate is identified, evaluation is straightforward. Exudates have a broader differential, but major concerns are bacterial infection, malignancy, inflammatory diseases, and tuberculosis. Effusions associated with pneumonia are common (parapneumonic effusions), and the clinician must determine if the effusion needs drainage or not. In general, a pleural fluid pH <7.20, low glucose, elevated LDH, and high neutrophil count indicates that the effusion needs drainage irrespective of the presence of bacteria on gram stain or culture. Malignant effusions are identified conclusively by cytology. Inflammatory effusions, such as those produced by rheumatoid arthritis, typically have a low glucose and may have low complement levels and an elevated rheumatoid factor. High lymphocyte counts are associated with lymphoma and tuberculosis. Elevated amylase can be seen with pancreatitis and esophageal rupture. Bloody effusions may be seen with pulmonary embolism (Am Fam Physician 2006;73:1211). Pleural fluid analysis in general has a poor diagnostic yield with respect to recovery of bacteria, mycobacteria, and malignant cells. A negative test in the face of high pretest probability for one of these conditions is undependable (Singapore Med J2006;47:609).

Complications: Major complications are bleeding, infection, pneumothorax, and postexpansion pulmonary edema. Rarely, laceration of visceral organs can occur if the needle is introduced in too low an interspace. Pneumothorax, the most common complication, is stated to occur anywhere between 4% and 30%

of the time without ultrasound guidance, and in the 2–3% range with ultrasound. Operator experience reduces complications. Small pneumothorax is managed with observation; larger pneumothorax may need either a pleural catheter with Heimlich valve or formal chest tube (Chest 2003;123:418).

Further Testing: Undiagnosed pleural effusions are managed by utilization of other diagnostic modalities (bronchoscopy, CT, etc.) or direct inspection of the pleural space with pleuroscopy or thoracoscopy. Yield of thoracoscopy is superior to closed needle biopsy of the pleura (Chest 1979;75:45).

2.9   Transthoracic Needle Biopsy (TTNB)

Clin Chest Med 1999;20:805

Introduction: TTNB is the procedure of choice for sampling peripheral lung lesions both for cytology and microbiology. The procedure can also be used for more central lesions in the hands of skilled operators. It complements, rather than replaces, fiber-optic bronchoscopy.

Physiology: Detailed imaging of the chest has become commonplace with CT, PET, and MRI techniques, and it is possible to define precisely the anatomic location of an abnormality. A needle introduced through the chest wall does not need to follow the path of a bronchus to reach its target, and it can be guided precisely in real time using CT or fluoroscopy. Accuracy of localization under these circumstances is high.

Description of Procedure: Once a decision is made to use TTNB, the patient is asked to refrain from the use of antiplatelet and anticoagulant drugs for an appropriate time period, usually 5–7 days. A final diagnostic image is made the day of the procedure to evaluate for intervening changes such as PTX, effusion, or even regression of the lesion. The abnormality is identified using the imaging system of choice (a high percentage of these procedures are performed under CT guidance). The patient is appropriately positioned and the skin site of puncture is anesthetized. Some centers will use conscious sedation as well. The selection of biopsy method is technical, but distills to the choice of a cutting/coring needle vs. an aspirating needle. Cutting needles, which provide a histologic specimen, are appropriate for larger more peripheral lesions. Aspirating needles can also provide a good specimen for the diagnosis of malignancy and are preferred for microbiologic sampling. The trajectory from the skin to the abnormality is planned to minimize traversal of lung tissue and to avoid vascular structures. When possible, point-of-care cytology evaluation of the specimen confirms adequate material and a preliminary diagnosis. Postprocedure care includes monitoring for pneumothorax and hemoptysis as the two serious common complications. Patients are rested with biopsy site down for 2 hours, X-rayed, held another 2 hours, re-X-rayed, and discharged. A small pneumothorax is managed conservatively, but a larger PTX or a symptomatic PTX requires a chest tube (either large bore or catheter, see **Tube Thoracostomy**). Some centers advocate rapid discharge if the patient is stable and does not develop a pneumothorax within an hour (Radiology 2001;219:247).

Indications for the Procedure: The procedure will be motivated by the presence of an imaging abnormality. Solitary pulmonary nodule, mediastinal mass, peripheral lung mass, pleural mass or thickening, or infiltrate suggestive of infection (cavity, opacities in immunocompromised host, etc.). Contraindications include intractable cough, inability to cooperate, uncontrolled bleeding diathesis, one working lung, mechanical ventilation, and severe COPD (increases morbidity associated with pneumothorax and increases risk of pneumothorax).

Interpretation of Results: A peripheral malignant lesion will be identified as malignant 80–90% of the time, often with accurate cell type identification. A definitive benign diagnosis cannot be obtained with equal reliability, and varies from condition to condition. A benign or inflammatory result of TTNB cannot exclude with certainty the presence of cancer if the pretest probability of malignancy is high. Bacterial, fungal, or mycobacterial species recovered from TTNB are by definition pathogens because there is no upper airway contamination of the specimen (Ugeskr Laeger 1995;157:6580, Respiration 1995;62:1).

Complications and Limitations: The major complications of the procedure are pneumothorax, hemorrhage, vasovagal instability, and rarely air embolism. Any of these events can precipitate cardiovascular instability or respiratory failure in the fragile patient. Incidence of complication is increased by the use of large-bore cutting needles, emphysema, and patient coughing/motion. A small pneumothorax can be managed conservatively; larger air collections may need catheter or large bore tube drainage. It is theoretically possible that malignant cells or infection could spread along the needle track and this is sometimes described with mesothelioma in particular. The procedure provides no information about bronchial anatomy, and the risk of pneumothorax is >10% if a cutting needle is employed.

Further Testing: TTNB is complementary to FOB, and a nondiagnostic TTNB may be followed by FOB, VATS, or OLB.

2.10 VATS, Open Lung Biopsy, and Mediastinoscopy

Murray and Nadel 2005;1:651

Introduction: These three procedures are used for diagnosis as well as treatment. The purpose of including these procedures in this book is not so much to provide technical detail, but to provide the clinician with some sense of how they are used and what the patient can expect.

Physiology: VATS (video-assisted thoracoscopic surgery) and OLB (open lung biopsy) breach the chest wall and enter the pleural space. The pleural space can be inspected and biopsied. The lung parenchyma can also be biopsied. The advantage of surgical lung biopsy (the collective term for VATS and OLB) over endoscopic lung biopsy is specimen size. This permits the pathologist to evaluate architecture and histology as well as cytology. Specimen size also reduces sampling error. The larger specimen permits a variety of tests including culture and specialized staining as well as simple H&E staining. In comparison to closed needle pleural biopsy (Abrams or Cope), pleural biopsy using VATS or OLB permits visual or tactile choice of the biopsy site, as well as a larger specimen. Directed biopsy is a great advantage, as pleural lesions often have large skip areas. Mediastinoscopy can be performed using a number of techniques, but the most common is anterior cervical mediastinoscopy. This procedure permits biopsy and inspection of mediastinal lymph nodes.

Description of Procedure: All three procedures require general anesthesia. Mediastinoscopy starts with a suprasternal incision and finger blunt dissection into the tissue planes of the mediastinum around the anterior trachea. An instrument similar in appearance to a laryngoscope is advanced into the mediastinum along the trachea. Lymph node biopsy is the usual goal of the procedure, although the surgical literature describes other uses of the technique. In the absence of complications, the patient recovers from general anesthesia and is discharged the same day. VATS requires double lumen tube endotracheal intubation so that the lung to be biopsied (or pleural space to be inspected) can be deflated. Usually, three stab wounds are made in the chest and instrumentation ports are placed. A telescope and instrumentation devices are introduced through the ports and specimens obtained. Lung biopsies are obtained using a stapling technique. After the procedure, a chest tube is inserted. The patient usually remains in the hospital at least one night to assure that there is no bleeding or air leak, after which the chest tube is removed and the patient discharged. OLB does not require deflation of the lung of interest, so a single lumen endotracheal tube is used. A small (6–8 cm, sometimes larger) intercostal incision is made, and the lung is delivered into the wound; a stapling gun-based biopsy can be obtained and the wound closed. As in VATS, a chest tube is inserted at least overnight to assure adequate hemostasis and pleural closure.

Indications for the Procedure: Mediastinoscopy is used primarily in two scenarios: evaluation of mediastinal lymphadenopathy, such as would be seen in sarcoidosis or lymphoma, and evaluation of mediastinal node status in a patient with lung cancer. Anterior cervical mediastinoscopy can access peritracheal nodes, some right mainstem bronchus nodes, and sometimes subcarinal nodes. If these nodal stations require evaluation, mediastinoscopy is an effective and relatively safe procedure. VATS can be used to sample the pleural space and the lung. Parenchymal lung biopsy, wedge resection of a specific lesion, and biopsy of the parietal pleura are all performed routinely. In the appropriate setting, the technique can biopsy the lateral wall of the mediastinum to assess lymph nodes inaccessible to the mediastinoscope. Open lung biopsy provides good access to lung tissue; ability to inspect the lung and pleural surface is more limited than VATS but still quite satisfactory. OLB may be the only choice for a patient who has extensive pleural adhesions preventing deflation of the lung. OLB is a faster procedure and physiologically less demanding on the patient because single lung ventilation is not required. For this reason, OLB may be favored as a "quick and dirty" biopsy in a severely ill, immunocompromised patient with pneumonia.

Interpretation of Results: The interpretation of the results of these procedures is highly dependent on the patient's problem, and is addressed in the disease-specific sections.

Limitations and Complications: Complications of mediastinoscopy such as bleeding are rare. Fibrosis of the mediastinum can prevent advancement of the instrument and increases the risk of tissue injury and bleeding. Nodal access is limited to the anterior paratracheal lymph nodes, very proximal right hilar lymph nodes, and some subcarinal lymph nodes. It is more difficult to predict the safety of OLB and VATS since the range of procedures and patients is much wider. In general, because of the smaller incisions, VATS is less painful postoperatively and patients return to activity more quickly. Patients undergoing lung biopsy with VATS are forewarned that the procedure may be converted to an open procedure if the lung cannot be deflated. With both VATS and OLB for DPLD, it is tempting for the surgeon to biopsy the very tip or edge of a lobe as this is technically simpler and safer. However, there is often nonspecific fibrosis present and the correct diagnosis can be missed. Often the pulmonary physician plans the site of biopsy with the surgeon.

Chapter 3

Pulmonary Therapeutics

3.1   Introduction

The lungs present a variety of challenges and opportunities in therapeutics:

- The lungs have a large surface area that is in constant contact with the environment. This encouraged use of inhaled medications, and they have become a mainstay of therapy.
- The lungs' most important task is the provision of oxygen to the rest of the body. Because oxygen has such a short half-life in the bloodstream, impaired oxygen uptake treated with supplementation of oxygen requires continuous inhalation of the enriched air mixture. This is inconvenient both for the patient and clinician and requires specialized equipment.
- The lungs depend upon a surrounding bellows mechanism for respiration; when this mechanism fails (either primarily or as a consequence of pulmonary disease), respiration can be supported mechanically. Providing support includes replacing the bellows mechanism and connecting the patient to the respirator.
- The primary defense mechanism of the respiratory system is mechanical clearance of infection and foreign material in the airway. This process is amenable to augmentation.
- Consequences of respiratory failure are catastrophic. Respiratory problems are common with thoracic and extrathoracic surgery. It is possible to identify patients at risk for poor outcomes and avoid or reduce complications.

- Patients with chronic lung disease become deconditioned, frustrated, and depressed. These problems can be addressed with graded exercise and counseling.

This chapter addresses the strategies used for aerosol therapy, physiotherapy, rehabilitation, surgery, interventional bronchoscopy, mechanical ventilation, and perioperative respiratory care. Common pulmonary medications are also reviewed.

3.2 Theory of Inhaled Medications

Introduction: The lung presents a unique opportunity for topical therapy. The alveolar and bronchial surfaces provide a large surface area for the absorption of medications into the systemic circulation. Alternatively, it is possible to apply poorly absorbed medications directly to abnormal pulmonary tissues, achieve a high local concentration, and have relatively little systemic effect. In practice, although it is possible to use the lung for systemic absorption (e.g., morphine, epinephrine, lidocaine) the majority of clinical applications aim for high local concentrations and high therapeutic ratios. Modern inhaled medications have been around since the late 1800s with the use of stramonium cigarettes and inhalation of jimson weed smoke for asthma (both plants are of the nightshade family and have substantial concentrations of belladonna alkaloids). Modern techniques use nebulizers, metered dose inhalers, and dry powder inhalers. Respiratory medications used in these systems include beta agonists (both long and short acting), topically active steroids of varying potency, atropine-like agents, and other anti-inflammatory medications such as nedocromil and cromolyn. Several products combine agents to improve ease of use and leverage the synergy of the mixtures. Some of these medications use inhalation because of rapid onset of effect (short-acting beta agonists); others medications, particularly the steroids, seek a high therapeutic ratio and limited systemic absorption. All of these medications must be nonirritating when inhaled, have topical activity, and be capable of aerosolization. The nebulizer systems must be relatively cheap, easy to use, deliver predictable amounts of medication, and deliver medication to the lungs with a minimum of drug deposited on other tissues. The lung and upper respiratory tract are designed to prevent deposition of particles in the lower respiratory tract. The nose and other upper respiratory tract structures are designed to filter out large particles, and very small particles (<2 μ) can be inhaled and exhaled while they stay in suspension. Particles appropriate to inhaled medications are between 2 and 5 μ, and these have a good chance of raining out in the bronchi and bronchioles as the velocity of the inspired air drops. Particle generators that create particles in this size range are described below. This section does not address the pharmacology of the drugs (see **Pulmonary Medications**).

Nebulizers

Nebulizers suspend a liquid medication containing solution in air. Ultrasonic nebulizers jiggle a standing body of liquid, breaking the surface layers off into the air in small particles. These particles are then inhaled. Updraft nebulizers use the Bernoulli effect to draw a thin column of fluid out of a reservoir by blowing a jet of air over a tube in the liquid. As the liquid is drawn up the tube, it is struck by the air jet and broken into small particles. Updraft nebulizers are much less expensive and far more common than ultrasonic units for delivery of medications. Many kinds of medications are available in forms that can be used in a nebulizer. The advantages of these units include the ability to deliver large amounts of medication quickly, a humidifying effect of the carrier solution, and no need to coordinate breathing with the machine; it presents a steady cloud of medication. Disadvantages include unfavorable particle distribution size with a preponderance of large particles that are absorbed transmucosally in the mouth and/or swallowed, significant systemic delivery of medication, the inconvenience of dependence on the nebulizer unit, the air compressor to drive it and a power source, and the length of treatment (usually 15–20 min). To use, the patient simply fills the reservoir with the medication solution, turns on the compressor, and slowly inhales the mist as it comes out of the mouthpiece. Children or patients with limited ability to cooperate will often take a nebulizer treatment through a face mask of the type used with mixer-delivered oxygen (see **Oxygen Therapy**). Often underappreciated but very real in daily practice is the psychological effect of the clouds of medicated mist. Systemic delivery of large amounts of medication, particularly beta agonists, adds a "kick" to the treatment that is often experienced as a positive by the patient. For these reasons, despite the inconvenience and the suboptimal physics of the device, nebulizers remain popular among patients. Newer units include breath-actuated nebulizers which are used to deliver inhaled medications over an extended period of time in an emergency room or hospital inpatient setting.

Metered Dose Inhalers

These devices are small pressurized metal canisters that contain a mixture of medication, various stabilizing and dispersing agents, and a propellant. The devices are structured in such a way so that pressing the stem into the body of the canister fills a small container within the device to a predetermined level (hence the named metered dose). Release of the stem permits the gas/liquid/medication mixture to leave the canister through the stem into a pinhole atomizer that is incorporated into the outside plastic carrier of the canister. As the pressure in the canister is lowered by the release of contents, more propellant boils off from liquid to gas phase and the unit is ready to deliver another dose (usually takes 20–60 seconds to reequilibrate). Like nebulizers, older metered dose inhalers suffer from poor particle distribution size, leading to mouth deposition of medication. Additionally, these units require coordination of activation and inhalation to get a full dose. For these reasons, there has been interest in devices to reduce velocity of the aerosol jet, permit rainout of the larger particles outside the mouth, and create a reservoir of aerosol to inhale so that coordination is not as critical. These devices are referred to colloquially as spacers. The convenience, portability, potency, and variety of medications available in MDIs makes this delivery system the leading mechanism for inhaling medication. However, at the end of 2008 chlorofluorocarbons (CFC), the propellant used in MDIs until now, will be banned. Hydrofluoroalkane-propelled MDIs (HFA inhalers) are already on the market and will replace the CFC-based units. These units are fundamentally better, with slower particle velocity and smaller, more uniform particle size. However, different physical characteristics of the particles can potentially interfere with the function of the spacers currently in use (http://www.touchbriefings. com/ pdf/890/PT04_peart.pdf 2003;2007). Because of slower particle velocity and better particle distribution size, spacer use may not be as critical. MDI use, with or without a spacer, consists of exhaling to below FRC as far as comfortable, placing the unit (or spacer) in the mouth, depressing and releasing the canister, and breathing slowly but steadily as the stream of medication is delivered. A 5–10 second breath hold is appropriate to permit rainout of medication in the airway.

Dry Powder Inhalers

Withdrawal of CFC-based MDIs from the market spurred interest in other delivery systems, and dry powder inhalers have been successfully developed and marketed. With this delivery system, a dry powder is made available for inhalation, and it is the inhalation itself that delivers the medication to the airways; there is no propellant. Once patients become accustomed to these units, they are generally well liked. Some patients have difficulty with the transition from MDIs to DPIs, but this can be overcome with teaching and preparation. Patients who have very advanced lung disease may not be able to generate sufficient inspiratory flow to deliver drugs to the lungs. In my personal experience, there appears to be a slightly higher (though still acceptable) incidence of hoarseness and cough in patients using this delivery system as compared to those patients using MDIs. Perhaps the greatest problem with this system is the lack of uniformity in mechanism. Each company has its own proprietary system for delivery of drug: Discus, Turbohaler, Aerolizer, HandiHaler, Rotacaps, and Twisthaler are all trade names for patented delivery systems for different agents. They are all effective, and all different. Patients must be taught carefully how to use these inhalers. In my consultative practice, approximately 5–10% of my newly referred patients are not using their DPI properly, and in this subset teaching is a big part of the remedy for "refractory disease" or "therapeutic failure." Studies suggest that this percentage may be conservative. Despite these problems, the DPI systems are well liked by patients because they are convenient, and many of the most effective drugs for asthma and COPD are delivered using one of these mechanisms. When a new DPI is introduced into a clinician's practice, package instructions should be reviewed prior to prescription, and this may be one of the times when a detailed interaction with a drug company representative may be of benefit to patients. All of these delivery systems have placebo units for demonstration, and the clinician or their staff should do a demonstration for the patient.

Indications: Inhaled medication therapy is indicated any time medication is to be applied topically to the airways.

Complications, Problems: DPIs and MDIs are often very expensive. Residue medication in the mouth can lead to irritation or thrush (steroids). Systemic effect is significant despite topical delivery (hypokalemia from albuterol, early cataracts and bone density loss from inhaled steroids). Patients tend to overmedicate with MDIs in particular and require careful teaching as part of their care plan (see **Asthma**) (MGMC Grand Rounds: A Geek's Guide to Inhalers; 2005).

3.3   Medications for Airways Disease

National Asthma Education and Prevention Program 2007, pp. 213–276. The NAEPP guidelines provide a host of further references and reading. The full study (as opposed to the executive summary) is a remarkable document.

Introduction

Several broad classes of medications are used for airways disease. These include β agonists (both long acting [LABA] and short acting [SABA]), atropine-like agents, corticosteroids (inhaled and systemic), methylxanthines, anti-IgE antibody, leukotriene modifiers, and mast cell stabilizers. Clinically relevant information about each medication class will be reviewed. The reader is urged to cross-reference to the sections on asthma and COPD. Two terms deserve definition because they are used extensively below. Controller medications are used on a scheduled basis to prevent symptoms and exacerbations. Rescue medications are used to terminate an acute exacerbation.

Beta Agonists

β agonists stimulate β receptors on smooth muscle, stimulating the production of cyclic AMP and promoting relaxation of airway constrictor muscles.

SABA agents are used as rescue medications. Commonly used inhaled agents include albuterol, levalbuterol (R-isomer of albuterol), metaproterenol, and pirbuterol. These agents are generally safe, and are considered first-line agents for acute relief of bronchospasm. Transition from CFC to HFA propellants for MDIs containing SABAs and other drugs is well under way (early 2008) and will be completed by the end of 2008. This change will not have a material effect on the efficacy of these medications (improvement, if anything). Common side effects include tremor, jitteriness, and occasionally palpitations. Large doses (overdoses) may cause arrhythmias and hypokalemia. Some authorities believe that levalbuterol offers an advantage in reduced side effects compared to mixed isomer β agonists, but the aggregate evidence is conflicting. Many clinicians monitor SABA use as one of several indicators of overall disease control (less SABA use implies better overall control).

LABA agents are considered to be controller medications. Only two members of this class are available, salmeterol and formoterol. Both agents bind more tightly to the β receptor sites and have bronchodilator effects for approximately 12 hours. Both are supplied as dry powder inhalers. Anecdotally, some of my older patients have found the salmeterol DPI easier to use than the formoterol DPI; the latter requires manipulation of a somewhat brittle capsule into a recess in the inhaler. The (R,R) isomer of formoterol, arformoterol, is available as a solution for nebulization that requires refrigerated storage until use. There is no doubt that these drugs are effective long-acting bronchodilators capable of reducing exacerbations. However, questions have arisen over the safety of LABA agents, particularly in asthmatics. Some studies have demonstrated increased death rates attributable to these agents; these studies have been refuted by other investigations showing no relationship between LABA use and excess mortality. Subgroup analysis suggested that mortality and exacerbation was associated negatively with inhaled corticosteroid (ICS) use and positively with high-dose LABA. There also appeared to be excess risk associated with African-Americans (although this may well be a proxy for poor access to care and adverse societal issues). Current recommendations advise against the use of LABA as a single agent (i.e., without coprescription of ICS) and strict adherence to dosing guidelines. Definitive research proving the protective effect of ICS coadministration is pending. Current (2007) National Asthma Education and Prevention Plan (NAEPP) guidelines continue to recommend the use of ICS/LABA combinations for more difficult to control asthma. Manufacturers have produced combined ICS/LABA preparations as salmeterol/fluticasone (available as MDI and DPI) and formoterol/budesonide (available as MDI), which largely addresses the need for coadministration of the drugs (and the clumsiness of the formoterol DPI!). Both combination agents are effective and well tolerated. Although I do not have the wide breadth of experience provided by a clinical study, my experience has been that my patients have benefited greatly from the LABA/ICS combinations. For some individuals the level of function and sense of well-being restored by the use of LABA/ICS has been nothing short of remarkable, and several patients have been fully weaned from chronic oral steroids. I have had no ill effects in my patient population. I would make the final observation that investigators (those both supporting and decrying the use of LABA agents) have not factored in the effect of increased physical activity (BMI, cardiovascular conditioning), weight bearing exercise (osteoporosis), and reduced systemic steroid exposure (multiple adverse effects) afforded by LABA/ICS therapy in their risk-benefit calculus.

Atropine-Like Agents

These agents currently include ipratropium and tiotropium. Both of these drugs are inhaled. These agents block muscarinic parasympathetic nervous system receptors. Ipratropium is relatively short acting (4–6 hours) and tiotropium is relatively long acting (~24 hours). Ipratropium is used adjunctively for asthma exacerbations and is often combined with albuterol both as an MDI and nebulizer solution. It is not recommended as a controller agent in asthma, but is used on a scheduled basis in many COPD patients. Tiotropium is distributed as a dry powder for inhalation contained in a capsule. It is indicated as a chronic medication for COPD. The inhaler device is generally user-friendly, although it still requires placing a capsule in a small well. Tiotropium has been very effective in some COPD patients, greatly increasing functional status and sense of well-being. Tolerance is generally good, with dry mouth a common side effect. Patients with glaucoma should be observed carefully, and the powder should not get in the patients' eyes. Urinary retention is also a possibility. Dosage is fixed at one capsule's contents inhaled per 24 hours.

Corticosteroids

Inhaled Corticosteroids: These drugs are the cornerstone of controller therapy for asthma and play a major role in the treatment of COPD. As the medications have evolved over the last 30 years, a wider variety of specific drugs has become available, and a greater range of dosing is possible. As described in the LABA section, fixed combination ICS/LABA therapy is also available. Higher-potency compounds have become commonplace, and many of these drugs have limited systemic bioavailability (poorly absorbed, experience first-pass hepatic metabolism, or both). Current ICS include triamcinolone, beclomethasone, budesonide, fluticasone, flunisolide, and mometasone. Ciclesonide was approved for use in the United States as this book was going to press; I am personally unfamiliar with this agent. The mechanism of asthma and COPD stabilization is incompletely understood, but reduction of inflammation by blocking cytokine release, eosinophil recruitment to the airways, and inflammatory mediator release has been documented. Use of ICS in asthma is associated with fewer exacerbations, higher FEV_1, and less bronchial hyperreactivity. ICS is the primary, preferred controller medication in asthma. ICS use in COPD decreases the number of exacerbations and appears to slow disease progression. Recent studies suggest that there may be a modest effect on survival as well, but that this protective effect is greatest with LABA/ICS combinations (N Engl J Med 2007;356:775). ICS use in adults is associated with accelerated cataract formation, reduced bone mineral density, dermal thinning, and changes in glucose metabolism. Local side effects include oral thrush, dysphonia, and occasionally reflex cough. Dosing is covered in disease-specific sections.

Systemic Corticosteroids: These drugs are used both for control and rescue in all airway diseases and many parenchymal lung diseases. Dosing regimens are disease specific. However, in all conditions the goal of therapy is to reduce dose and duration of steroid to the lowest possible level consistent with control of the disease. This usually includes introduction of various steroid-sparing strategies, which again are disease specific. Asthma strategies, for example, would include introduction of LABA/ICS inhalers, leukotriene modifiers, and/or IgE antibodies. Systemic steroid side effects are well described, including adrenal suppression, dermal thinning, hypertension, glucose intolerance, Cushing's syndrome, cataracts, muscle weakness, and immune incompetence, the latter making the patient susceptible to opportunistic infection and reactivation TB.

Methylxanthines

Aminophylline and theophylline have been available for decades. As phosphodiesterase inhibitors, they increase cyclic AMP levels in bronchial smooth muscle. They have modest potency as bronchodilators, and investigations demonstrate multiple anti-inflammatory properties. They also appear to augment respiratory muscle function. The drugs have a narrow therapeutic ratio and even when in therapeutic concentration are frequently poorly tolerated; the most common reason for stopping the drug was dyspepsia. Toxicity includes arrhythmias and seizures. Dosing is driven by blood concentration measurements, and many clinicians' target serum concentration is 5–10 mg/L. Some authorities recommend concentrations as high as 10–20 mg/L. Theophylline metabolism varies widely among patients, is influenced by underlying illness, and is influenced by drug interactions. Depending upon the preparation (immediate release or extended release), kinetics can vary widely among specific medications, and often days of therapy are needed to achieve a new steady state concentration after dose change. Aminophylline and theophylline are not considered first-line therapy for either asthma or COPD, but may be useful as adjuncts. If unfamiliar with the use of methylxanthine therapy, review of the general principles of therapy and understanding of the kinetics of the specific product to be used is appropriate (Drugs Today [Barc] 2004; 40:55).

Nedocromil and Cromolyn

These chemically different agents have similar effects, stabilizing mast cells and preventing eosinophil recruitment. Cromolyn started its clinical life as an irritating inhaled powder; it is now available as an MDI. Nedocromil has always been available as an MDI. Nedocromil is more potent, and after a 30-day run-in period, can be used twice daily rather than four times; cromolyn requires continued qid dosing. Both agents are less potent than other controllers such as ICS. They may, however, be used as adjuncts in asthma (they are not considered first-line therapy) and also may be used as a hybrid rescue/controller agent when used as a pretreatment for exercise or unavoidable allergen exposure. In my clinical practice, patients who have a significant allergic component to their asthma appear to benefit more from these drugs.

Leukotriene Modifiers

Montelukast, zafirlukast, and zileuton are the leukotriene modifiers available in the United States. Montelukast and zafirlukast are leukotriene-receptor antagonists (LTRA); zileuton is a 5-lipoxygenase inhibitor. All three drugs may improve FEV_1 in asthmatics. They do not have a role in the treatment of COPD unless there is a prominent asthmatic component to the patient's condition. They are oral systemic medications. Collectively, they are less potent than ICS and are considered adjunctive therapy; they may also be used as the primary controller medication in patients with mild to moderate asthma who cannot or will not use ICS. These drugs, in my experience, are not uniformly effective. Some patients will have tremendous relief of symptoms, and others have no improvement. Patients who are aspirin sensitive or have a significant allergic component seem to be more likely to benefit. Zileuton has drug interactions and requires routine hepatic monitoring; NAEPP guidelines suggest this renders the drug less desirable, and I agree. Zafirlukast and montelukast do not require laboratory monitoring. Zafirlukast is a twice-daily drug, and montelukast is once a day, taken in the late afternoon or evening. My clinical experience is that the incidence of LTRA side effects (headache and nausea) is higher with zafirlukast. Overall, this plus once-a-day dosing would make montelukast a better choice. Patients should be given a several weeks' clinical trial before assessing success or failure of these drugs. Finally, there are reports of association between LTRA and Churg-Strauss syndrome (see **Pulmonary Vasculitis**). It is not clear if this is causal or if the LTRA has an "uncovering" mechanism revealing Churg-Strauss, rather than asthma, as the underlying condition.

Anti-IgE Therapy

Omalizumab is a recombinant DNA-derived human monoclonal antibody to IgE. Binding to the Fc portion of the molecule, IgE is prevented from binding to mast cells and basophils. Studies also show reductions in bronchial and sputum eosinophils. The drug is given by injection subcutaneously, with dose and frequency determined from a manufacturer-provided dosing chart that is based on patient weight and IgE level. Interestingly, the manufacturer did not study treatment of patients with very high IgE levels or weights, and treatment of patients who are very heavy, have very high IgE levels, or both, is technically off-label. Therapy with omalizumab is considered in patients with moderately severe or severe persistent asthma who have elevated IgE levels and evidence (RAST or skin test) of an allergic component to their asthma. Patients should receive the medication for several months before deciding that treatment is successful or not. There are reports of ~0.1% of patients receiving the medication having an anaphylactic reaction to the medication. It is recommended (black box warning) that the patient be observed around the time of the injection and that they have an epinephrine self-injection device for possible late reaction. My personal experience with this medication has been generally very positive, and omalizumab has been an excellent steroid-sparing agent. The majority of patients have experienced great benefit. Most third-party payors enforce rigid eligibility guidelines because of the expense involved, and patients chafe at supervised injections. My greatest frustration has been the IgE level and weight restrictions in the FDA-approved labeling; a number of patients with markedly elevated BMIs and/or IgE levels have been denied access to this drug because treating them would be off-label (and hence outside the contractual obligations of the third-party payor).

3.4 Chest Physiotherapy: Lung Expansion Therapy and Bronchial Hygiene

Egan's Fundamentals of Respiratory Care 2003, Chapters 36 and 37, pp. 863–910.

Introduction: Lung expansion therapy and bronchial hygiene therapy are adjuncts used in the treatment of numerous conditions. Their utility and implementation should be understood by clinicians. Lung expansion therapy refers to therapy directed at preventing and/or reversing pulmonary atelectasis. Bronchial hygiene therapy refers to treatment directing at improving bronchial drainage.

Indications for Therapy: Mechanical clearance of the airways is the first line of host defense for the lungs, more so than cellular or humoral immune mechanisms. This is accomplished by coughing, deep breathing, and raising sputum. Augmenting and restoring these functions helps prevent postoperative complications, maintains quasi-normal lung function in chronically impaired patients, and ameliorates symptoms in patients with excessive sputum production. Lung expansion therapy is indicated for the prevention and treatment of atelectasis. Typically, the patient will have undergone recent surgery and/or be receiving pain medications or sedatives. Pain-induced or drug-induced shallow respiration causes atelectasis with fever and potential for infection and impaired gas exchange. Patients with upper abdominal and thoracic incisions are at greatest risk, as are patients who received general anesthesia. Patients with neuromuscular disorders have ineffective cough leading to atelectasis and infection. Additionally, some patients with diseases associated with high sputum volumes (bronchiectasis, CF, Kartagener's) have better performance status and better gas exchange with scheduled bronchial hygiene therapy to reduce sputum burden. Patients at risk (smokers, elderly, preexisting cardiac/pulmonary disease) typically are placed on a program of expansion therapy perioperatively. Patients who have excessive sputum production, atelectasis, and/or ineffective cough are good candidates for bronchial hygiene therapy.

Technique: Therapies for bronchial hygiene and lung inflation have considerable overlap. The simplest intervention is coughing and deep breathing. The patient is asked to take deep breaths and cough, and is encouraged to do so. If the exercises are performed, it is an effective intervention. Pain and sedation can interfere with execution. Incentive spirometry uses a device that allows the therapist to set an inspiratory volume goal. The patient is then asked to inhale slowly and steadily until that inflation goal has been met. This is repeated several times a day until the patient is unlikely to have atelectasis, which usually corresponds to initiation of sustained and generally unassisted ambulation. An older lung inflation therapy is IPPB, intermittent positive pressure breathing. The patient is asked to synchronize breathing with a device that senses inspiration and delivers a large, pressurized volume of air. Although popular in the past, this intervention has no benefit over incentive spirometry or coughing and deep breathing and is used uncommonly. Lung inflation is also enhanced with several passive devices that produce positive end expiratory pressure (PEEP). Trade names include TheraPEP and Acapella. These devices, along with similar units, force the patient to exhale against a partially closed airway several times in succession, several times a day. By producing PEEP, the devices prevent atelectasis. Some units allow exhaled air to escape so as to produce an oscillating air column that promotes cough. Patients find them easy to use, and the oscillating air column is very tolerable. CPAP alone used postoperatively in high-risk patients has also been shown to be effective in reducing atelectasis. (Chest 2005;128:821). Although not strictly a respiratory intervention, pain control without sedation, such as that achieved with epidural analgesia, is effective at reducing postoperative respiratory complications (Anesthesiol Clin North America 2000;18:407). Early ambulation also appears to be an effective intervention. See **Pulmonary Complications of Surgery.** Techniques used to promote bronchial hygiene center around promoting cough and improving mucus flow. Many of these techniques use oscillating or vibrating airflow. The most common and simplest technique is percussion and postural drainage. The patient (if tolerated) is positioned to maximize drainage from a particular portion of the lungs and the therapist percusses the patient manually. Vibratory therapy uses a vibrating instrument applied to the chest wall to stimulate mucus drainage. Extensive use is made of supervised coughing with assist and forced expiratory technique (huffing—coughing from mid lung volume without closing the glottis), termed *active cycle breathing* (ACB). More sophisticated techniques for patients who can develop an effective cough include high-frequency chest wall oscillation (The Vest), which consists of a vestlike garment filled with air bladders attached to an insufflator that rapidly fills and empties the bladders in the vest to apply high frequency compression to the chest wall. A device called the Flutter Valve consists of a steel ball in a cup attached to a mouthpiece. Depending upon the angle at which the device is held, more or less effort is needed to overcome the resistance of the ball. This sets up an oscillating air column within the airways, which is also effective. For patients who cannot develop an effective cough, such as patients with neuromuscular disease, the technique of abdominal thrusts (essentially a Heimlich maneuver performed from the bedside) provides assistance with airway clearance. More sophisticated equipment includes mechanical insufflation-exsufflation units that rapidly inflate the lungs and then actively reduce airway pressure to mimic a cough. These devices can be helpful for patients with quadriplegia. The well-trained, experienced respiratory care practitioner has assessment skills and a knowledge base that can help the clinician plan and execute therapy; their advice should be sought.

Complications: These interventions are generally safe. Hypoxia, discomfort or injury from percussion (esp. patients with osteoporosis, metastatic disease of the ribs, preexisting rib fractures), reduction of cardiac output during cough, and/or retching/vomiting may occur. The potential exists for an abdominal wound to open from excessive coughing. Pneumothorax, pneumomediastinum, or subcutaneous emphysema can also occur. Patients with unstable head, neck, or spine injuries should receive chest physiotherapy cautiously if at all. Patients with elevated intracranial pressures should not receive this therapy. Patients with highly communicable respiratory disease (e.g., tuberculosis) pose a risk to personnel.

Alternatives: Patients with either refractory atelectasis and/or difficulty clearing secretions and coughing may require translaryngeal suctioning, endotracheal intubation, or even tracheostomy if the problem is permanent.

3.5   Oxygen Therapy

Introduction: Oxygen therapy is ubiquitous in the inpatient setting and increasingly used in the outpatient setting. Outpatient use will no doubt continue to rise as the population ages and medicine becomes more skilled at the management of chronic illness. In the hospital, oxygen can be applied by mask, nasal prongs, directly to the trachea, as a component of invasive or noninvasive mechanical ventilation, and in a face tent. The gas can be humidified, pure, mixed with air, mixed with helium, warmed, cooled, at atmospheric pressure and at hyperbaric pressures. (Hyperbaric oxygen therapy will not be discussed. Review reference: QJM 2004;97:385.) Outpatient oxygen (also referred to as domiciliary oxygen) potentially can be provided with equally dizzying complexity. Practically, the vast majority of patients use nasal oxygen, simple mask systems, and/or as part of mechanical ventilation. Adequate tissue oxygenation is critical to normal metabolism and life of the patient. A discussion of the biochemical oxidation of carbon and hydrogen in humans is beyond the scope of this book. In practical terms, acute global hypoxia short of critical oxygen starvation has a multitude of adverse effects on mentation, cardiac function, renal function, and pulmonary function. Cardiac inotropes don't work, patients can't think straight, they retain fluid, diuretics don't work, they have arrhythmias, they have pulmonary hypertension, and they develop splanchnic ischemia. Any and all of these can lead to death. Chronic hypoxia has similar effects and additionally will have stimulation of erythrocyte production. Some changes associated with chronic oxygen deprivation cannot be reversed with restoration of normal oxygen levels. Although acute use of oxygen in a vast number of illnesses is automatic, I could not find randomized, controlled trials to support this practice in all settings. Chronic use of oxygen has been well studied, particularly in patients with chronic obstructive pulmonary disease, and a survival benefit is documented (Ann Intern Med 1980;93:391, Lancet 1981;1:681). Delivery of oxygen is usually as a low flow of pure, desiccated oxygen or oxygen mixed with air. High-flow pure oxygen may be required in refractory or critical situations. In all of these situations, the gas must be adequately humidified prior to application to the trachea, otherwise mucosal damage can occur. The desired level of oxygen in the blood relates to the oxygen hemoglobin dissociation curve. Since the goal of oxygen therapy is to promote adequate oxygen delivery to the tissues, there should be as high an oxygen content of the blood as is feasible and safe. Because the curve flattens out after 90% saturation, there is usually little value to trying to achieve saturations of 95% or 100%. Generally, a PaO_2 sufficient to achieve a saturation of 90% or greater is considered adequate. Oxygen in high concentration has been shown to be toxic to alveolar tissue (Chest 1985;88:900). In patients who are chronically hypercarbic, hypercarbic respiratory drive can be depressed and ventilation may be driven by hypoxia. Excessive use of oxygen, so as to suppress hypoxic drive, can precipitate respiratory failure (Am Rev Respir Dis 1991;144:526). This mechanism is often misunderstood by house officers with concern expressed that an excessive FIO_2 rather than a high PaO_2 is the problem. It is not the FIO_2 that suppresses respiration; there are no oxygen receptors in the lungs. Rather, it is the PaO_2 sensed at the carotid body that is critical, and PaO_2 should not be allowed to rise to more than 70–75. It should also be noted that deliberate reduction in FIO_2 below safe levels to produce hypoxia so as to promote ventilation is dangerous and ill considered.

Indications for Therapy: In the acute setting, supplemental oxygen is provided as part of initial treatment of almost any serious illness. Continued use of oxygen is driven by arterial blood gas determinations and oximetry (see **Arterial Blood Gases** and **Oximetry**). Oxygen is administered to maintain saturations higher than 90–92%. Supplementation is increased or decreased to achieve that goal. Some practitioners will try and achieve higher saturations in cardiac illness or acute brain injury, but there is no data to support this practice. Many hospital respiratory care departments have a protocol, usually implemented as a policy and/or procedure to have the respiratory care practitioner adjust oxygen flow or FIO_2 as needed to achieve the stated saturation goals. As the patient improves, oxygen is gradually weaned off. In some cases, oxygen is continued into the home setting. Because of the expense and inconvenience, most third-party payors in the United States have clearly delineated requirements for prescription of domiciliary oxygen. While many clinicians bridle at the restrictions imposed by Medicare and other insurance programs (and sometimes rightly so), the coverage requirements imposed by Medicare are grounded in the data from the NOTT trial and the British MRC trial (Ann Intern Med 1980;93:391, Lancet 1981;1:681). To receive oxygen benefits under Medicare the following criteria must be met:

- The patient must have a severe lung disease that impairs gas exchange.
- Symptoms consistent with hypoxemia
- Must be clinically stable, with all other reasonable measures in place
- If the patient has a PaO_2 55 mmHg or less, or a saturation of 88% or less, that person qualifies for 24/7 supplemental oxygen
- If the patient has a PaO_2 55 mmHg or less or a saturation of 88% or less during sleep, that person qualifies for oxygen supplementation during sleep.
- If the patient has a PaO_2 55 mmHg or less or a saturation of 88% or less during exercise, that person qualifies for oxygen supplementation during exercise.
- If the patient has a PaO_2 56–59 mmHg or a saturation of 89%, oxygen may be prescribed if there is concomitant evidence of cor pulmonale, dependent edema, or erythrocytosis.

Because of the way Medicare is administered, it is possible that a local carrier can impose additional restrictions or requirements. The outline above should not be taken as definitive (http://www.cms.hhs. gov/mcd/viewncd.asp?ncd_id=240.2&ncd _version=1&basket=ncd%3A240%2E2%3A1%3AHome+Use +of+Oxygen 1999; 2007).

Technique: Oxygen institutionally is usually provided by a large tank of liquid oxygen that is converted to a high pressure gas distributed by infrastructure piping. At the point of care pressure is reduced and flow determined by a regulator. Oxygen can be provided as a low flow to the patient through a nasal cannula. This system is well tolerated, easy to implement, and cheap. FIO_2 cannot be set exactly, and can vary depending upon the patient's pattern of breathing. Nasal oxygen can be defeated completely if the patient mouth breathes. At flows above ~5 lpm, the stream is uncomfortable and drying. As a rule of thumb, each 1 lpm increases the FIO_2 by about 3%. Venturi masks use a relatively low flow of oxygen that jets through a small orifice. This creates a Venturi effect and draws air along with the oxygen. The result is a high-flow, fixed FIO_2 system that uses relatively little oxygen. The therapist changes nozzles and flow rates to set different FIO_2s. This is effective for mouth breathers, and where a precise FIO_2 (e.g., CO_2 retaining patients) is necessary. The high flow can be uncomfortable, and the inspired gas is difficult if not impossible to humidify. Mixers mix air and oxygen at high flow. The gas is easily humidified and is well tolerated. The equipment is wasteful of oxygen and requires large corrugated tubes to bring the gas to the patient. The mixture can be presented through a face mask, a face tent (similar to a mask, but does not cover the nose—used in claustrophobic patients) or can be connected to a tracheostomy tube. Oxygen is mixed into gas delivered by mechanical ventilation by a mixer internal to the ventilator. NIPPV devices vary, and can require a bleed-in technique (oxygen injected into the airstream without a precise FIO_2, patient oximetry is monitored for effect) or a mixer. In the outpatient setting oxygen is stored at the point of care. Liquid oxygen systems can provide high flow if needed (chronic ventilator patients, patients with advanced lung disease requiring a high flow rate, etc.) and are valued by ambulatory patients for the lightweight, high-capacity portable systems. Liquid systems constantly boil off oxygen so there is loss of product even when the unit is not in use. The patient is committed to receiving deliveries of LOX at specified intervals, and overnight travel is difficult. Compressed gas systems are rarely used as the primary stationary system, but a large tank of compressed gas is always left in the home for emergencies.

Compressed gas with a conserving system is an attractive, less expensive alternative to a liquid system for portable use. Oxygen concentrators use zeolite canisters to adsorb nitrogen and provide oxygen-enriched air. Commercial home units can easily achieve a gas that is 95% oxygen (http://www.nda.ox.ac.uk/wfsa/html/u01/u01_009.htm 1992;2007). Maximum flow is usually 5 lpm. Although favored by insurance companies (the patient pays for the electricity, major cost of use) they are noisy, use a lot of electricity, and create a lot of heat. Nonetheless they are the mainstay of stationary home systems. Oxygen is generally delivered by nasal prongs. Oxygen can also be used in tracheostomy systems, home ventilators, and other specialized mechanisms. Some clinicians advocate transtracheal oxygen where a small catheter is percutaneously inserted into the trachea, and oxygen is delivered directly to the lower respiratory tract (Clin Chest Med 2003;24: 489, Eur Respir J 1997;10:828). Although researchers have found this to be a safe and effective means of treatment in the properly chosen patient, I have never had a patient who wanted this means of therapy. Oxygen-conserving devices deliver oxygen only during inspiration. These are generally electronic flow/pressure monitoring devices (there are some passive units still in operation, using a reservoir system) and sense inspiratory flow. The length, frequency, and flow rate of the pulse of oxygen can be adjusted to meet the patient's oxygen supplementation needs. These units do not work well with mouth breathers. I have watched patients' saturations drop steadily as they speak, and rise steadily as they listen. Battery failure results in a default constant flow state, and there are other safety features present as well. In general, these units are well liked and reduce oxygen consumption; a small, lightweight tank permits many hours of independent activity or travel. Heliox is a helium–oxygen mixture sometimes used to treat asthma or COPD. The lower density of the gas mixture effectively lowers airway resistance because of different flow characteristics of the gas. However, there is no convincing evidence that this intervention influences outcome (Cochrane Database Syst Rev 2006;CD002884).

Complications: Improper use of oxygen can cause CO_2 retention in susceptible individuals and in high FIO_2 situations may cause oxygen toxicity. Oxygen is an oxidizing accelerant gas under pressure, and both institutional and domiciliary users must respect the potential destructive power of the tanks and the fire hazard of the oxygen itself. Clinicians should reflect carefully before prescribing home oxygen for patients who continue to smoke as facial burns and even house fires can result from smoking while using oxygen.

Alternatives: If the patient's medication, rehabilitation, and sleep-disordered breathing has all been optimized, there is no alternative to oxygen supplementation.

3.6 Pulmonary Rehabilitation

These are excellent, succinct reviews of the subject: Am J Respir Crit Care Med 1999;159:1666, Thorax 2001;56:827

Introduction: One of the goals of chronic pulmonary disease management is to help the patient maximize functional status and emotional well-being with his or her remaining physical and emotional resources. Pulmonary rehabilitation is a multidisciplinary program of assessment, graded exercise therapy, and education to improve the quality of life and functional status of patients with pulmonary disease. The process is an adjunct to, and does not replace, medical management. Because it is not possible to perform sham rehabilitation, blinded randomized controlled studies are not available to support the use of this treatment. However, good quality clinical studies including non-blinded randomized allocation of therapy support the observations of reduced cost of care, better functional status, and improved quality of life.

Indications for Therapy: The British Thoracic Society suggests that pulmonary rehabilitation is appropriate when the patient starts to become impaired by their pulmonary disease. The American Thoracic Society agrees with this, suggesting that many referrals to rehabilitation programs occur too late in the course of the illness to benefit the patient maximally. Pulmonary rehabilitation should be considered when the patient starts to have respiratory-related anxiety about activity; dyspnea with activity; limitation of social, personal care, or leisure function; and loss of independence. Pulmonary rehabilitation is useful in patients with COPD and other forms of chronic lung disease, and is a major component of treatment of advanced lung disease with LVRS and lung transplantation.

Technique: Rehabilitation begins with a comprehensive assessment of the patient's medical status including pulmonary function studies. Evaluation of educational needs and identification of any cognitive impairment is important. Identification of coexisting depression and anxiety in patients with advanced lung disease is common, and an effort should be made to identify these problems if present. These patients frequently have nutritional problems, and nutritional status should be assessed. As a compromise between cost and precision, many programs use a 6-minute walk to assess exercise capacity objectively. Formal cardio-pulmonary exercise testing is more exact (see **Cardiopulmonary Exercise Testing**). Once exercise capacity is quantified, endurance training is the foundation of therapy. ATS guidelines recommend 20–45 minutes of exercise that produces a heart rate of 60–90% predicted or an oxygen uptake of 50–80% maximum 3–4 times per week. Endurance improves only in those muscle groups trained, so most programs provide upper and lower extremity training. Strength training outcomes have not been as comprehensively studied, but strength training is a part of most programs. Respiratory muscle training can produce an increase in respiratory muscle strength, but this does not translate to improved pulmonary function or clinical improvement. Training effect decays rapidly and retention of improvement requires that the patient maintain an exercise program. Most exercise programs funded by Medicare are 4 weeks in duration. The educational component consists of breathing strategies, energy conservation, smoking cessation, basic anatomy and physiology, pharmacology at the patient level, and discussion of end-of-life issues. Nutritional assessment and counseling can be provided in groups and/or individualized. Group and patient-specific self-assessment and care skills provide genuine empowerment and reduce unnecessary utilization of services. Patient outcomes are assessed with exercise tests (6-minute walk and CPET when appropriate), health status questionnaires, and dyspnea assessment.

Complications: A carefully designed and administered pulmonary rehabilitation program poses little risk to the patient. It is possible to precipitate a cardiac event such as infarction/angina or induce an arrhythmia. Precipitation of a pulmonary exacerbation is possible but unusual. Some patients do not have the financial or personal resources to complete the program.

Alternatives: Severely impaired patients may not benefit from this intervention as much as those patients with more limited impairment. Severely impaired patients may benefit from lower intensity intervention in the home. Although programs are usually held on an ambulatory outpatient basis, some or all components of rehabilitation may be provided to the patient while they are inpatients in a physical rehabilitation unit or in a skilled nursing facility.

3.7 Pulmonary Complications of Surgery

Introduction: The respiratory system has a high rate of complication after surgery, even with nonthoracic surgery. General anesthesia and paralysis cause atelectasis, and poor control over and weakness of the upper airway can lead to aspiration. Postoperatively, pain may inhibit coughing and deep breathing, and narcotics used to control pain may in themselves cause hypoventilation and atelectasis. In older studies of surgery involving upper abdominal incisions, postoperative pneumonia occurred in some populations 50% of the time. Pulmonary resection leads to the same problem of atelectasis and pneumonia, and adds the additional dimension of permanent removal of lung tissue. If more lung tissue is removed than the patient can tolerate, chronic respiratory failure may be the consequence. For this reason, efforts have been made to identify high-risk populations, define appropriate interventions, and accurately judge the consequences of pulmonary resection in someone whose breathing may already be compromised. This appropriate tendency toward conservatism must be balanced against the need to provide life-saving surgery in patients with few alternatives to an operation.

Indications: Almost all forms of surgery without pulmonary resection can precipitate respiratory complications, and these complications can happen in anyone. However, the greatest risk has been shown repeatedly to occur in the elderly, patients with preexisting COPD, CHF, patients who cannot fully provide their own ADLs, and ASA Class II or greater. Hypoalbuminemia has surprising predictive power for postoperative complications. Prolonged anesthesia, thoracic incisions, and upper abdominal incisions markedly increase the risk of pneumonia and atelectasis. Neurosurgery, head and neck surgery, and vascular surgery are also associated with increased risk. Interestingly, smoking (when separated from pulmonary dysfunction) poses little incremental risk, and obesity similarly has less effect than might be predicted.

Controlled asthma appears to generate no incremental risk in this setting. Obstructive sleep apnea has recently been recognized as a major risk factor for operation and anesthesia, but does not affect the lung directly. (See **Obstructive Sleep Apnea.**) Preoperative chest X-rays and spirometry (except, perhaps to confirm or deny the presence of obstructive lung disease) do not appear to play a role in identifying high-risk patients (Ann Intern Med 2006; 144:575, Am J Respir Crit Care Med 2005;171:514). In contrast to surgery without pulmonary resection, patients being considered for pulmonary resection must have a careful, objective data-driven evaluation of preoperative and predicted postoperative pulmonary function (see **Bronchogenic Carcinoma**).

Technique: Patients may be assigned to low-risk and high-risk categories based on the kind of surgery considered, their medical history, and straightforward examination. If there is any question regarding pulmonary status, spirometry to confirm or deny the presence of COPD is appropriate. These patients should be taught coughing and deep breathing exercises or use other forms of lung expansion therapy (see **Chest Physiotherapy**). Adequate pain control, early ambulation, and when appropriate epidural analgesia (Anesthesiol Clin North America 2000;18:407) may all be helpful. Active pulmonary exacerbations should be treated preoperatively, nutrition should be optimized, and cardiovascular status should be optimized. Although there is little or no evidence to support it, smoking cessation prior to surgery is encouraged. Patients undergoing pulmonary resection need careful assessment prior to operation (Chest 2003;123:105S). A variety of assessments based on pulmonary function and exercise capacity have been proposed and validated. Using pulmonary function testing, an FEV_1 of 2 liters or greater, or an FEV_1 of 80% predicted or greater indicates an ability to withstand pneumonectomy, and no further testing is needed. If the FEV_1 is >1.5 liters, the patient is suitable for lobectomy, and no further testing is required. Patients with values lower than these require further evaluation, usually in the form of quantitative lung perfusion testing. In this test, radioactively tagged albumin is injected into the patient. Regional and total counts for the lungs are measured, and the ratio of regional/total counts correlates strongly with the fraction of the measured FEV_1 contributed by that region. Patients who have a predicted postoperative FEV_1 of 40% or less have a high rate of complication and death. Measurement of the DLCO is recommended if there is any suggestion of interstitial lung disease. Again, a predicted postoperative DLCO of <40% is associated with a high rate of death and complication. CPET-based testing depends on Vo_2 max. Values above 20 ml/kg/min are not associated with excess mortality or complication. Values below 10 ml/kg/min are associated with very high excess mortality and complication. Intermediate values require careful review and integration with other pieces of physiologic data. Stair climbing, 6-minute walks, and shuttle walks can also be used. If a patient cannot climb one flight of steps, the risk of complication is very high, and if he or she can climb more than 3–5 flights of steps, the risk of complication is low. These tests are disliked by investigators because they are poorly standardized. However, they may be quite useful in clinical practice. Arterial blood gases are valuable in the treatment of the patient, but both $Paco_2$ and Pao_2 have no predictive value in lung resection outcomes. In patients undergoing pulmonary resection, lung expansion therapy, good analgesia, and early ambulation are vital. Perioperative cardiac evaluation and management are also key to good outcomes, as the risk of cardiac complication in these patients in general is high (J Am Coll Cardiol 1996;27:910).

Complications: Interpretation of some of the risk data that has been cited is difficult. Many of the study were performed in the 1970s, 1980s, and early 1990s. Marked improvements in perioperative management have occurred between these observations and the present, and it is possible that some recommendations regarding acceptable risk and outcomes are too conservative. LVRS in this context is counterintuitive, as many of these patients would be considered at tremendous risk for lung resection yet do well. This effect is often put to use when justifying surgery on a patient with a small lung cancer but who has poor pulmonary function. If the lesion is in a region of severe emphysema, pulmonary function may actually improve postoperatively. Finally, techniques of wedge and segmental resection using VATS may have value as interventions in patients with marginal lung function. This also changes the selection process for patients with malignant lung lesions. In the end, however, there is a requirement that the patient retain a minimum ventilatory capacity to survive; unfortunately this simply is not always possible, and some patients can't have pulmonary resection of any degree.

Alternatives: Lung cancer patients who have potentially curable lesions may require nonsurgical management if lung function is inadequate, reducing their chance of cure. Patients with advanced lung disease generally should have nonoperative management of all diseases whenever possible. Patients with truly life-threatening illness who need nonpulmonary surgery for survival may wish to hazard surgery. Many of these patients may have complications and a difficult course, but ultimately survive and do not require chronic ventilator support. Care can be withdrawn humanely and with dignity if chronic respiratory failure ensues and this is not acceptable to the patient (see **Palliative Care**).

3.8   Respiratory Assistance Devices

Introduction

Pulmonary physicians and physiologists recognize hypoxic and ventilatory failure. Hypoxic failure is intuitive; the lung is unable to provide adequate oxygen for the body. Ventilatory failure occurs when the respiratory system is unable to excrete carbon dioxide sufficiently to maintain homeostasis. Hypoxia can occur for many reasons (see **Hypoxia**), but ventilatory failure occurs only because the respiratory system is unable to maintain adequate minute ventilation. Ventilatory failure, either acute or chronic, occurs because: (1) the intact bellows mechanism is not receiving appropriate signals from the brain (narcosis, brain injury, injury to spinal cord or phrenic nerves), (2) the intact bellows mechanism cannot generate an adequate minute ventilation to compensate for abnormal lung function, or (3) the bellows mechanism itself has failed (muscular dystrophy, myasthenia gravis, etc.). These categories are not mutually exclusive, and multiple pathologies can coexist. In addition, patients with ventilatory failure may have failure of oxygenation as well. Respiratory assistance devices provide three services to the failing respiratory system: (1) they create a mechanism whereby ventilation is maintained, (2) they provide a means of delivering supplemental oxygen in the context of ventilation, and (3) they provide end-expiratory pressure in excess of atmospheric pressure to improve oxygenation.

The range of devices is broad and ingenious. The two common forms of respiratory assistance in the United States today are invasive and noninvasive positive pressure ventilation. There are a variety of different strategies for taking over for the patient's breathing, synchronizing with the patient's breathing, helping a little, helping a lot. The primary difference between invasive and noninvasive ventilation, however, is that invasive ventilation uses a connector directly to the trachea, and noninvasive ventilation uses a mask or similar device that attaches to the patient's mouth and/or nose and uses the natural upper airway. In addition to treating respiratory failure, NIPPV is used extensively for the treatment of sleep-disordered breathing.

Negative pressure ventilation is increasingly uncommon, but mimics the bellows mechanism in that the lungs are inflated by creating negative pressure around the lungs, outside the chest wall.

The final mechanism is direct stimulation of the diaphragm. This is used for primary ventilatory failure (Ondine's curse), phrenic nerve injury, and spinal cord injury.

Mechanical ventilation is a field of strong opinion, many experts, much discussion, much innovation, and many right answers. Positive pressure ventilation dominates research and clinical practice. Much of the newer research is technology driven: microprocessors and electronic sensors permit respiratory strategies and equipment inconceivable 20 years ago. In our excitement over technology and theory, it is sometimes easy to lose perspective and forget that the laws of physics, chemistry, thermodynamics, and physiology still apply. Boyle's law has not taken a holiday, no flow occurs in an occluded tube, and a severely damaged alveolus deprived of its blood supply cannot participate in gas exchange. The discussion regarding acute mechanical ventilation for respiratory failure is about strategies and devices to eke out the last bit of function from a failing organ in the hope that enough time can be purchased so that the body can heal itself. Most ventilated patients who die do not die of respiratory failure, but of complications of treatment or the underlying illness.

Airway Management

Introduction: Airway management permits reliable access to the lower respiratory tract for hygiene and ventilation. Endotracheal intubation and tracheostomy are the most common means of accessing the lower airway, bypassing the upper respiratory tract. These techniques are used in the management of the unstable patient in a critical care setting and are used in anesthesia and head and neck surgery as well. Medical and critical care perspectives will be discussed. These techniques permit maintenance of airway patency, allow lower airway hygiene, and deliver positive pressure ventilation. Specialized techniques such as laryngeal mask airway (LMA) are not used routinely in an ICU or chronic setting and will not be covered.

Endotracheal Intubation

Technique: Standard adult-size endotracheal tubes have a large, main airway and a small caliber channel for inflation of a sealing balloon at the distal end of the tube. Some tubes have a third port for continuous suction of secretions that pool above the cuff. These tubes reduce VAP (Am J Med 2005;118:11) but are expensive. Tubes are passed through the nose (nasotracheal) or mouth (orotracheal) under direct vision (rarely blindly) with a blade laryngoscope or fiberscope. Position in the trachea below the larynx and above the main carina is confirmed by CO_2 sensors and direct inspection or chest X-ray. Specific techniques of intubation vary and are beyond the scope of this book. Sedation and paralysis protocols are not fully standardized, but do not vary widely (Anaesthesia 2004;59:675). Endotracheal intubation is dangerous and operator dependent. It is estimated that trainees must perform ~50 intubations to have a 90% probability of successful intubation (Anesthesiology 2003;98:5).

Indications: Maintain airway patency (coma, injury, infection); prevent aspiration (neurologic disease); maintain lower airway hygiene (suctioning, lavage); permit connection to means of mechanical ventilation for ventilation and oxygenation.

Contraindications: Severe upper airway injury (consider tracheostomy); intubation and mechanical ventilation are often the prelude to extensive resuscitation and the patient's advance directives should be considered; operator inexperience (get help!).

Complications: Dental injury; laryngeal injury; esophageal intubation with failure to ventilate/oxygenate; failure of intubation. Cardiovascular instability at the time of emergency intubation should be anticipated (medications, vagal stimulation, transient worsening hypoxia, and transition to positive pressure ventilation are the precipitating factors). Tracheal injury can occur over time from interruption of capillary blood flow at the site of the sealing balloon if cuff pressure is too high. Laryngeal injury also can occur with protracted intubation. The endotracheal tube bypasses the defense mechanisms of the upper airway and plays a major role in the development of VAP.

Alternatives: NIPPV (see **Noninvasive Positive Pressure Ventilation**); Laryngeal mask (Anesthesia and Analgesia 1998;87:5); tracheostomy. When prolonged airway maintenance is anticipated, transition to tracheostomy is appropriate. Timing of transition is not standardized. Most practitioners will consider referral for tracheostomy after 7–14 days of ET intubation. Evidence exists that late tracheostomy (>21 days) is associated with less favorable outcome (Crit Care Med 2005;9:R46, Clin Chest Med 2003;24:10).

Tracheostomy

Technique: Conventional surgical and percutaneous techniques are available. The conventional surgical approach is standardized (Clin Chest Med 2003;24:10). A percutaneous technique is preferred by some (Clin Chest Med 2003;24:8). Both can be done bedside or in a procedure suite. Local anesthesia with sedation or general anesthesia are used, the latter particularly if other procedures (e.g., gastrostomy) are performed simultaneously. A variety of tracheostomy tubes (cuffed, uncuffed; fenestrated, nonfenestrated; plastic, metal; foam cuff) are available, and the choice is beyond the scope of this book. The first tube inserted immediately after the tracheostomy is created is usually a cuffed nonfenestrated plastic tube with a removable inner cannula. A nonpermanent tracheotomy will usually seal itself in 24–48 hours after the tracheostomy tube is removed.

Indications: Primary emergent tracheostomy is uncommon, TV shows notwithstanding: upper airway injury, severe epiglottitis, wedged foreign body, failure of intubation. Elective tracheostomy is performed in the context of long-term airway management for ventilation, secretions, and aspiration. It is still used rarely for

PULMONARY THERAPEUTICS

obstructive sleep apnea. Tracheostomy may also play a role in the treatment of head and neck tumors.

Contraindications: Uncontrolled bleeding diathesis, severe neck injury/abnormality.

Complications: Extensive bleeding from anatomic vascular variant; injury to thyroid; tracheal stenosis. Speech requires a specialized tracheostomy tube and teaching. The swallowing mechanism is impaired by the presence of the tracheostomy tube and often forces placement of some form of feeding tube. Chronic bronchitis and tracheitis are common. Long-term outpatient tracheostomy is a significant challenge to patient and family (N Eng J Med 1983;308:2). Percutaneous tracheostomy has been associated with perforation of the posterior membraneous sheath of the trachea.

Alternatives: Prolonged endotracheal intubation. There are few alternatives for long-term airway management.

3.9 Noninvasive Positive Pressure Ventilation (NIPPV)

Crit Care Clin 2007;23:22

Introduction: NIPPV has turned sleep apnea from a curiosity to a treatable disease, reduced morbidity and mortality of acute pulmonary edema, and permitted management of other forms of respiratory failure without intubation and mechanical ventilation. It has extended the life and well-being of patients with neuromuscular disease, and provided comfort and reduction of breathlessness to those who cannot be cured.

NIPPV supports respiration through several different mechanisms. Because it is applied to the nose or nose and mouth, the pressurized column of air acts as a pneumatic splint to maintain upper airway patency. This is the primary mechanism of treatment used in obstructive sleep apnea. End-expiratory pressure, either bilevel or continuous, prevents end-expiratory alveolar collapse and shifts FRC to a higher volume, placing a stiff, non-compliant lung on a more advantageous segment of the lung's compliance curve. Both of these effects decrease the work of breathing and improve oxygenation. In studies of congestive heart failure treated by NIPPV, CPAP and bilevel PAP are equally effective; probably the end-expiratory effect is dominant. Differential inspiratory and expiratory pressures, referred to as *bilevel positive pressure ventilation*, inflate the lung to an initial pressure and the airway pressure is then dropped. The lung deflates passively by elastic recoil. This mechanism also reduces the work of breathing and can effectively ventilate the lung if there is inadequate muscle strength. If there is no spontaneous respiration, the unit can provide ventilation if it has a backup rate. Because the column of air is applied to the upper airway, there is a pressure gradient from the nose or mouth to the alveoli. Particularly in the case of patients with obstructive apnea or other upper airway abnormalities, there can be a considerable dissipation of pressure proximal to the larynx. For this reason, alveolar end-expiratory pressure tends to be relatively low and unpredictable when delivered through NIPPV. Upper airway pressure gradients, mask seal, and intrinsic limitations of the dedicated NIPPV units also limit the utility of NIPPV for patients with very stiff lungs needing high inspiratory pressures. The mechanism of NIPPV in COPD probably relates to both reduction in the mechanical work of breathing and overcoming intrinsic PEEP (J Pain Symptom Manage 2000;19:378).

Indications for Therapy: NIPPV can be used in both acute and chronic conditions. Acute application of NIPPV has been shown to improve outcomes in cardiogenic pulmonary edema (Postgrad Med J 2005;81:637) and acute exacerbation of COPD (Indian J Chest Dis Allied Sci 2000;42:105). NIPPV has been shown to prevent reintubation in patients with marginal respiration recovering from general anesthesia and who have been extubated.

PULMONARY THERAPEUTICS

NIPPV may also prevent reintubation if a patient weaning from mechanical ventilation has been extubated prematurely. NIPPV can be used acutely to treat asthma and neuromuscular respiratory failure, and can be used to reduce dyspnea in patients receiving palliative care. CPAP has been used to treat postoperative atelectasis. Use of NIPPV requires a cooperative (or at least passive) patient with a patent airway (no trauma, bleeding), who does not have excessive secretions, and is not at high risk for regurgitation. Patients who are hemodynamically unstable, who require emergent intubation, who have critically abnormal oxygenation not responding to therapy, or in whom therapy is expected to last more than 24–48 hours should be considered for conventional mechanical ventilation. Patients with noncardiogenic pulmonary edema often present a difficult ventilation scenario and are poor candidates for NIPPV. Chronic application of NIPPV is standard therapy in the treatment of obstructive and central sleep apnea. NIPPV is effective in patients with obesity hypoventilation syndrome. Long-term nocturnal respiratory support for patients with chronic neuromuscular respiratory failure is effective and improves quality of life, daytime function, and reduces hypercarbia (Thorax 1995;50:604). Use of NIPPV nocturnal ventilation for patients with COPD appears to improve symptoms but is not associated with survival benefit (Cochrane Database Syst Rev 2002;CD002878). Chronic ventilation also requires a cooperative patient without excessive secretions and with a relatively normal upper airway. In both acute and chronic settings NIPPV is contraindicated if interruption of mechanical ventilatory assistance would be life threatening; the patient must have some intrinsic (albeit inadequate) ventilatory capacity remaining.

Technique: Acute application of NIPPV is provided in a critical care setting in many institutions. Some authors feel that use on a general medical floor or intermediate care unit is also appropriate.

Although some conventional mechanical ventilators can be configured to provide NIPPV, dedicated acute NIPPV units are more common and less expensive. Unlike home units for chronic ventilation or sleep apnea, these machines have more sophisticated alarms, can estimate delivered tidal volume, are more easily configured, and some have integrated oxygen mixers (older and/or simpler models may not). Full face (nasal/oral) or nasal mask is applied and adjusted by the RCP. Adjustments are made iteratively, starting with an inspiratory pressure in the 8–12 cm H_2O range and an expiratory pressure in the 4–6 cm H_2O range. FIO_2, IPAP (inspiratory pressure), and EPAP (expiratory pressure) are adjusted to patient comfort, saturation, and tidal volume (usually 400–600 cc range). Arrival at effective settings is associated with symptom relief and is an indicator of successful adjustment. Unlike invasive mechanical ventilation, symptoms may resolve quickly while $PaCO_2$ falls slowly. Slow resolution of blood gas abnormalities is not in itself an indication of treatment failure. Weaning from NIPPV depends upon etiology of respiratory failure. Patients with pulmonary edema often use the device for 2–4 hours and then change directly to supplemental oxygen. Patients with other forms of respiratory failure may use the device gradually less over the course of days. At some point in the hospitalization the patient is switched to supplemental oxygen (if needed) alone. Patients with persistent symptoms may be candidates for long-term support: invasive mechanical ventilation, chronic nocturnal NIPPV, etc., depending on the situation.

PULMONARY THERAPEUTICS

Selection of patients for chronic NIPPV is driven by clinical and financial indications. The most common indication for NIPPV in the United States is treatment of obstructive sleep apnea. At present, almost all insurers require a polysomnogram with EEG information to qualify for NIPPV. CMS regulations regarding the type and setting of polysomnograms to qualify for NIPPV have recently changed (March, 2008). These changes undoubtedly will drive a variety of changes in testing requirements.

An RDI of 5 or greater in patients with target organ signs or symptoms or an RDI of 15 is usually required for treatment. Once a diagnosis has been made and the patient has met qualifying criteria, the patient is fitted for a mask, airway pressure is applied, and the patient's sleep monitored. CPAP is generally used first. Pressure is increased to maintain saturation, abolish apneas, and reduce or eliminate snoring (snoring implies persistent excessive intrapleural pressure swings). If apneas are abolished but hypoxia persists, supplemental oxygen is added. The patient will be changed to bilevel PAP for equipment intolerance or complex sleep apnea. OSA is most pronounced when the patient is supine and in REM stage. Most technologists feel that a titration is complete when no respiratory events are seen when the patient is in supine REM. Initiation of chronic NIPPV in patients with chronic respiratory failure is less defined, and there is no uniform protocol. The patient can be titrated in a sleep laboratory, in a hospital bed, or as an outpatient. The mask is fitted, and IPAP and EPAP are set to patient comfort and a tidal volume in the 400–600 ml range. Assessment of outcome is based on resolution of signs and symptoms and improvement in daytime arterial blood gases.

There are a wide variety of nasal masks, oral/nasal masks, nasal pillows (connect directly to nostrils), hoses, head straps, and compressors. Fitting and titration of NIPPV is as much a talent as a science, and a comfortable mask and correct titration are prerequisites to patient compliance. Effective and competent NIPPV technologists should be encouraged, nurtured, and jealously guarded from rival institutions.

Complications: The greatest concern regarding acute NIPPV is progressive deterioration of the patient despite therapy. Patients and clinicians should anticipate this possibility and determine if the patient would be a candidate for invasive ventilation or not (see **Positive Pressure Mechanical Ventilation, Palliative Care**). Excessive secretions, regurgitation, and loss of airway control are other potential complications; some patients also complain of air swallowing. Long-term therapy patients typically may have problems with skin irritation on the face, mask fit, and/or nasal congestion. Other patients may have difficulty with a sense of oppression from the airflow. Addressing these problems is largely symptomatic and to some degree, art. Humidification of the air column, nasal steroids, alternative mask styles, and switch to bilevel therapy can all be helpful. I have found that an unhurried, detailed, patient-driven description of the precise obstacle to tolerance is very helpful and can point the clinician toward the correct intervention; "I can't stand the %$#@ thing!" is unhelpful and should not be the patient's final say on the matter. Compliance is a chronic issue, and studies indicate that average NIPPV use is 4 hours per night. Many newer home therapy units have compliance-recording mechanisms that permit medicolegal documentation of therapy and clinically can serve as a launching point for discussions regarding outcome and compliance.

Alternatives: Acutely, the patient may be offered invasive ventilation or simple oxygen. Chronic alternatives depend upon the underlying diagnosis and include invasive ventilation for respiratory failure. Patients with sleep apnea have surgical and dental options as well as weight loss and simple oxygen supplementation.

BiPAP vs. Bilevel PAP: BiPAP is a registered trademark of the Respironics Corporation. Its use to describe bilevel PAP is ubiquitous, somewhat akin to the use of the term Kleenex to describe soft paper facial tissue. This book prefers the vendor-neutral term *bilevel PAP.*

3.10 Positive Pressure Mechanical Ventilation

Crit Care Clin, Mechanical Ventilation 2007;23, # 2. This issue of *Critical Care Clinics* is a superb point of departure for further reading.

Introduction: Positive pressure invasive mechanical ventilation is the mainstay of ICU care of acute respiratory failure. Invasive positive pressure mechanical ventilation is also used in selected patients for the treatment of chronic respiratory failure. This article is by necessity a survey of the field and more conceptual than practical. My hope is that the reader will have a framework upon which to undertake further reading and self-education.

Mechanical ventilation supports failing oxygenation and failing ventilation. Failing oxygenation is treated by raising the FiO_2 in inspired air to overcome ventilation perfusion mismatch in functioning alveoli, increasing ventilation to lower alveolar CO_2 (and raising the oxygen partial pressure by the alveolar air equation), and recruitment and retention of marginally functioning alveoli through application of positive (i.e. supra-atmospheric) end expiratory pressure (PEEP). Failed ventilation is treated by substituting mechanical delivery of fresh inspired gas mixture to functioning alveoli at a sufficient minute ventilation to allow adequate carbon dioxide excretion. These two concepts are the basics; all modes of mechanical ventilation in one way or another simplify to these concepts. It has been identified by researchers and clinicians that secondary effects are critical: flow rate in inspiratory gas, synchronization with patient effort, how much oxygen, how much pressure, positioning of the patient, hemodynamic status of the patient, and many other parameters can be adjusted and optimized to eke the last bit of function out of the failing lung. However, all modes must respect the need for mass transfer of oxygen and carbon dioxide, and that sick, stiff alveoli once collapsed are hard to open again, especially if there is no surfactant present.

Excluding high-frequency jet ventilation and high-frequency ventilation, conventional ventilatory modes classify into volume-cycled and pressure-cycled ventilation. These terms refer to how the inspiratory component of the breathing cycle terminates. Volume-cycled ventilators stop delivering gas after a target volume is reached; pressure-cycled units stop delivering gas after a target pressure is achieved. Both modes in practice have multiple layers of alarms and termination conditions to end an inspiration if delivery of the target volume or pressure will create a hazard. Volume-cycled ventilation for many practitioners is more intuitive: set a volume, set a frequency, set an oxygen content, set an end-expiratory pressure, and call me in an hour with the blood gases. For the majority of patients, volume-cycled ventilation is safe, effective, and easy to administer and is the mode of choice in the United States. Pressure-cycled ventilation (PCV) requires more thought and attention. A target pressure is set, and the patient must then be observed for the resultant tidal volume. Theoretical advantages of PCV suggest that overall airway pressure should be lower, and that gas distribution throughout the lungs will be more uniform. My own observation is that PCV forces the clinician to stand at bedside micromanaging the initiation of ventilation. I suspect that personal observation and attendance accounts for at least a component of the perceived superiority of PCV in difficult cases. Microprocessors, inexpensive flow and pressure sensors, high-speed precision gas valves, and miniaturization have permitted a reduction in size of ventilators and an increase in monitoring capability as well as modes of support. Some modes, such as pressure support, are of genuine value (excellent patient synchronization and comfort, self-regulation of blood gases), while other modes are answers in search of a question.

Successful termination of mechanical ventilation requires the underlying process that led to respiratory failure to have resolved. This requirement for successful weaning sometimes is overlooked. Once it is clear that the patient is recovering, the patient should demonstrate sufficient strength and return of lung function to generate adequate gas exchange with a natural airway and spontaneous, unassisted bellows function. Weaning strategies are diverse and controversial. Weaning consists of testing and conditioning. The testing component assesses cooperation, respiratory muscle strength, reserve, and gas exchange. Protocols range from tests of muscle strength to having the patient breath spontaneously through their artificial airway and seeing if they get into distress or not. If the patient passes the testing component, the airway is removed and the patient returns to spontaneous breathing. If the patient does not demonstrate adequate function for weaning, the conditioning component comes into play. The patient is asked to gradually take on a greater and greater component of the work of breathing over time, presumably strengthening their respiratory muscles as this happens. Conditioning can take the form of short (and increasing) periods of spontaneous ventilation (T-piece trials), a mixture of spontaneous and assisted breaths (intermittent mandatory ventilation), or modes where each breath has spontaneous and assisted work components (pressure support). It seems to me that little in the world of pulmonary medicine creates more heat and less light than discussions regarding weaning. Biases and opinions are strong. Lots of strategies work. In the end, when the patient is ready to come off the ventilator, he or she will let you know. They will look stronger, their oxygenation will be better, they'll make eye contact, and whatever testing component used will often show an unequivocal result. Use whatever strategy you and your colleagues feel works.

Two of the more fruitful areas of recent investigation regarding mechanical ventilation have to do with reduction in complications and prevention of ventilator-associated lung injury. Attention to detail regarding nutrition, control of infection, thromboembolism prophylaxis, hemodynamic management (including blood products if necessary), early mobilization, and prevention of VAP are critical to successful outcomes. Many critical care units have "ventilator order bundles" that implement the most widely accepted interventions (orogastric tube, head of bed up 30°, etc.) automatically. Prevention of lung injury has taken a step forward with the recognition that the injured lung can be further injured by the shear forces induced by large volume ventilation. Protocols to use low-volume ventilation and permitting hypercapnea are safe, effective, and are associated with good outcomes (see **Adult Respiratory Distress Syndrome**). Oxygen toxicity has been recognized for many decades, and avoiding excessive oxygen concentration has always been a goal of therapy.

Long-term mechanical ventilation uses different, less sophisticated equipment and takes place in the home or long-term care environment. The populations using this intervention are diverse, including spinal cord injury patients, neuromuscular disease patients (ALS, Guillain-Barré), and COPD patients. For the properly motivated patient and family, long-term mechanical ventilation can be an appropriate component of an effective care plan providing longevity and good quality of life. For others, the experience is a misery.

Indications for Therapy: Acute respiratory support with a mechanical ventilator is indicated for patients suffering from hypercarbic and/or hypoxic respiratory failure. The patient should be an appropriate candidate for aggressive management, and should have some realistic hope for recovery from the underlying process. Initiation of critical care inappropriately is a medical tragedy that can leave painful memories for the healthcare team and surviving family.

Long-term ventilatory support is less of an abrupt decision. The scenario is that of initiation of acute mechanical ventilation, resolution or partial resolution of the underlying precipitating cause, but the patient cannot be weaned from support. Long-term ventilator dependence is established after weeks or months of rehabilitation, support, and therapy. Patient, caregivers, and family must evaluate and accept the responsibilities associated with this therapy in the community, which include tracheostomy care, ventilator care, restrictions on mobility and travel, and the like.

Technique: Initiation of mechanical ventilation requires establishment of an artificial airway (see **Airway Management**). The patient is usually sedated to comfort while on mechanical ventilation. Practice varies among institutions, but some degree of physical restraint is also common. Placement of an arterial catheter is usual. Establishment of adequate oxygenation rather than adequate ventilation is the first priority, and initial ventilator settings reflect attempts at aggressive oxygenation and relatively modest efforts at ventilation (abrupt alkalosis is poorly tolerated by the critically ill patient). An iterative process of blood gas determination, interpretation of results, and ventilator adjustment occurs until there is satisfactory gas exchange. Treatment of the underlying condition and comorbidities are undertaken simultaneously. Depending upon acuity of the patient and the underlying illness, blood gases and clinical status are monitored periodically to assure stability. If the patient worsens, more aggressive therapy is provided. Improvement permits reduction in therapy. At some point, usually when the patient's FIO_2 is 50% or less, and PEEP is 5 cm H_2O or less, evaluation of suitability for weaning is initiated. If the patient can be weaned, further recovery happens with a natural airway and spontaneous ventilation. If weaning is not possible, the patient is often given a tracheostomy and an institution-specific program of rehabilitation is started. Depending upon the setting, this may occur in a stepdown unit, the ICU itself, or a long-term care facility. If the patient is judged ventilator bound, development of a long-term care plan using portable, home-based equipment is initiated. This chain of events is difficult, complicated, and painful, yet sometimes rewarding. Weaning takes anywhere from days to months and requires the diligence and hard work of many talented professionals.

Complications: Invasive mechanical ventilation is inherently dangerous. Ventilator-associated pneumonia, often with resistant pathogens, is the greatest concern. Barotrauma, both tension pneumothorax and alveolar shearing injury, are recognized complications. Positive pressure ventilation can reduce cardiac output and produce cardiovascular collapse. Airway management, nutrition, and vascular access are also associated with complications, and all of these ancillary interventions are required for positive pressure ventilation.

Alternatives: Negative pressure ventilation, noninvasive positive pressure ventilation, palliation.

3.11 Negative Pressure Mechanical Ventilation

Respir Care Clin N Am 2002;8:545, Eur Respir J 2002;20:187

Introduction: Negative pressure mechanical ventilation (NPMV) has been largely replaced by positive pressure ventilation. However, some patients continue to be treated with this method. Negative pressure ventilators were first introduced in the 1920s with Drinker's iron lung. Use of this technology during the 1950s polio epidemic permitted survival of thousands of patients. Less cumbersome and less isolating means of creating negative pressure were developed in later years. However, convenience and survival advantage made positive pressure ventilation the intervention of choice. All NPMV units create a negative intrapleural pressure mimicking normal breathing. Various modes of ventilation permit greater or lesser degrees of inspiratory assistance, synchronization with patient efforts, and expiratory assistance.

Indications: Theoretically, any patient requiring long-term mechanical ventilatory assistance could be considered for NPMV. Practically speaking good candidates for NPMV should have normal upper airways (NPMV can worsen OSA by increasing the upper airway pressure gradient). Comorbid conditions that require frequent access to the torso would be a relative contraindication. NPMV is less effective than positive pressure ventilation when providing support for diseased lungs (as opposed to an ineffective bellows mechanism).

Technique: Because this mode of ventilation is used so infrequently, there are no well-defined choices or algorithms for therapy. Currently available devices include the original iron lung, cuirass, and jacket ventilator. The iron lung is a cylinder closed at one end. The patient is placed in the cylinder, and the patient's head protrudes from the open end of the cylinder. A rubber seal around the neck permits development of a negative pressure with respect to atmosphere within the chamber. Access ports permit attendance to the patient. The cuirass has the appearance of a turtle shell. The device is strapped around the torso and a bladder interposed between the patient and the hard shell inflates and deflates, producing negative intrapleural pressure. The poncho wrap consists of an (relatively) airtight jacket worn under a rigid frame. Air is pumped in and out of the jacket to produce negative intrapleural pressures sufficient to ventilate the patient. In all of these systems, pressure swings (both positive and negative), frequency of ventilation, and sensitivity to patient effort can be varied and will determine tidal volume, respiratory frequency, and minute ventilation. These parameters are adjusted to patient comfort and correction of blood gas abnormalities.

Complications: NPMV can exacerbate sleep apnea. NPMV can cause musculoskeletal pain and skin breakdown from areas of contact with the equipment and prolonged positioning.

Alternatives: Noninvasive positive pressure ventilation, invasive positive pressure ventilation, diaphragm pacing, rocking beds, frog breathing.

3.12 Diaphragmatic Pacing

Chest Surg Clin N Am 1998;8:331, J Am Paraplegia Soc 1991;14:9

Introduction: Diaphragmatic pacing is a means of providing diaphragm activation for patients who have central nervous system or very high cervical lesions causing failure of ventilation. The technique has been available since the late 1960s, but is used infrequently due to cost, complexity, and the small number of patients who can benefit.

Indications: Diaphragm pacing is appropriate in patients who have an intact diaphragm and phrenic nerve. Patients who have central alveolar hypoventilation and high cervical cord injuries (C2 and above) are the most appropriate candidates. Patients with intact airways and pulmonary parenchyma are appropriate candidates, as the paced diaphragm can only provide a fraction of the work of a normal diaphragm. Since the units are considerably more complex than cardiac pacemakers, the patient and caregivers must be motivated and able to provide some component of self-care.

Technique: Initial evaluation for diaphragm pacing includes testing for phrenic nerve integrity and diaphragm function. Once the patient is felt to be an appropriate physiologic candidate, the unit is implanted. Unlike a cardiac pacemaker, the implanted device is passive. A subcutaneous antenna receives RF energy radiated from the external stimulator and converts it to an electrical stimulus. Larger amounts of energy and longer trains of pulses are required to pace this larger muscle, and an implanted battery is impractical.

There are currently three commercially available units on the market, all of which stimulate the phrenic nerve rather than the diaphragm and use a transmitter/receiver technology. Incisions are made either in the neck or in the upper thorax, and the stimulating electrodes are placed appropriately. The receiving antenna is placed subcutaneously on the lower thorax. Once the

PULMONARY THERAPEUTICS

patient has healed, pacing parameters (intensity of stimulation, length of pulse train, etc.) are adjusted to provide adequate ventilation and patient comfort. Continued monitoring is necessary to assure adequate function, and alignment of receiver and transmitter antennas on the body surface. Particularly in patients with primary, central alveolar hypoventilation, diaphragmatic pacing can lead to improvement in functional status and lifestyle. In patients in whom the diaphragm has been inactive, conditioning may be required before there is effective contraction.

Complications: As with any electromechanical implanted device, there are potential complications of infection and inflammation. Perhaps the greatest disappointment for some patients is the need for continued tracheal access, either with a capped tracheostomy or a tracheostomy button. Some authorities feel that this aspect of diaphragmatic pacing has been underemphasized.

Alternatives: The main alternative to this method of ventilation is positive pressure ventilation.

3.13 Therapeutic Bronchoscopy

Introduction: Over the past 2 decades the fiber-optic bronchoscope has become recognized as a therapeutic tool. Rigid bronchoscopy has been used for many decades for foreign body extraction and other procedures in the airway. Miniaturization, improved tools, and better bronchoscopes have made new therapeutic interventions feasible.

Indications for Procedure: Therapeutically, the bronchoscope is used to remove secretions and foreign bodies, debulk malignancies blocking the major airways, deploy stents, and treat small cancers definitively. Bronchoscopy is used frequently in the postoperative setting to resolve atelectasis caused by proximal mucus plugging, despite questions remaining about the precise role of this intervention (Chest 2003;124:344). Although chest physiotherapy (see **Chest Physiotherapy**) is the initial treatment of choice, severely compromised patients or patients failing to respond to noninvasive therapy may be lavaged clean with bronchoscopy. Fiber-optic bronchoscopy is used successfully in adults and children for foreign body extraction (Eur Respir J 1999;14:792). Tumors in the large airways can impair gas exchange and lead to postobstructive pneumonia. Bronchoscopy can deliver a coagulating probe (electrocautery, cryosurgical, or most frequently near-infrared laser) to the tumor, and the mass reduced in size and removed so that a stent to maintain airway patency can be deployed. In patients with small visible tumors confined to the mucosal surface of the airway who are not surgical candidates, physical ablation with lasers or similar devices or photodynamic therapy can be considered (Semin Respir Crit Care Med 2004; 25:387). The choice of intervention depends upon the operator, the precise location and size of the obstruction, and the patient's overall prognosis, and is best left to the interventional pulmonary physician or thoracic surgeon (Respiration 2006;73:399). Minimally invasive lung volume reduction surgery has been performed with fiber-optic bronchoscopy as well (see **Lung Volume Reduction Surgery**).

Technique: Please see **Diagnostic Bronchoscopy** for the general approach to fiber-optic bronchoscopy. In many instances, the patient will have an orotracheal tube in place and may be under light general anesthesia because the bronchoscope must be removed and inserted repeatedly. Bronchoscopy for bronchial toilet and atelectasis may be the main exception to the orotracheal tube rule. The airway is evaluated diagnostically. The operator then decides to use a rigid or flexible bronchoscope and chooses the appropriate instruments. Bronchial toilet and foreign body extraction are generally straightforward and involve suction and/or grasping of foreign body/material and removal. Laser coagulation involves placing a fiber-optic guide in the operating channel of the scope. The scope and fiber bundle are brought into contact with the tumor and energy is applied. After the tumor is coagulated, a forceps instrument is passed into the operating channel and the tumor is debrided. This procedure is repeated until there is a satisfactory bronchial lumen. A metal mesh stent is often deployed after this procedure to maintain airway patency. Stents can also be used in patients with benign strictures. Ablation of small microinvasive airway tumors can be performed with coagulating units such as those already described or with photodynamic therapy. In the latter technique, a porphyrin derivative taken orally by the patient is selectively concentrated in tumor tissue. This chemical acts as a photosensitizing agent and appropriate spectrum light is applied to the tumor, resulting in cell destruction. Tumor destruction can also be attempted with brachytherapy and cryotherapy.

Complications: Any bronchoscopic procedure can be associated with hypoxia and arrhythmia. It is possible to lose control of a foreign body and drive it deeper into the airways, requiring surgical extraction. Tissue destruction procedures can be associated with bronchial perforation, bleeding, or pneumothorax. Bronchial perforation can lead to mediastinitis, which may have catastrophic results. Uncontrollable bleeding from a systemic pressure bronchial artery can lead quickly to asphyxiation. Stents may migrate.

Alternatives: Rigid bronchoscopy, surgery, external beam radiation therapy, chemotherapy, palliative management.

3.14 Tube Thoracostomy

Mastery of Surgery 2001;1:630

Introduction: Chest tubes are used for the therapeutic drainage of the pleural space. Chest tubes may also be used to introduce medications or other agents for treatment of the pleural space. Air, pleural fluid, and blood may require different devices and strategies for evacuation and drainage. In the absence of pleural air or liquid, the pleural space is a potential space that has a net negative pressure with respect to atmosphere. Once the pleural space is opened to atmosphere from a procedure or trauma, air is drawn into the pleural space and the lung collapses. If a drainage tube (chest tube) is placed, air will flow freely in and out of the pleural space and the bellows mechanism that inflates the lung will be defeated. Once a tube is placed there must be some way to isolate the drainage tube from the atmosphere and allow only one-way travel of gas and liquid. The three chamber chest drainage system commonly seen in US hospitals consists of a collection chamber for pleural fluid, the water seal chamber, and the pressure regulation chamber. The schematic is seen in Figure 3.1. The collection chamber is a container for drained pleural fluid that is in communication with the water seal chamber. As the patient inhales, water will be drawn up the submerged tube, preventing an inrush of air into the pleural space. The height of the column of water above the waterline in the tube during inspiration is an indication of the negative pressure within the pleura. If the pressure in the pleura becomes positive because of air or fluid, it can be

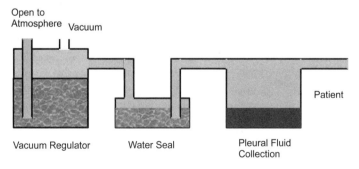

Figure 3.1 Tube thoracostomy drainage system.

expelled out the chest tube when the pressure is greater than the depth of the tube submersed in the water seal chamber. The tube is usually submerged only 2 or 3 cm, implying a positive pleural pressure of only 2 or 3 cm H_2O. The final chamber is the pressure regulation chamber. Irrespective of the level of vacuum applied at the vacuum port, the negative pressure in the chamber will only be negative to the depth that the tube in communication with the atmosphere is submersed. The wild bubbling that is often seen in a chest drainage system is useless, and just a thin stream of bubbles in the regulation chamber means that regulated vacuum has been achieved. Bubbling to any degree in the water seal chamber, however, indicates an air leak in the pleural space or in the drainage system. Some newer systems use a dry vacuum regulator. Another system used to evacuate the pleural space is a one-way valve. Because of the tendency of pleural fluid to gum up the works, valve systems are generally only used for pneumothorax, although some liquid-tolerant systems are available. The most common of these systems is the Heimlich valve.

Technique: Surgical tube thoracostomy is usually performed under local anesthesia (hopefully generous) and sterile conditions. The procedure can be performed at the bedside. The tube is placed high in the chest for pneumothorax (anteriorly in the 2nd intercostal space), and low in the chest for liquid (5th intercostal space in the anterior axillary line). An incision is made one interspace below the selected interspace for introduction into the chest cavity. Blunt dissection is used to make a subcutaneous tunnel, and the pleural cavity is entered with either the finger, a trochar, or a hemostat. Most surgeons prefer a blunt approach rather than a trochar. The tube is then inserted into the pleural cavity and directed either apically or basally. The tube is sutured in place and petrolatum gauze is used to further enhance the air seal. A heavy dressing is placed over the wound. The tube is connected to a chest drainage system as described above.

Radiologists, intensivists, or surgeons may place a small bore pigtail catheter for control of a spontaneous or procedure-related pneumothorax. This is also performed under local anesthesia, and the catheter is directed apically. A Heimlich valve is often used for evacuation of the air. The drainage system is removed when there is no further air leak, or fluid drainage is minimal. Satisfactory lung expansion is confirmed with a chest X-ray. There is some local variation in technique, with some surgeons permitting water seal only for 12–24 hours (no vacuum connected to chest drainage system) before removing the tube or catheter. A decision to place a chest tube vs. a pigtail will often depend on local skills and the distress of the patient. When the tube is removed, the drainage wound heals by secondary intention and is not sutured closed.

Indications for the Procedure: Pleural drainage is used for large, recurrent effusions, blood, empyema, and large air leaks. Because many pneumothoraces are related to procedures, there is interest in determining who needs a chest tube/catheter/nothing (observation). One study suggests that the majority of procedure-related pneumothoraces can be treated with an 8Fr pigtail catheter with a Heimlich valve or observation (Radiology 2001;219:247). Conventional chest tubes usually should be inserted for fluid drainage. Chest tubes can also be inserted for pleurodesis to ablate the pleural space. Pro-inflammatory materials are put in the pleural space, allowed to coat the pleura, and the residua removed. This procedure is performed less frequently now that VATS-directed talc poudrage is available and appears to be more effective.

Complications: Bleeding and infection are potential complications of any surgical procedure. Injury to the intercostal neurovascular bundle may take place. Lung laceration or laceration of abdominal contents can also occur. Laceration of the pericardium and/or left ventricle is rare but may also happen, particularly with inexperienced operators. Misplacement of the chest tube can lead to inefficient drainage. Although some chest tubes are delivered with a sharp trochar for insertion, complications are probably more common when this technique is used. Rapid decompression of the atelectatic lung may lead to reexpansion pulmonary edema.

3.15 Advanced Lung Disease

Introduction

Many chronic lung diseases are progressive, rendering the patient increasingly dyspneic and impaired. Activity is sharply restricted, and frustration increases, as does depression. Dyspnea, inability to perform self-care, and marked exercise limitation are the hallmarks of advanced lung disease. Patients reach a point where medicines don't work, oxygen doesn't work, and symptoms are constant. The patient is faced with difficult choices: chronic ventilation, structuring a plan of palliative management, or use of advanced interventions that carry their own risks and problems. Ventilation and palliation are not disease dependent. Chronic ventilation may appeal particularly to patients with neuromuscular respiratory failure, because relatively simple ventilators are effective, and because therapy directed at augmenting or replacing the pulmonary parenchyma will have no effect. Chronic ventilation may also appeal to some patients with emphysema. Again, relatively simple ventilators can provide support. For all patients, initiation of long-term mechanical ventilation requires considerable physical, financial, and emotional resources. Success requires residence in a long-term care facility or the constant assistance of family and attendants in the home. For some patients, perhaps many patients, this is not an attractive choice, and it is common (at least in my experience) to have patients choose a program of palliation rather than home ventilation. Even when advanced techniques are available, palliation may be an attractive alternative. Patients with severe parenchymal destruction, either through inflammation and fibrosis or emphysema, may avail themselves (if qualified) of advanced techniques such as lung transplantation and lung volume reduction surgery. This section will address basic issues of palliation, LVRS, and lung transplantation as they relate to the primary care physician. Chronic positive pressure ventilation is covered in **Positive Pressure Mechanical Ventilation.**

Lung Volume Reduction Surgery (LVRS) and Bullectomy

The decision memorandum from CMS is comprehensive, thoughtful, and readable: http://www.cms.hhs.gov/determination process/downloads/id96.pdf 2003;2007, COPD 2005;2:363 is an excellent, relatively recent general review.

Introduction: LVRS, also referred to as reduction pneumoplasty, improves the physiological function of patients with emphysema by removing emphysematous lung to permit the remaining, more healthy lung to function more efficiently. The resected lung is diseased, but without dominant, large bullae. This is in contrast to bullectomy, where easily identified giant bullae are resected. Both procedures have been associated with improvement in physiologic measurements of lung function and functional capacity. In general, the risk–benefit ratio of bullectomy appears more favorable than that of LVRS. The mechanism of action of lung volume reduction surgery is not fully understood. There is a spectrum of physiologic effect, including improvement in elastic recoil and radial traction on alveoli, improvement in diaphragm function by reducing hyperinflation, and changes in cardiopulmonary interdependence. Bullectomy, particularly where the bulla(e) takes up more than 1/3 of the hemithorax and is associated with sustained, significant improvement in survival, functional status, and physiology. Bullectomy reduces FRC, improves elastic recoil, improves dynamic compliance, and improves lung-diaphragm interaction (makes the diaphragm more efficient).

After the initial description in the mid-1990s of LVRS, the procedure was applied wholesale, unselectively, to large numbers of Medicare beneficiaries. Due to the cost involved, and the large number of fatalities, Medicare placed a moratorium on payment for this procedure (classical bullectomy was not subject to this moratorium) and the National Emphysema Treatment Trial was started. Patients were randomized to receive aggressive medical therapy and rehabilitation alone, or with LVRS as well. As the trial progressed, a subset of individuals at high risk for poor outcome after LVRS was identified, and the trial proceeded with this subgroup excluded. At the conclusion of the trial, US Medicare agreed to pay for LVRS for appropriately screened and selected individuals provided that the surgery was done at a center of excellence (distributed through the country). Current therapy reflects the outcome of this trial and its recommendations (N Engl J Med 2003;348:2059).

Emphysema is a common illness, and the primary clinician will often see patients with advanced COPD. Although complex, it is worth understanding the selection process for patients so that appropriate referrals can be made.

Indications for Therapy: LVRS: Patients with an FEV_1 <20% predicted, DLCO <20% predicted, and homogeneous emphysematous changes (not upper lobe predominant) have an unacceptable mortality and are excluded from operation. Patients with upper lobe predominant emphysema and a low exercise capacity benefit from LVRS the most, and have a survival as well as functional advantage. Selection criteria are designed to exclude the first group and maximize inclusion of the second. (See Table 3.1, [http://www.cms.hhs.gov/transmittals/downloads/R44NCD.pdf 2005;2007]). Bullectomy does not have as rigid guidelines, but patients who appear to benefit the most include patients with a preserved FVC, FEV_1 >40% predicted, who are dyspneic, and who have bulla(e) taking up over 30% of the hemithorax (Eur Respir J 2004;23:932).

Technique: The most common surgical approach is either median sternotomy or VATS. In the absence of complications, patients are discharged rapidly and resume their previous activities. Multiple

Table 3.1   Inclusion/Exclusion Criteria for Lung Volume Reduction Surgery under US Medicare Guidelines. All criteria must be met. Capitalized conjunctions are logical operators. Cotinine is a metabolic breakdown product of nicotine.

General	Undergo pulmonary rehabilitation History and exam consistent with emphysema BMI <31.1 for men and <32.3 for women
Imaging	Emphysema must be demonstrated by HRCT Emphysema must be upper lung zone predominant
Pulmonary Function	FEV <45% pred. (AND >15% if >70 y.o.) IF FEV_1 <20% pred. THEN DLCO >20% pred. required TLC >100% pred. AND RV > 150% pred.
Cardiac	No active cardiac ischemia Ejection fraction > 45%
Room Air Arterial Blood Gases	P_{CO_2} <60 (<55 if >1 mile above sea level) AND P_{O_2} >45 (>30 if 1 mile above sea level)
Exercise Capacity	Post rehab 6 min walk must be >140 m. EXCLUDE high exercise capacity (>25 watts , >40 watts) AND non-upper-lobe emphysema
Tobacco	Arterial COHb <2.5% OR Serum cotinine <13.7 ng/ml

studies have demonstrated improvements in exercise tolerance, 6-minute walk, FEV_1, and reduction in need for supplemental oxygen. Outcomes depend upon physiologic parameters at the time of presentation, but 50–75% of patients had more than 12% increase in FEV_1, which as a point of reference is considered to be a significant response to inhaled bronchodilator on PFT testing.

Complications: The advance that has permitted successful surgery is use of bovine pericardium strip buttressing of the suture line; this greatly reduced postoperative prolonged air leak. Despite this, perioperative morbidity and mortality for this procedure are high. Air leak > 7 days is ~40–50%. Perioperative mortality is ~4%. Surgical complication requiring reoperation is ~8%. In my limited experience, and drawing on the experience of other pulmonary physicians, the positive effect of LVRS will last 3–5 years before the patient becomes severely symptomatic again. A debate regarding LVRS continues, albeit at a low level, because the relatively modest, short-term gains are at the cost of considerable expense and risk.

Alternatives: The main alternative to LVRS is lung transplantation if age and functional criteria for transplantation can be achieved. Patients who underwent lung transplantation appeared to have better functional and physiological outcomes. LVRS has been considered by some as a bridging procedure, and LVRS is not a contraindication to subsequent lung transplantation. Under development is bronchoscopic lung volume reduction, where one-way valves are introduced by bronchoscope into the upper lobes, inducing partial or complete atelectasis of the emphysematous lung. Physiologic effect appears to be less than that of LVRS. However, there is good relief of dyspnea, the procedure has low morbidity, and is reversible (J Thorac Cardiovasc Surg 2007; 133:65, Chest 2004;126:238).

Lung Transplantation

Introduction: Lung transplantation is reserved for patients with advanced lung disease who otherwise are relatively (emphasizing relatively) healthy. Because of the dearth of donor lungs, selection criteria are stringent. Even with aggressive attempts to procure organ donors and less rigorous standards for donor lungs, the number of potential recipients outstrips donor lungs available, and this will be the case for the foreseeable future. Seventeen hundred transplants were performed in 2003. In any given year, approximately 7000 organ donors are available. Mechanism of death (thoracic injury) and delay in defining the patient as an organ donor (leading to contamination of the lungs or ARDS) leave only 20% of these donors as lung donors. Approximately 4000 people were on the transplant waiting list in that same year (J Heart Lung Transplant 2005;24:956). On the positive side, surgical technique, improved selection algorithms, and improved posttransplant immunosuppression have enhanced outcomes greatly. Two interesting features of lung transplantation are the use of different selection criteria and transplant technique depending on the underlying disease, and the standardization among centers of selection of recipients so as to create an equal playing field among centers and potential recipients. Additionally, this aids analysis of outcomes.

Indications: Four classifications of disease states are considered for transplantation: obstructive lung disease, fibrotic lung disease, bronchiectatic lung disease (including cystic fibrosis), and pulmonary vascular disease. Common among all groups are certain requirements. The patient must not have osteoporosis (immunosuppressive regimens all induce osteoporosis—patient must go into this with calcium reserve). There must be no active substance abuse or tobacco abuse for at least 6 months, and the patient must submit to appropriate random drug/nicotine testing. Severe musculoskeletal disease affecting the thorax is an absolute contraindication, as is body weight >130% or <70% of ideal. Patients must have sufficient psychosocial resources to withstand the transplant process. Renal insufficiency (creatinine clearance <50 ml/min) is a contraindication. HIV infection, active hepatitis B (antigen detectable), and hepatitis C are also contraindications. Patients must be free of malignancy for at least 2 years, and patients with higher-stage colon, breast, melanoma, or renal cancer conceivably should be disease free for 5 years.

PULMONARY THERAPEUTICS

Patients receiving heart-lung transplants should be <55 years old, double lung 60 years, and single lung 65 years. Patients with obstructive lung disease must have optimum medical management with oxygen, rehabilitation, and appropriate bronchodilator therapy. Neither steroids nor previous LVRS are absolute contraindications to transplantation. For patients with COPD, FEV_1 should be <25% predicted, associated with cor pulmonale, and/or hypoxia and/or hypercarbia ($PaCO_2$ >55). Patients with multiple features deteriorate rapidly and are given preference. Patients with bronchiectatic lung disease are primarily patients with cystic fibrosis. Panresistant organism colonization or chronic infection is a relative contraindication to transplantation. CF patients are considered for transplant when their FEV_1 is <30% predicted, or their trajectory of deterioration is very rapid with a higher FEV_1. $PaCO_2$ of 50 or greater and PO_2 of 55 or less on room air are poor prognostic factors indicating need for transplant, as is being young and female. Idiopathic pulmonary fibrosis occurs in older patients, often with a smoking history. As such, they should be screened for comorbidities such as cancer and coronary disease carefully. The notoriously rapid decline of these patients indicates that transplant should be considered early, with FVC 60–70% predicted and DLCO 50–60% predicted. Increasing symptoms should also be an indication for transplantation. Patients with fibrotic lung disease as a consequence of systemic illness should have quiescent systemic illness. Patients with pulmonary hypertensive disease should be NYHA Class III or IV. This is the only requirement for patients with congenital heart disease causing PAH. Patients with idiopathic pulmonary artery hypertension should have failed optimum medical management including pulmonary vasodilators, and should have evidence on right heart catheterization of a pulmonary artery mean pressure of 55 or greater, a reduced cardiac output (2.2 l/min/m^2), and elevated right atrial pressure (>15) (Am J Respir Crit Care Med 1998; 158:335, Chest 2005;127:1006).

Technique: Transplantation is done only at transplant centers. A candidate patient is presented for evaluation to the center usually by his or her local specialist. Screening to review indications and contraindications is conducted. Once accepted as a candidate, time on the waiting list varies from weeks to years depending upon diagnosis, condition at presentation, trajectory of illness, and luck (histocompatibility with a potential donor). Choice of operation and operative technique is complex and will not be reviewed in detail. Patients with severe, combined heart and lung disease receive heart-lung transplantation. Patients with pure emphysema, primary pulmonary hypertension, and fibrotic lung disease are eligible for either single or double lung transplant. Patients with bronchiectasis and chronic respiratory colonization are better served with double lung transplants. For patients eligible for either single or double lung transplantation, decisions are made at the time of donor availability.

Once the transplant has been performed, the patient is subjected to vigorous immunosuppression. Approximately half of centers use some form of induction therapy followed by chronic immunosuppression. Induction regimens include antithymocyte and antilymphocyte globulin and anti-IL2. Maintenance immunosuppression is provided with a variety of agents. The most common combination (but only by a few percent) is prednisone, mycophenolate, and tacrolimus. Other agents such as cyclosporine and azathioprine are used as well. All centers use combination therapy.

Posttransplant monitoring consists of surveillance for rejection, damage from immunosuppressive agents, and infection. Approximately 2/3–3/4 of centers perform surveillance bronchoscopy and biopsy. Prophylaxis for fungal and viral (CMV) disease is provided by most centers.

PULMONARY THERAPEUTICS

Survival varies slightly by procedure. However, 1-month survival is 80–85%, 1-year survival 65–75%, 2-year survival 55–65%, and 3-year survival 50–55%. Bilateral lung transplant appears to have the best prognosis. Patients with cystic fibrosis appear to have the most benefit from the procedure. Patients with pulmonary fibrosis appear to derive relatively little benefit from the procedure. Quality of life for survivors of the procedure is better, but the rate of return to work is not high (Am J Respir Crit Care Med 1997;155:789).

Complications: Patients who receive lung transplantation are unstable at the time of operation and there is a perioperative mortality of 15–20%. If the patient survives the initial phase, major problems include acute and chronic rejection, opportunistic infection, and complications caused by immunosuppressive regimen. A high percentage of patients will experience an episode of acute rejection, which is usually treated with high-dose steroids. Chronic rejection takes the form of bronchiolitis obliterans or evidence of chronic vascular rejection with progressive dyspnea and loss of function. Both conditions are diagnosed and monitored with fiber-optic bronchoscopy and transbronchial lung biopsies. Chronic rejection remains a source of morbidity and mortality long term despite improvements in short-term survival after transplant (Eur Respir J 2003;22:1007). Opportunistic infection is of great concern. Bacterial pneumonia is the most common lung infection, followed by cytomegalovirus infection. Ganciclovir is the most commonly used agent for both prophylaxis and treatment of CMV. Other viral infections, fungal infections, and PCJ are concerns as well. Mycobacterial infection occurs, but is less common (Chest 1993;104:681).

Alternatives: There are few alternatives to lung transplantation. For patients with COPD, consideration can be given to LVRS (see **Lung Volume Reduction Surgery**). For other patients, institution of palliation may be the best course.

Palliative and End-of-Life Care

Introduction: All therapy does not meet with success. We all must die, for this is the natural state of things. The weariness, exhaustion, and pain of chronic illness and the reality of incurable disease prompt clinicians and patients to ask how they can undertake the terminal phases of care with success, equanimity, and grace. Ending unsuccessful curative treatment is not a bad thing. It stops pain, gives rest, and allows survivors to go on to other things. However, the practitioner is not released from his or her obligation to comfort, to relieve suffering, and alleviate pain. As care focuses away from cure and toward palliation, the clinician takes on a new set of responsibilities that can be as exacting as any attempt at cure. This section does not emphasize ethics and legal issues, but addresses some of the specific interventions and methods that can be used for end-of-life symptom relief.

Palliation does not expect cure, but seeks to control unpleasant or painful symptoms while permitting the patient to interact with family and loved ones and maintain autonomy and dignity. Palliation begins with recognition on the part of all concerned that cure or significant delay of treatment failure is no longer possible. Once that decision is made, regular testing, monitoring, and medications used for primary control of the underlying disease are stopped or reduced, and greater emphasis is placed on medications to control pain, discomfort, and similar noxious sensations. Although these medications are not held back from the patient when undergoing attempts at curative treatment, there is a greater willingness to use larger doses of medications that can depress consciousness or depress respiration. In ICU or hospital-based settings, withdrawal of active therapy may accelerate the dying process because the patient is so dependent upon external support.

Ideally, end-of-life care and palliation are the results of an ongoing dialog among the clinicians, the healthcare team, the patient, and his or her loved ones. This discussion is based on legal and ethical principles that permit the patient to declare his or her intentions and have them respected and followed. Medical ethical standards in the United States are based on autonomy, beneficence, and nonmaleficence. That is to say, the physician or other clinician is obligated to involve the patient in decision making and to respect their wishes, to act in the best interests of the patient, and not to harm the patient. This ethical position is coupled with statutory and case law that has repeatedly supported and upheld the right of the patient to decline treatment as an expression of personal liberty and autonomy. This same body of law protects the physician from accusations of assault, negligence, and homicide if the practitioner assists his or her patient in halting therapy so long as the intent of the assistance is the amelioration of suffering rather than hastening the patient's death. This topic is introduced elegantly and succinctly in this reference: Critical Care Clin 2007;23:21.

Indications for Therapy: Palliative therapy and end-of-life care are appropriate when it is agreed that attempts to control the disease process are no longer appropriate and that attention to comfort and relief of symptoms is paramount. In the outpatient setting, where the disease process has evolved slowly, initiation of the palliative phase of care is sometimes unnoticed by patient and clinician; there is a tacit understanding that treatment is not going well, and it is time for palliation. In other outpatient situations, the transition is specific and proactive with an emphasis on facts, statistics, and efforts to assess survival probability and an evaluation of medical futility. In my own rural Maine practice, surrounded by matter-of-fact patients with whom I have a long-standing relationship, I have had patients ask me simply, "Is it time?" This is a question that allows one to explore how the patient feels and if he or she is ready to enter the terminal phases of their illness.

In a hospital setting, the decisions tend to be more objective. The patient is in the hospital because of or for active treatment. Withdrawal of active treatment is more likely to be associated with rapid deterioration of the patient, and there is less opportunity for reversing the decision. The discussion tends to be more complex, more emotionally charged, and more fact based.

Technique: Once a decision to limit care has been reached, the patient's medications are reviewed. Drugs not essential to comfort are stopped, as is laboratory testing and X-rays. Patients with advanced lung disease face pain, anxiety, and dyspnea as their major problems. Techniques for control of pain in palliative settings are well described and revolve around scheduled, preemptive (rather than reactive) opiate use with provision for breakthrough pain as well. The use of potentiating agents such as phenothiazines or anxiolytics is also standard. Treatment of anxiety can be accomplished with benzodiazepines. Dyspnea has been successfully treated in many trials with opiates (Thorax 2002;57:939). Intravenous, subcutaneous, and immediate and controlled release oral opiates can be used in both home and institutional settings. Nebulized morphine does not appear to have an advantage of morphine given by other routes (J Pain Symptom Manage 2005;29:613). Routine use of oxygen has not been found to be effective (Respir Med 2004;98:66). Bilevel positive pressure ventilation has been used for palliation of dyspnea (Cancer J 2006;12:365).

Other major physical problems include depression, skin breakdown, and constipation (particularly with the use of high-dose opiates.) Although situational depression is appropriate, disabling depressive symptoms defeat the purpose of palliative care and deserve treatment with antidepressants and antipsychotics if appropriate. Skin breakdown is prevented with careful and frequent positioning and repositioning. Immediate control and

clean-up of incontinence coupled with use of skin barrier oint-
ments also preserve skin integrity. Most patients will require some
form of bowel regimen, which should consist of both a stool soft-
ener (bisacodyl) and promotility agent such as senna or an
osmotic agent such as lactulose or polyethylene glycol.

Social problems include isolation and progressive inability to
provide self-care. Involvement of family and friends helps the
patient maintain dignity and independence. Many patients also
see this period in life as an opportunity for introspection and
greater spirituality, and religious figures may play an important
role for the patient. Help may be provided by local hospice programs and inpatient-based hospice programs as well (Chest 2002;
121:220).

Complications: The greatest concern of most practitioners is the inadvertent hastening of death or disability in the hope of providing
comfort. Gross negligence or malificence notwithstanding, there
are substantial civil and criminal protections for the physician or
other clinician acting in good faith with the intent to treat suffering rather than hasten death. Implicit in the change to a palliative mindset is the permission of the patient and their loved ones
to err on the side of too much, rather than too little, medication.

Alternatives: Some patients and families cannot accept failure or the
inevitability of death and will resist palliation. Some physicians
are uncomfortable declaring medical futility. If there is a profound difference of philosophy and outlook between the treating
practitioner and patient, it is best to end the relationship while
everyone is on speaking terms and help the patient find a more
suitable partner in their medical endeavors.

Additional Reading: In-depth article on treatment and pathophysiology
of dyspnea in COPD (J Pain Symptom Manage 2000;19:378).

Chapter 4

Airway Diseases

4.1 Asthma

NAEPP NAEPP (National Asthma Education and Prevention Program 2007). This document is a treasure. All tables, figures, and forms are in the public domain. The document is heavily referenced and is an excellent source for further reading.

Epidemiology: Asthma is a common illness, with prevalence rates thought to be ~5% of the adult population. The illness tends to cluster in families. Research indicates that incidence rates are higher in inner-city populations, and adult asthma occurs more frequently in women. Inner-city African-Americans have a much higher death rate from asthma than whites. Certain occupations also predispose to asthma.

Pathogenesis and Natural History: The pathogenesis of asthma is incompletely understood, and the clinical syndrome of asthma is probably a final common pathway of several different mechanisms. Allergen exposure, viral infection, host factors, genetic predisposition, and presumably as yet unidentified other factors combine in some way to trigger the clinical syndrome. In the past, emphasis was placed on the allergic Type I immune response with eosinophils and IgE felt to dominate pathogenesis. Recent investigations suggest a more complex process with neutrophils, lymphocytes, and a variety of mediators of inflammation playing a role. The inflammatory response, irrespective of etiology, is responsible for the clinical syndrome. The NAEPP defines four

167

characteristics of clinical asthma. First, there are *symptoms*. The classic tetrad is cough, wheeze, sputum, and dyspnea. Not all asthmatics have all components all the time, which is one of the difficulties with diagnosis. Second, there is *airway obstruction*. Bronchial smooth muscle constriction causes reduction of airway caliber, as does mucus hypersecretion and airway wall edema. The obstruction is measurable and often a critical component of diagnosis. Obstruction is reversible (or at least partially so) with treatment. Third, there is *inflammation*. Airways are hyperemic, there are inflammatory cells in sputum and bronchial washings, and use of anti-inflammatory agents such as corticosteroids resolve symptoms. Finally, there is *bronchial hyperresponsiveness*. Irritants, cold air, and other triggers will cause more cough, more sputum, and more bronchoconstriction in a patient with asthma than in a normal individual. Testing for hyperresponsiveness is sometimes a component of diagnosis. Some patients with asthma will experience airways remodeling, causing irreversible obstruction. Patients with asthma tend to lose lung function at a faster rate than normals as they age. Occupational exposures are of concern as well. Some occupational exposures (e.g., isocyanates) can precipitate *de novo* asthma. General irritants may not necessarily precipitate asthma, but can produce exacerbations and make the disease more difficult to control. One of the questions facing researchers is whether early intervention can prevent airways remodeling and accelerated loss of lung function. This issue has not been resolved.

Patients with fully reversible asthma will experience long periods that are symptom free punctuated by exacerbations. The cause of these exacerbations may or may not be identifiable. The inflammatory response causes bronchoconstriction, airways edema, mucus hypersecretion, and enhanced susceptibility to further inflammation and symptoms. Patients with incompletely reversible asthma have persistent inflammation of varying degrees and are chronically symptomatic unless receiving treatment. They too are susceptible to episodes of exacerbation precipitated by environmental factors and infections. Typical triggers for intermittent and persistent asthma include viral respiratory infections, bacterial respiratory infections, air pollution and other environmental irritants, allergen exposure, tobacco smoke, cold air, gastroesophageal reflux, and exercise. Patients with occupational asthma will react to substances encountered in the workplace, but will also have reaction to nonspecific exacerbating factors. Most patients have onset of asthma in childhood or adolescence, but a significant number of patients may have onset in later life as well.

During an exacerbation, airway caliber is reduced by bronchoconstriction, mucus, and edema. Patients will cough from airways irritation, and the sputum may contain plugs and eosinophils. Because airways obstruction is greater during expiration than inspiration, air trapping occurs, and the lungs become hyperinflated. This, along with the increased airways resistance, is one of the primary mechanisms of dyspnea. Additionally, there is evidence that there is active participation of respiratory muscles in aiding the hyperinflation. Overinflating the chest places the respiratory system on a different point on the compliance curve and can aid exhalation. Because of muscle activation during inhalation and active, muscle-assisted exhalation (as opposed to normal passive expiration), there is an elastic load placed on the respiratory system as well as a resistive load. Usually, the noxious stimulus of bronchoconstriction with excess mucus production and cough produces mild to moderate hyperventilation with reduced P_{CO_2}. V/Q mismatching occurs quickly in asthma, and hypoxia is common during exacerbation or poorly controlled persistent symptoms. Wheezing is produced by high-velocity airflow through irregular airways. Absence of wheezing in a patient with a severe attack is a bad prognostic sign implying little or no airflow, and return of wheezing may actually indicate that the patient is improving. In severe, life-threatening exacerbations, progressive bronchoconstriction and hyperinflation lead to respiratory muscle fatigue and no gas exchange; death occurs from respiratory failure. The drive to hyperventilation in severe exacerbations is very strong; a normal (much less elevated) $PaCO_2$ in a patient with clinically severe disease is an ominous sign.

Symptoms: The cardinal symptoms of asthma are cough, wheeze, sputum, dyspnea, and chest tightness. Symptom variability over time also characterizes the disease; all asthmatics have symptoms that fluctuate over time. Patients who have long periods (weeks to months) when they are symptom free are said to have inter-mittent asthma. Patients with incomplete clearing of symptoms, or who have symptoms every few days, have persistent asthma. The distinction is important because of the different manage-ment. Variability may be circadian (nocturnal asthma), due to other organ dysfunction (cardiac asthma, gastroesophageal reflux), or due to external, environmental stimuli; see Table 4.1 for common exacerbating factors. *Not all patients will manifest all five symptoms when they have an exacerbation.* Cough as the sole presenting symptom of asthma is recognized (N Engl J Med 1979;300:633), and many patients will have dyspnea and wheeze

---

Table 4.1 Common Sources of Asthma Exacerbation

Exercise
Viral infection
Animals with fur or hair
House-dust mites (in mattresses, pillows, upholstered furniture, carpets)
Mold
Smoke (wood or tobacco)
Pollen
Changes in weather
Strong emotional expression (laughing or crying)
Airborne chemicals or dusts
Menstrual cycles

2007 NHLBI Expert Panel Report 3: Guidelines for the Diagnosis and Management of Asthma. The work of the Expert Panel is gratefully acknowledged.

without much chest tightness, cough, or sputum. Nocturnal cough without other symptoms can be an indication of incomplete control in a patient with chronic symptoms. Most patients can identify their triggers of exacerbation, especially with some prompting. Examination will vary as well. A patient with intermittent asthma in a symptom free period will have a normal exam. Someone in a severe exacerbation may not be able to finish a sentence. The chest will appear hyperexpanded, and often the patient will not want to lie down. Diaphoresis is common in a severe exacerbation. Some patients may want to rest their arms or hands on a table in front of them, similar to a COPD patient (see **Chronic Obstructive Pulmonary Disease**). Hyperpnea is uniformly present and tachycardia is almost always present. Accessory muscle use for breathing is usually seen, and pulsus paradoxus can be detected when taking the patient's blood pressure. Wheezes and rhonchi (low pitched wheezes) will be heard throughout the chest. The wheezes have multiple dominant frequencies indicating that they are generated at multiple sites in the lung. Common coexisting conditions may include eczema (atopy) and nasal polyps.

Patients with less dramatic presentations may complain of vague chest tightness or cough with exercise or when they walk into a room with smokers. Nocturnal cough or chest tightness is a common presenting complaint, as is reduced exercise tolerance. Other patients may complain of wheezing or coughing for months after a viral infection. With a delayed diagnosis of asthma, patients may give a retrospective history of many episodes of "bronchitis" in childhood. Another feature of adult asthma is that many patients had asthma as a child that "went away" in their late teens or early 20s, and returned with a vengeance in the patient's 30s or 40s. There is not reliable transmission of asthma from generation to generation, but it does cluster in families. History of asthma in relatives should raise clinical suspicion. Patients will often be able to identify exacerbating factors, particularly if the clinician offers various suggestions and a list from which to pick.

Certain occupations carry a high risk of asthma (Am J Respir Crit Care Med 2005;172:280). Hundreds of sensitizing agents have been identified (http://asmanet.com/asmapro/ agents.htm 1999; 2007). Patients who have occupational asthma will be worse when exposed to the offending agent(s) at work and will be better when away from work. (How do you feel Sunday night as opposed to Friday afternoon?) Table 4.2 lists common sensitizers.

Table 4.2   Common Sensitizers and Related Occupations Seen in Occupational Asthma

Diisocyanates	Auto body workers Insulation installers Painters Carpenters and woodworkers
Wood dusts (e.g., western red cedar)	Sawmill workers Woodworkers and carpenters
Latex (natural rubber)	Healthcare workers Rubber manufacturing
Anhydrides	Plastics industry
"Raw" organic dusts (animal, plant allergens, unprocessed)	Farmers Laboratory workers
Enzymatic cleaners	Cleaners Laboratory workers
Food proteins (egg, wheat dust)	Food processors
Flour	Bakers
Solder flux	Electronics workers
Persulfates	Hairdressers

Metal dusts
    Chromium
    Nickel
    Platinum salts
	Specific occupation
	    Concrete workers
	    Welders
	    Platinum refinery workers

Modified from Mapp, 2005

Course/Prognosis/Complications: Widely variable. Most patients with access to competent health care are able to lead productive, mostly symptom free lives provided that they offer in return a modicum of compliance with medical therapy and can communicate effectively with their practitioners. A small number of patients have a very severe course with frequent exacerbations and chronic systemic steroids despite everyone's efforts. Patients who die of their asthma usually do so because of reasons other than the severity of their asthma. That is to say, their asthma may be severe but other patients of equal severity seem to do better. Risks of fatal outcome include frequent hospitalizations, previous near-fatal attack (intubation), low socioeconomic status, poor access to health care, mental illness, inability to assess the severity of an attack, and inability of the clinician to assess the severity of the exacerbation. Better access to health care, protocol-based management, aggressive education, savvy patients, and diligent clinicians should reduce asthma morbidity and mortality.

Imaging: Findings on X-ray are usually not prominent. There may be some increased lung volumes, and there may be air trapping. Some patients may have accentuation and thickening of bronchial walls, termed *peribronchial cuffing*. Mucus plugging may lead to atelectasis, either small plates of atelectasis or whole lobe or even whole lung, although the latter two occurrences are uncommon. The presence of parenchymal damage, fibrosis, pneumonia-like infiltrates, bronchiectasis, or bullae indicates the presence of a complication or comorbid condition.

Laboratory: There is no specific laboratory test associated with asthma. Eosinophilia and elevated IgE levels suggest associated allergy and atopy. RAST tests and skin tests may be used for allergy testing. Patients with ABPA (see section on **Aspergillus** in **Opportunistic Fungal Infections**) may have presence of *Aspergillus* precipitins. Patients in exacerbations may have elevated WBC counts because of stress and/or steroids. Pulmonary function testing will show an obstructive pattern that is partially or fully reversible to inhaled bronchodilators. There may be modest air trapping. Many patients, even when between exacerbations and feeling well, may have a normal FEV_1 but a reduced $FEF_{25\%-75\%}$. Patients with asthma will also respond to provocative testing, lowering their FEV_1 in excess of that of normals in response to inhaled methacholine (or in some labs, histamine or cold air).

Diagnosis: I consider these to be the three cornerstones of asthma diagnosis:

1. Asthma is a diagnosis *suggested* by clinical observations and complaints, *confirmed* by spirometry, and *supplemented* by laboratory testing.
2. Asthma is a *chronic* condition, and a diagnosis of asthma should not be based on a single episode of bronchospasm.
3. The diagnosis of asthma is a *life-changing diagnosis* with implications for future activity, employment, and commitment to long-term medication use and monitoring. The diagnosis must be accurate.

The diagnosis of asthma should be considered when the key indicators described in Table 4.3 are present. There are no set number of indicators that need to be present. The NAEPP recommends the use of spirometry to ascertain objectively whether or not reversible airway obstruction is present. Significant reversibility is usually defined by a >12% increase in FEV_1 from baseline provided that the absolute change is >200 ml. Some authors feel that a change ≥10% of predicted FEV_1 has better discriminatory function. If reversible obstruction is not identified with spirometry (i.e., the patient is in a period of normal lung function) bronchoprovocation may be helpful. Additional testing may be required (complete pulmonary function testing, chest X-ray, allergy testing, echocardiography) to complete evaluation and differential diagnosis. Common alternative diagnoses are in Table 4.4. Table 4.5 and Table 4.6 provide a guide for initial diagnosis and assessment. A common asthma presentation that is often misdiagnosed is cough variant asthma, where cough is the primary (and

Table 4.3   Key Indicators for Considering a Diagnosis of Asthma

Consider a diagnosis of asthma and performing spirometry if any of these indicators are present. These indicators are not diagnostic by themselves, but the presence of multiple key indicators increases the probability of a diagnosis of asthma. Spirometry is needed to establish a diagnosis of asthma.

Wheezing: high pitched whistling sounds when breathing out—especially in children. (Lack of wheezing and a normal chest examination do not exclude asthma.)

History of any of the following:
Cough, worse at night
Recurrent wheeze
Recurrent difficulty in breathing
Recurrent chest tightness

Symptoms occur or worsen in the presence of
Exercise
Viral infection
Animals with fur or hair
House-dust mites (in mattresses, pillows, upholstered furniture, carpets)
Mold
Smoke (wood or tobacco)
Pollen
Changes in weather
Strong emotional expression (laughing or crying)
Airborne chemicals or dusts
Menstrual cycles

Symptoms occur or worsen at night, awakening the patient.

2007 NHLBI Expert Panel Report 3: Guidelines for the Diagnosis and Management of Asthma. The work of the Expert Panel is gratefully acknowledged.

Table 4.4   Common Differential Diagnostic Possibilities for Asthma in Adults

Cystic fibrosis (late diagnosis)
Congestive heart failure
Pulmonary embolism
Mechanical airway obstruction (tumor)
Pulmonary infiltrates with eosinophilia
ACE inhibitor–induced cough
Vocal cord dysfunction

2007 NHLBI Expert Panel Report 3: Guidelines for the Diagnosis and Management of Asthma. The work of the Expert Panel is gratefully acknowledged.

AIRWAY DISEASES

Table 4.5   A Detailed Medical History of the New Patient Who Is Known or Thought to Have Asthma Should Address the Following Items

1. **Symptoms**
   Cough
   Wheezing
   Shortness of breath
   Chest tightness
   Sputum production

2. **Pattern of symptoms**
   Perennial, seasonal, or both
   Continual, episodic, or both
   Onset, duration, frequency (number of days or nights, per week or month)
   Diurnal variations, especially nocturnal and on awakening in early morning

3. **Precipitating and/or aggravating factors**
   Viral respiratory infections
   Environmental allergens, indoor (e.g., mold, house-dust mite, cockroach, animal
       dander or secretory products) and outdoor (e.g., pollen)
   Characteristics of home including age, location, cooling and heating system,
       wood-burning stove, humidifier, carpeting over concrete, presence of molds or
       mildew, characteristics of rooms where patient spends time (e.g., bedroom
       and living room with attention to bedding, floor covering, stuffed furniture)
   Smoking (patient and others in home or daycare)
   Exercise
   Occupational chemicals or allergens
   Environmental change (e.g., moving to new home; going on vacation; and/or
       alterations in workplace, work processes, or materials used)
   Irritants (e.g., tobacco smoke, strong odors, air pollutants, occupational chemi-
       cals, dusts and particulates, vapors, gases, and aerosols)
   Emotions (e.g., fear, anger, frustration, hard crying or laughing)
   Stress (e.g., fear, anger, frustration)
   Drugs (e.g., aspirin; and other nonsteroidal anti-inflammatory drugs, beta-
       blockers including eyedrops, others)
   Food, food additives, and preservatives (e.g., sulfites)
   Changes in weather, exposure to cold air
   Endocrine factors (e.g., menses, pregnancy, thyroid disease)
   Comorbid conditions (e.g., sinusitis, rhinitis, GERD)

4. **Development of disease and treatment**
   Age of onset and diagnosis
   History of early-life injury to airways (e.g., bronchopulmonary dysplasia,
       pneumonia, parental smoking)
   Progression of disease (better or worse)
   Present management and response, including plans for managing exacerbations

Table 4.5   (continued)

Frequency of using SABA
Need for oral corticosteroids and frequency of use

5. Family history

History of asthma, allergy, sinusitis, rhinitis, eczema, or nasal polyps in close
   relatives

6. Social history

Daycare, workplace, and school characteristics that may interfere with adherence
Social factors that interfere with adherence, such as substance abuse
Social support/social networks
Level of education completed
Employment

7. History of exacerbations

Usual prodromal signs and symptoms
Rapidity of onset
Duration
Frequency
Severity (need for urgent care, hospitalization, ICU admission)
Life-threatening exacerbations (e.g., intubation, intensive care unit admission)
Number and severity of exacerbations in the past year
Usual patterns and management (what works?)

8. Impact of asthma on patient and family

Episodes of unscheduled care (ED, urgent care, hospitalization)
Number of days missed from school/work
Limitation of activity, especially sports and strenuous work
History of nocturnal awakening
Effect on growth, development, behavior, school or work performance, and lifestyle
Impact on family routines, activities, or dynamics
Economic impact

9. Assessment of patient's and family's perceptions of disease

Patient's, parents', and spouse's or partner's knowledge of asthma and belief in
   the chronicity of asthma and in the efficacy of treatment
Patient's perception and beliefs regarding use and long-term effects of medications
Ability of patient and parents, spouse, or partner to cope with disease
Level of family support and patient's and parents', spouse's, or partner's capacity to
   recognize severity of an exacerbation
Economic resources
Sociocultural beliefs

* This list does not represent a standardized assessment or diagnostic instrument.
The validity and reliability of this list have not been assessed.
2007 NHLBI Expert Panel Report 3: Guidelines for the Diagnosis and Management of
Asthma. The work of the Expert Panel is gratefully acknowledged.

AIRWAY DISEASES

Table 4.6   Sample Questions* for the Diagnosis and Initial Assessment of Asthma

A "yes" answer to any question suggests that an asthma diagnosis is likely.

In the past 12 months . . .

☐ Have you had a sudden severe episode or recurrent episodes of coughing, wheezing (high-pitched whistling sounds when breathing out), chest tightness, or shortness of breath?

☐ Have you had colds that "go to the chest" or take more than 10 days to get over?

☐ Have you had coughing, wheezing, or shortness of breath during a particular season or time of the year?

☐ Have you had coughing, wheezing, or shortness of breath in certain places or when exposed to certain things (e.g., animals, tobacco smoke, perfumes)?

☐ Have you used any medications that help you breathe better? How often?

☐ Are your symptoms relieved when the medications are used?

In the past 4 weeks, have you had coughing, wheezing, or shortness of breath . . .

☐ At night that has awakened you?

☐ Upon awakening?

☐ After running, moderate exercise, or other physical activity?

*These questions are examples and do not represent a standardized assessment.
2007 NHLBI Expert Panel Report 3: Guidelines for the Diagnosis and Management of Asthma. The work of the Expert Panel is gratefully acknowledged.

sometimes sole) presenting manifestation of asthma. Investigation, however demonstrates the presence of bronchoreactivity, triggers, etc. The differential diagnosis of isolated cough is discussed elsewhere (see **Cough**). It is a disservice to the patient to make a diagnosis of asthma without objective spirometric confirmation of the clinical impression.

Treatment: Treatment of asthma as of this edition is based on the 2007 NAEPP guidelines. This document, which provides much of the information in this section, is the most recent iteration of an effort to improve and standardize asthma care by applying scientific principles of diagnosis and management:

1. The diagnosis should be confirmed through objective means before undertaking treatment if at all possible.

2. Initial evaluation of the patient should develop a comprehensive profile of lifestyle, support mechanisms, and other resources necessary to the care of a chronic illness as well as identification of triggers of exacerbation.

3. The patient should be classified as to severity and pattern of illness.

4. Medical therapy should be based on the severity and pattern of illness.

5. Environmental interventions should be undertaken as appropriate.

6. The patient should be educated as to the nature of the illness and taught self-management including self-monitoring (with or without peak flow monitoring), a general asthma care plan, and an emergency action plan.

7. The clinician should "close the loop" by endeavoring to achieve maximum control of the illness by monitoring the effects of therapy and adjusting therapy to achieve greatest benefit.

Asthma is currently classified as intermittent or persistent; persistent is subclassified as mild, moderate, and severe. Criteria for severity classification both prior to and during long-term treatment are provided in Table 4.7. Severity classification while on treatment is assessed by the intensity (step number) of therapy required to maintain control.

Current practice appropriately places emphasis on self-care; the clinician is a guide and mentor, helping the patient develop good self-care habits, safe independence in self-evaluation and treatment, and setting the overall goals and boundaries of therapy. This requires the patient to have an understanding of the disease, how to self-monitor, and how to respond to changes in his or her condition. Many hospitals and organizations have asthma education programs, which can be used very successfully. However, it is the responsibility of the clinician to reinforce this teaching and provide the medical component. This last piece

Table 4.7 Classifying Asthma Severity in Youths >12 y and Adults

Classifying severity for patients who are not currently taking long-term control medications

Components of Severity		Classification of Asthma Severity (Youths >12 y and adults)			
				Persistent	
		Intermittent	Mild	Moderate	Severe
Impairment	Symptoms	2 days/week	>2 days/week but not daily	Daily	Throughout the day
Normal FEV$_1$/FVC 8–19 y 85% 20–39 y 80% 40–59 y 75% 60–80 y 70%	Nighttime awakenings	<twice/month	3–4/month	>1/week but not nightly	Often 7/week
	Short acting beta$_2$ agonist use for symptom control	<2 days/week	>days/week but not >1/day	Daily	Several times/ day
	Interference with normal activity	None	Minor limitation	Some limitation	Extremely limited
	Lung functon	Normal FEV$_1$ between exacerbations FEV$_1$ >80% pred. FEV$_1$/FVC normal	FEV$_1$ >80% predicted FEV$_1$/FVC normal	FEV$_1$ >60% but <80% pred. FEV$_1$/ FVC reduced 5%	FEV$_1$ >60% pred. FEV$_1$/ FVC reduced >5%
Risk	Exacerbations requiring oral systemic corticosteroids	0–1/year	>2/year		
		Consider severity and interval since last exacerbation. Frequency and severity may fluctuate over time for patients in any severity category.			
		Relative annual risk of exacerbations may be related to FEV$_1$			

Level of severity is determined by assessment of both impairment and risk. Assess impairment domain by patient's/caregiver's recall of previous 2–4 weeks and spirometry. Assign severity to the most severe category in which any feature occurs.

At present, there are inadequate data to correspond frequencies of exacerbations with different levels of asthma severity. In general, more frequent and intense exacerbations (e.g., requiring urgent, unscheduled care, hospitalization, or ICU admission) indicate greater underlying disease severity. For treatment purposes, patients who had ≥2 exacerbations requiring oral systemic corticosteroids in the past year may be considered the same as patients who have persistent asthma, even in the absence of impairment levels consistent with persistent asthma.

Classifying severity in patients after asthma becomes well controlled, by lowest level of treatment required to maintain control.

	Classification of Asthma Severity		
	Intermittent	Persistent		
		Mild	Moderate	Severe
Lowest level of treatment required to maintain control	Step 1	Step 2	Step 3 or 4	Step 5 or 6

2007 NHLBI Expert Panel Report 3: Guidelines for the Diagnosis and Management of Asthma. The work of the Expert Panel is gratefully acknowledged.

consists of a plan of self-monitoring using either peak flow monitoring or symptom-based assessment; a means of communication with the clinician for consultation and/or emergency care as well as regular assessment; a foundation medical regimen of controller medications; a superimposed layer of therapy for exacerbation; and a plan for emergency self-treatment, including activation of community EMS services if appropriate. Sample asthma action plans are provided in the NAEPP document; these are in the public domain and may be freely reproduced.

Environmental factors may play a role in the management of asthma. This may include evaluation of allergy with skin tests or RAST testing and mitigation of environmental factors when possible. Table 4.8 and Table 4.9 address investigation of various environmental factors and possible interventions, respectively.

Medical therapy is based on prevention of symptoms and exacerbations with the use of controller medications and resolution of symptoms and exacerbations with rescue medications. Airway medications are discussed in detail elsewhere (see **Medications for Airways Disease**). Short-acting beta agonists, ipratropium, and systemic steroids are the primary rescue medications. Inhaled steroids are the cornerstone of controller therapy in adults, supplemented by long-acting beta agonists, leukotriene modifiers, methylxanthines, mast cell stabilizers, and anti-IgE therapy. Initial therapy is based on the assessment of the patient's severity at presentation. Reassessment increases or decreases the intensity of intervention as needed. A summary of step therapy is provided in Figure 4.1. Recommended starting step level correlated to severity is shown in Table 4.10.

Control of symptoms is assessed collaboratively between the patient and clinician(s). Inadequate control of symptoms should prompt intensification of therapy. Patients who are rendered symptom free with therapy should have their controller therapy gradually reduced under supervision to find the minimum amount

Table 4.8   Inhalant Allergens

Does the patient have symptoms year-round? (If yes, ask the following questions. If no, see next set of questions.)

- ☐ Does the patient keep pets indoors? What type?
- ☐ Does the patient have moisture or dampness in any room of his or her home (e.g., basement)? (Suggests house-dust mites, molds.)
- ☐ Does the patient have mold visible in any part of his or her home? (Suggests molds.)
- ☐ Has the patient seen cockroaches or rodents in his or her home in the past month? (Suggests significant cockroach exposure.)
- ☐ Assume exposure to house-dust mites unless patient lives in a semiarid region. However, if a patient living in a semiarid region uses a swamp cooler, exposure to house-dust mites must still be assumed.

Do symptoms get worse at certain times of the year? (If yes, ask when symptoms occur.)

- ☐ Early spring? (trees)
- ☐ Late spring? (grasses)
- ☐ Late summer to autumn? (weeds)
- ☐ Summer and fall? (*Alternaria, Cladosporium,* mites)
- ☐ Cold months in temperate climates? (animal dander)

Tobacco Smoke

- ☐ Does the patient smoke?
- ☐ Does anyone smoke at home or work?
- ☐ Does anyone smoke at the child's daycare?

Indoor/Outdoor Pollutants and Irritants

- ☐ Is a wood-burning stove or fireplace used in the patient's home?
- ☐ Are there unvented stoves or heaters in the patient's home?
- ☐ Does the patient have contact with other smells or fumes from perfumes, cleaning agents, or sprays?
- ☐ Have there been recent renovations or painting in the home?

Workplace Exposures

- ☐ Does the patient cough or wheeze during the week, but not on weekends when away from work?
- ☐ Do the patient's eyes and nasal passages get irritated soon after arriving at work?
- ☐ Do coworkers have similar symptoms?
- ☐ What substances are used in the patient's worksite? (Assess for sensitizers.)

(continues)

Table 4.8 (continued)

Rhinitis

☐ Does the patient have constant or seasonal nasal congestion, runny nose, and/or postnasal drip?

Gastroesophageal Reflux Disease (GERD)

☐ Does the patient have heartburn?

☐ Does food sometimes come up into the patient's throat?

☐ Has the patient had coughing, wheezing, or shortness of breath at night in the past 4 weeks?

☐ Does the infant vomit, followed by cough, or have wheezy cough at night? Are symptoms worse after feeding?

Sulfite Sensitivity

☐ Does the patient have wheezing, coughing, or shortness of breath after eating shrimp, dried fruit, or processed potatoes or after drinking beer or wine?

Medication Sensitivities and Contraindications

☐ What medications does the patient use now (prescription and nonprescription)?

☐ Does the patient use eyedrops? What type?

☐ Does the patient use any medications that contain beta-blockers?

☐ Does the patient ever take aspirin or other nonsteroidal anti-inflammatory drugs?

☐ Has the patient ever had symptoms of asthma after taking any of these medications?

2007 NHLBI Expert Panel Report 3: Guidelines for the Diagnosis and Management of Asthma. The work of the Expert Panel is gratefully acknowledged.

of therapy needed for control. Table 4.11 classifies the level of control through objective and subjective means of assessment. Table 4.12 is one of several documents in the NAEPP that offer assessment strategies.

Patients evaluated and treated for exacerbation should be questioned carefully to try and identify the cause of the decompensation. Noncompliance, viral infections, GERD, postnasal drip, and environmental changes (animals, work, bedding, temperature, humidity) are common problems. Older patients or patients with preexisting cardiovascular disease may suffer from heart failure. The clinician must distinguish between a transient setback requiring rescue or a fundamental change in the character or severity of the asthma requiring modification of the foundation manage-

Table 4.9 Summary of Measures to Control Environmental Factors That Can Make Asthma Worse

Allergens

Reduce or eliminate exposure to the allergen(s) the patient is sensitive to, including:

☐ **Animal dander:** Remove animal from house or, at a minimum, keep animal out of the patient's bedroom.

☐ **House-dust mites:**

—**Recommended:** Encase mattress in an allergen-impermeable cover; encase pillow in an allergen-impermeable cover or wash it weekly; wash sheets and blankets on the patient's bed in hot water weekly (water temperature of >130 °F is necessary for killing mites): cooler water and detergent and bleach will still reduce live mites and allergen level. Prolonged exposure to dry heat or freezing can also kill mites but does not remove allergen.

—**Desirable:** Reduce indoor humidity to at or below 60%, ideally 30–50%; remove carpets from the bedroom; avoid sleeping or lying on upholstered furniture; remove carpets that are laid on concrete.

☐ **Cockroaches:** Use poison bait or traps to control insects, but intensive cleaning is necessary to reduce reservoirs. Do not leave food or garbage exposed.

☐ **Pollens (from trees, grass, or weeds) and outdoor molds:** If possible, adults who have allergies should stay indoors, with windows closed, during periods of peak pollen exposure, which are usually during the midday and afternoon.

☐ **Indoor mold:** Fix all leaks and eliminate water sources associated with mold growth; clean moldy surfaces.

Consider reducing indoor humidity to or below 60%, ideally 30–50%. Dehumidify basements if possible.

☐ It is recommended that allergen immunotherapy be considered for patients who have asthma if evidence is clear of a relationship between symptoms and exposure to an allergen to which the patient is sensitive.

Tobacco Smoke

Advise patients and others in the home who smoke to stop smoking or to smoke outside the home. Discuss ways to reduce exposure to other sources of tobacco smoke, such as from daycare providers and the workplace.

Indoor/Outdoor Pollutants and Irritants

Discuss ways to reduce exposures to the following:

☐ Wood-burning stoves or fireplaces

☐ Unvented gas stoves or heaters

☐ Other irritants (e.g., perfumes, cleaning agents, sprays)

☐ Volatile organic compounds (VOCs) such as new carpeting, particle board, painting

2007 NHLBI Expert Panel Report 3: Guidelines for the Diagnosis and Management of Asthma. The work of the Expert Panel is gratefully acknowledged.

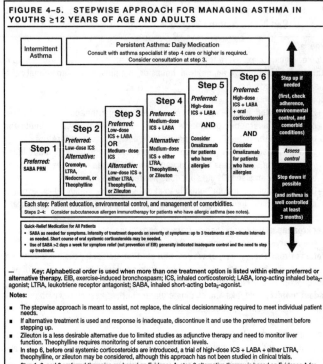

FIGURE 4-5. STEPWISE APPROACH FOR MANAGING ASTHMA IN YOUTHS ≥12 YEARS OF AGE AND ADULTS

Intermittent Asthma	Persistent Asthma: Daily Medication
	Consult with asthma specialist if step 4 care or higher is required.
	Consider consultation at step 3.

Step 1
Preferred:
SABA PRN

Step 2
Preferred:
Low-dose ICS
Alternative:
Cromolyn, LTRA, Nedocromil, or Theophylline

Step 3
Preferred:
Low-dose ICS + LABA
OR
Medium- dose ICS
Alternative:
Low-dose ICS + either LTRA, Theophylline, or Zileuton

Step 4
Preferred:
Medium-dose ICS + LABA
Alternative:
Medium-dose ICS + either LTRA, Theophylline, or Zileuton

Step 5
Preferred:
High-dose ICS + LABA
AND
Consider Omalizumab for patients who have allergies

Step 6
Preferred:
High-dose ICS + LABA + oral corticosteroid
AND
Consider Omalizumab for patients who have allergies

Step up if needed
(first, check adherence, environmental control, and comorbid conditions)

Assess control

Step down if possible
(and asthma is well controlled at least 3 months)

Each step: Patient education, environmental control, and management of comorbidities.
Steps 2–4: Consider subcutaneous allergen immunotherapy for patients who have allergic asthma (see notes).

Quick-Relief Medication for All Patients
- SABA as needed for symptoms. Intensity of treatment depends on severity of symptoms: up to 3 treatments at 20-minute intervals as needed. Short course of oral systemic corticosteroids may be needed.
- Use of SABA >2 days a week for symptom relief (not prevention of EIB) generally indicated inadequate control and the need to step up treatment.

— **Key:** Alphabetical order is used when more than one treatment option is listed within either preferred or alternative therapy. EIB, exercise-induced bronchospasm; ICS, inhaled corticosteroid; LABA, long-acting inhaled beta$_2$-agonist; LTRA, leukotriene receptor antagonist; SABA, inhaled short-acting beta$_2$-agonist.

Notes:

- The stepwise approach is meant to assist, not replace, the clinical decisionmaking required to meet individual patient needs.
- If alternative treatment is used and response is inadequate, discontinue it and use the preferred treatment before stepping up.
- Zileuton is a less desirable alternative due to limited studies as adjunctive therapy and need to monitor liver function. Theophylline requires monitoring of serum concentration levels.
- In step 6, before oral systemic corticosteroids are introduced, a trial of high-dose ICS + LABA + either LTRA, theophylline, or zileuton may be considered, although this approach has not been studied in clinical trials.
- Step 1, 2, and 3 preferred therapies are based on Evidence A; step 3 alternative therapy is based on Evidence A for LTRA, Evidence B for theophylline, and Evidence D for zileuton. Step 4 preferred therapy is based on Evidence B, and alternative therapy is based on Evidence B for LTRA and theophylline and Evidence D for zileuton. Step 5 preferred therapy is based on Evidence B. Step 6 preferred therapy is based on (EPR–2 1997) and Evidence B for omalizumab.
- Immunotherapy for steps 2–4 is based on Evidence B for house-dust mites, animal danders, and pollen; evidence is weak or lacking for molds and cockroaches. Evidence is strongest for immunotherapy with single allergens. The role of allergy in asthma is greater in children than in adults.
- Clinicians who administer immunotherapy or omalizumab should be prepared and equipped to identify and treat anaphylaxis that may occur.

Figure 4.1 Stepwise approach for managing asthma in youths >12 years of age and adults. 2007 NHLBI Expert Panel Report 3: Guidelines for the Diagnosis and Management of Asthma. The work of the Expert Panel is gratefully acknowledged.

Table 4.10   NAEPP Treatment Recommendations by Step and Severity

Severity	Initial Step
Intermittent	1
Persistent, mild	2
Persistent, moderate	3*
Persistent, severe	4 or 5*

*Consider a short pulse of oral steroids to effect prompt control and relief of symptoms.
2007 NHLBI Expert Panel Report 3: Guidelines for the Diagnosis and Management of Asthma. The work of the Expert Panel is gratefully acknowledged.

ment program. The underlying reason for decompensation must be sought and addressed.

Patients sufficiently ill to require hospitalization and/or emergency room therapy may be treated with aggressive interventions including intravenous steroids and frequent (or continuous) α agonist nebulization. Some experts continue to advocate intravenous aminophylline. Patients should not be discharged from the emergency room without a postencounter care plan, and a tapering course of steroids markedly reduces the probability of relapse.

An asthma attack severe enough to warrant hospital admission should prompt reassessment of the foundation care plan. A patient in severe distress (diaphoresis, unable to speak, large pulsus paradoxus, can't lie down) should be admitted to a critical care unit. Such patients should have an arterial blood gas analysis; a normal $PaCO_2$ or higher is ominous and may indicate the need for intubation and ventilation. Some patients may be helped by NIPPV, but patients in this state can fail rapidly, and intubation and mechanical ventilation should not be delayed if the patient is obviously failing. The mechanical ventilation of the asthmatic in extremis is one of the most difficult clinical problems in pulmonary medicine, and consultation is mandatory. Most of these patients require deep sedation or paralysis (with sedation) to reduce elastic load and static compliance. Hypercarbia is tolerated while steroids and bronchodilators take effect. The ventilator is adjusted to provide as high an

Table 4.11 Assessing Asthma Control in Youths >12 y and Adults

		Classification of Asthma Control (Youths >12 y and Adults)		
Components of Control		**Well Controlled**	**Not Well Controlled**	**Very Poorly Controlled**
Impairment	Symptoms	<2 days/week	>2 days/week	Throughout the day
	Nighttime awakenings	<twice/month	1–3/week	>4/week
	Short-acting beta2 agonist use for symptom control	<2 days/week	>2 days/week	Several times/day
	Interference with normal activity	None	Some limitation	Extremely limited
	FEV$_1$ or peak flow	>80% predicted/ personal best	60–80% predicted/ personal best	<60% predicted/ personal best
	Validated Questionnaires			
	ATAQ	0	1–2	3–4
	ACQ	<0.75	>1.5	N/A
	ACT	>20	16–19	<15

Risk	Exacerbations	0–1/year	>2/year
	Progressive loss of lung function	Evaluation requires long-term follow-up care	
	Treatment-related adverse effects	Medication side effects can vary in intensity from none to very troublesome and worrisome. The level of intensity does not correlate to specific levels of control but should be considered in the overall assessment of risk.	

ACQ values of 0.76–1.4 are indeterminate regarding well-controlled asthma

Notes:

The level of control is based on the most severe impairment or risk category. Assess impairment domain by patient's recall of previous 2–4 weeks and by spirometry/or peak flow measures. Symptom assessment for longer periods should reflect a global assessment, such as inquiring whether the patient's asthma is better or worse since the last visit.

At present, there are inadequate data to correspond frequencies of exacerbations with different levels of asthma control. In general, more frequent and intense exacerbations (e.g., requiring urgent, unscheduled care, hospitalization, or ICU admission) indicate poorer disease control. For treatment purposes, patients who had ≥2 exacerbations requiring oral systemic corticosteroids in the past year may be considered the same as patients who have not-well-controlled asthma, even in the absence of impairment levels consistent with not-well-controlled asthma.

2007 NHLBI Expert Panel Report 3: Guidelines for the Diagnosis and Management of Asthma. The work of the Expert Panel is gratefully acknowledged.

Table 4.12　Sample Questions for Assessing and Monitoring Asthma Control

Ask the patient:

Has your asthma awakened you at night or early in the morning?

Have you needed more quick-relief bronchodilator medication (inhaled short-acting beta2-agonist) than usual?

Have you needed any urgent medical care for your asthma, such as unscheduled visits to your doctor, an urgent care clinic, or the emergency department?

Are you participating in your usual and desired activities?

If you are measuring your peak flow, has it been below your personal best?

Actions to consider:

Assess whether the medications are being taken as prescribed.

Assess whether the medications are being inhaled with correct technique.

Assess lung function with spirometry and compare to previous measurement.

Adjust medications, as needed; either step up if control is inadequate or step down if control is maximized, to achieve the best control with the lowest dose of medication.

2007 NHLBI Expert Panel Report 3: Guidelines for the Diagnosis and Management of Asthma. The work of the Expert Panel is gratefully acknowledged.

inspiratory flow rate as possible (and therefore as short an inspiratory time as possible) with a prolonged expiratory phase. A relatively small tidal volume is used, and respiratory rate, flow rate, flow waveform, and other parameters are adjusted to prevent breath stacking (incomplete exhalation). Stacking can lead to dangerous hyperinflation with reduced venous return and hypotension; pneumothorax, the most feared complication of asthmatic mechanical ventilation, could be fatal in this setting.

4.2　Chronic Obstructive Pulmonary Disease (COPD)

www.goldcopd.org 2006;2007, http://thoracic.org/sections/copd/resources/copddoc.pdf 2004;2007.

Epidemiology: Chronic obstructive pulmonary disease (COPD) along with lung cancer is one of the great medical tragedies of the 20th and 21st centuries. In large part preventable, it is the fourth leading cause of death in the United States and an enormous cost and drain on the economy and the welfare of the populace. The Global initiative on Obstructive Lung Disease (GOLD) estimates that the identified prevalence of COPD is between 6% and 10%, and that true prevalence (using their aggressive definition and counting patients who are at present without symptoms) is two or three times that. The developing world is not spared; places such as China have a rate of smoking in men as high as 60%. The burden of disease that will be placed on individual countries and the world as these younger populations age is staggering. In the United States, COPD used to be a male disease, but as more women smoke, the male preponderance has disappeared. COPD is primarily a disease of the older middle aged and elderly, although patients with genetic predisposition or heavy smoke exposure may have earlier symptomatic disease.

Pathogenesis: COPD is caused primarily by first-person smoking. The health effects of smoking are well recognized, and a complete discussion of the diseases caused by tobacco use is beyond the scope of this book. Two main processes cause obstructive lung disease. First, a complex series of inflammatory events lead to the destruction of alveolar tissue with deleterious effects on V/Q matching as alveoli coalesce into large, relatively ineffective airbags that have unfavorable surface to volume ratios (volume increases with respect to surface area, rendering gas exchange ineffective). The same destruction of parenchymal tissue reduces radial traction on the airways during expiration, causing collapse of airways during exhalation and obstruction. Alveolar destruction also leads to loss of elastic recoil, making exhalation less efficient. This process is emphysema. In extreme cases, large numbers of alveoli may coalesce into large, thin-walled structures termed bullae. These spaces do not participate in gas exchange. Chronic bronchitis is an inflammatory condition with airways inflammation and mucus hypersecretion with reduction of airway caliber as a direct consequence of edema, inflammation, and mucus.

Additionally, many patients have a component of reactive airways disease. It is uncommon that a patient will have a "pure" case of emphysema or chronic bronchitis; adult smoking-related lung disease is usually a mix of two or three of these basic components. The term *COPD* is used as an umbrella term, encompassing all three processes in whatever proportion they occur. Unlike asthma, complete normalization of airway function *never* occurs.

The mechanism of pulmonary injury by tobacco smoke (and other forms of injury) is a subject of interest and research. Amplified inflammatory response to inhaled particles, oxidative stress, and creation of protease-antiprotease imbalance are all thought to play a role. Researchers have proposed an appealing model of development of COPD being related to the total burden of inhaled particles. In this paradigm, smoking tobacco will deliver a high burden of particles. However, this model also accounts for the component of COPD caused by industrial exposures, air pollution (indoor and outdoor), and environmental tobacco smoke. In developing countries, burning of biomass (refuse, wood, dung) in poorly ventilated or unventilated dwellings is responsible for a significant share of COPD (and affects women disproportionately because of cooking and domestic responsibilities). The genetics of COPD is poorly understood. Inherent susceptibility to the effects of tobacco smoke varies. Individuals with low levels of α-1-antitrypsin often develop severe emphysema at a very early age; this is an inherited disease with identified phenotypes and genotypes. However, there are also clusters of patients in families with emphysema where a clearly abnormal phenotype is not identified.

Chronic airway obstruction leads to predictable physiologic consequences. As work of breathing increases and V/Q matching becomes less favorable, exercise intolerance develops, eventually leading to dyspnea at rest. Similarly, V/Q mismatching is initially preserved at rest and only becomes apparent with exercise, with exercise-induced hypoxia preceding hypoxia at rest. Additionally,

V/Q mismatching may occur as a consequence of position. Smoking-related emphysema tends to occur in the upper lung zones; blood flow in the low pressure pulmonary system is influenced by gravity and when the patient is vertical there is preferential blood flow to the healthier lower lobes. When the patient is recumbent there is blood flow to the lung bases and apices, interfering with V/Q matching. Shunt physiology as a consequence of uncomplicated COPD does not occur.

Regulation and excretion of carbon dioxide in COPD are of clinical interest and sometimes misunderstood (please forgive a short detour into a general discussion of the mechanisms of hypercarbia). Hypercarbia is the consequence of CO_2 production in excess of CO_2 elimination; in COPD excess production is rarely the problem. CO_2 elimination is directly proportional to alveolar ventilation. Because of the difference in the body's handling of oxygen and carbon dioxide (carrier molecule vs. dissolved gas respectively), an increase in ventilation despite unfavorable V/Q relationships will increase or at least maintain adequate CO_2 elimination. This is why most pathological pulmonary conditions are not associated with hypercarbia, even shunt. As the severity of COPD increases, airways obstruction may become so severe that it reduces minute ventilation; expiration takes so long that the number and/or volume of breaths becomes too low to maintain adequate alveolar ventilation. There may be destruction of so many alveolar capillary units that there are not enough alveoli to ventilate, by definition reducing alveolar ventilation below a critical minute volume. Reduction of minute ventilation by both mechanisms can also be seen in other forms of very advanced parenchymal lung disease as well as airway disease. Hypercarbia may occur as a consequence of bellows and controller dysfunction. Expansion and contraction of the lungs to generate alveolar minute ventilation require adequate function of the control mechanism (brain and CO_2

receptors), intact transmission of the control impulses (intact nervous system), and functional bellows (respiratory muscles and rib cage). See **Neuromuscular and Ventilatory Control Conditions.** In COPD, malnutrition and chronic hyperinflation can reduce bellows efficiency by reducing muscle strength and mechanical efficiency, respectively. Chronic hypercarbia blunts the control mechanism with an impaired, lower-amplitude increase in ventilation in response to an increase in CO_2. These patients, unlike normal individuals, will depend upon hypoxia rather than hypercarbia to stimulate ventilation. If patients are rendered hyperoxic by too much supplemental oxygen, they may become more hypercarbic, become acidotic, and suffer respiratory arrest. Fortunately, suppression of respiratory drive does not occur until PaO_2 level is in the 80 mmHg range or greater. The fear that many physicians and ancillary professionals harbor regarding "CO_2 retainers" is often misapplied with a concern that supplemental oxygen itself (i.e., increased FIO_2) rather than elevated PaO_2 will trigger respiratory arrest. As will be discussed further in treatment, defense of oxygenation is more important than prevention of hypercarbia, and oxygen should be used, along with assisted ventilation as necessary to maintain tissue oxygenation. Careful titration of supplemental oxygen to prevent hyperoxia ($PaO_2 > 80$) will not trigger CO_2 retention in the vast majority of cases. If supplemental oxygen is provided and $PaCO_2$ increases while PaO_2 decreases, this is a manifestation of treatment failure rather than an iatrogenic effect of supplemental oxygen.

This short physiologic diatribe complete, patients with advanced obstructive lung disease, usually with FEV_1 measurements <40% predicted, may have obligatory CO_2 retention because of an *inability* to generate adequate minute ventilation. Other patients may have respiratory control problems with preserved ability to generate minute ventilation from a lung and bellows perspective, but *failure of the controller mechanism* to generate adequate instructions for maintenance of ventilation. The reason for this is not known. My own belief is that many of the latter group have sleep-disordered breathing.

Obliteration of alveoli by emphysema reduces the cross-sectional area of the lungs' vascular bed leading to pulmonary hypertension on a mechanical basis. Hypoxia leads to hypoxic pulmonary vasoconstriction, also leading to pulmonary hypertension. Elevated pulmonary pressures and elevated right ventricular load lead to right-sided congestive heart failure and right ventricular dilatation. This further impairs exercise intolerance and may cause fluid retention.

Many patients will lose muscle mass during the course of their disease. Loss of appetite, difficulty breathing and eating simultaneously, and an increased basal metabolic rate secondary to the increased work of breathing lead to a combination of malnutrition and muscle wasting, further impairing gas exchange and resistance to infection.

Patients with COPD are susceptible to exacerbations. Viral or bacterial infection, left- or right-sided congestive heart failure, excessive physical activity, environmental changes (e.g., air pollution) can lead to an abrupt and acute worsening of pulmonary function and performance status. Exacerbations may occur in the absence of an identifiable stimulus. Severity of an exacerbation may vary from a few days of mild discomfort to a requirement for a steroid pulse to hospitalization with intubation and mechanical ventilation. Many patients, particularly when their disease is advanced, will not return to previous baseline even after successful treatment of the exacerbation. Even in the absence of exacerbations, accelerated loss of lung function is relentless.

Symptoms: Cough, sputum, wheezing, dyspnea on exertion. Patients with advanced disease will have dyspnea at rest. Patients with right-sided CHF will have edema. Cyanosis is seen only in patients with hypoxemia. Orthopnea is common. One peculiarity of COPD is the sensitivity of the patient to dyspnea produced by arm work rather than leg work. On examination, patients may have a relatively normal exam in the early stages of illness. As the disease progresses, dyspnea may become more prominent, with dyspnea at rest observed even in the absence of an exacerbation. Breath sounds become more distant and wheezing may be heard on auscultation. Accessory respiratory muscle use becomes more apparent. Many patients will use pursed lip breathing to produce higher end-expiratory pressures and prevent airway closure. Some patients may also be observed to rest their arms on furniture or a cart; this improves chest cage mechanical advantage in the presence of hyperinflation (for some reason, it reminds me of a bird's posture and I call this position perching; the more common term is "tripodding"). Patients may have sudden chest pain in the presence of a pneumothorax when a bulla ruptures.

Course/Prognosis/Complications: Prior to current therapy, prognosis could be predicted from FEV_1. Prognosis has been harder to define with the advent of evidence-driven oxygen therapy; there is early evidence that ICS therapy may have an effect on prognosis as well. Lung transplantation can also prolong life; LVRS does not. NIPPV therapy is not thought to prolong life. Patients are at risk of chronic respiratory failure with a very poor quality of life. Cor pulmonale is another common complication. Patients with >20 pack-year tobacco use history are at risk for multiple comorbidities including atherosclerotic disease and malignancy. Patients with COPD appear to have an enhanced risk of pulmonary malignancy. This is a bad disease to die from. The course is long, uncomfortable, frightening, and frustrating.

Imaging: "Classic" smoking-related emphysema demonstrates hyperlucency in the upper lung zones, sometimes with identifiable bullae (thin, delicate line separating airspaces with no lung markings). There is crowding of lung markings and remaining lung tissue to the lung bases. The pattern is reversed in α-1-antitrypsin deficiency (more disease at the base of the lungs). On CT scans, emphysema has the appearance of black holes in the gray-black parenchyma. Subtle degrees of emphysema may be visible in the lower lobes on CT that are not apparent on plain film. Patients with less of an emphysema component to their COPD may have a relatively normal chest X-ray or just some modest hyperexpansion. Patients with concomitant nonspecific pulmonary fibrosis or respiratory bronchiolitis may have increased lung markings. Patients with fluid overload or right-sided CHF may have prominent septal lines and pleural effusions as well. Imaging results of patients with COPD should be reviewed carefully. The patient with COPD is fertile ground for pneumonia, heart failure, and pulmonary malignancy. Important changes can be missed in these patients with complex X-rays. Comparison to old films, when available, is helpful.

Laboratory: Pulmonary function testing is used for treatment and diagnosis. For a diagnosis of COPD, patients *must* have obstruction demonstrable, with an FEV_1/FVC ratio of 70% or less. Typically COPD patients will also have some degree of hyperinflation demonstrated by an elevated RV and/or TLC and/or FVC. With obliteration of the pulmonary capillary bed from emphysema, the blood content of the lung is reduced producing a lowering of the DLCO. Cardiopulmonary exercise testing may be of value in patients who have dyspnea in excess of what would be expected for their pulmonary function testing. Hypoxemia on blood gases is common. Hypercarbia is seen in patients with advanced disease or who have faulty CO_2 regulation (so-called blue bloaters). Stable patients with elevated $PaCO_2$ levels from either etiology will present an acid-base picture of compensated respiratory acidosis. A mixed acid-base picture may also be present because of comorbidities and diuretics. Patients with acute exacerbations may manifest acidosis with acute-on-chronic respiratory acidosis. Use of the acid-basis nomogram presented in the section on

Arterial Blood Gases is recommended. Chronic severe hypoxemia can lead to stimulation of erythropoietin production and erythrocytosis with elevated hemoglobin. (In my practice, an elevated hemoglobin is unusual. Most patients with COPD have a sufficient number of comorbidities to have low or normal hemoglobin.) WBC elevations may be seen from steroid use or infection. Electrolyte abnormalities are common from steroid use, diuretic use, or even SIADH. Patients with α-1-antitrypsin deficiency will have low α-1-antitrypsin levels. If a low level is identified, phenotyping of the molecule is indicated to determine if the patient is a homozygote or heterozygote. Although heterozygotes have an abnormally low level of protein, they largely retain protection of lung tissue (as long as they don't smoke or otherwise incur a high particulate burden). Homozygous patients have a much worse prognosis and should be considered for α-1-antitrypsin replacement. Echocardiography may be used to determine the presence of right ventricular dysfunction and/or pulmonary hypertension. Nutritional assessment with proalbumin levels may be occasionally indicated.

Diagnosis: Diagnosis of COPD is a clinical diagnosis confirmed by pulmonary function testing. The diagnosis should be considered in patients with chronic cough, dyspnea, and/or sputum production with appropriate risk factors/exposures. Spirometry should demonstrate FEV_1 measurements below 80% predicted and an FEV_1/FVC ratio of <70%. Reversal of flow limitation is incomplete, and symptoms as described above are chronic. Severity stratification will be discussed below in the treatment section. A common mistake of frontline practitioners is to label anyone with cough and a smoking history as having COPD. The differential diagnosis of COPD includes asthma, bronchiectasis, congestive heart failure, tuberculosis, early interstitial pneumonitis, and various forms of obliterative bronchiolitis. Many of these alternative diagnoses may be confirmed or eliminated with spirometry and a chest X-ray.

Treatment: Treatment goals for COPD are designed to prolong life, maximize functional status, maintain independence, and preserve pulmonary function. Interventions are based on disease severity. Broadly speaking, the foundation of treatment rests on:

1. Resolution of risk factors, specifically initiation and maintenance of tobacco abstinence
2. Development of a plan of medical therapy, including supplemental oxygen and surgical intervention as appropriate
3. Intensive education to develop and maintain the patient's ability for self-assessment and self-care
4. Maximization of physical strength and endurance
5. Periodic assessment by the patient's clinician to adjust therapy as the patient's baseline changes
6. Vigorous identification of and response to exacerbations
7. Proactive, early confrontation of end-of-life issues and care in the context of advanced disease

Most authorities recommend some manner of severity classification. Table 4.13 presents a matrix adapted from the 2006 GOLD document outlining spirometric definitions of severity associated with expected level of symptoms. Some readers may recall an earlier version of GOLD (2001) that described a stage 0 of patients with normal function but at high risk. This classification stage has been withdrawn. Readers should also note that all stages of illness require the presence of obstruction: the FEV_1/FVC ratio is less than 0.7 postbronchodilator administration indicating the presence of nonreversible abnormal expiratory flow limitation.

Smoking cessation is a necessary but sometimes frustrating component of COPD care. Smoking cessation reduces risk, slows progression of disease, and improves the quality of life. That said, it is often very difficult for patients to break this habit/addiction.

Table 4.13   COPD Severity Classification

Stage	FEV₁/FVC	FEV₁ % Pred.	Cough	Sputum	Dyspnea	Exercise Intolerance	Exacerbation Frequency	Respiratory Failure
I—Mild	<.70	≥80%	$\pm$	$\pm$	$\pm$	Not appreciated by patient	Infrequent	Not present
II—Moderate	<.70	≥50%, <80%	+	+	+	Slight	Infrequent but a problem	Not present
III—Severe	<.70	≥30%, <50%	++	++	+++	Impairs activity	Frequent	Not present, may occur w/exac
IV—Very Severe	<.70	<30%*	+++	++/ +++	++++	Impairs ADLs	Frequent	Often present on chronic basis

*May be ≤ 50% if Sx of resp failure are present: $Po_2 < 60$, $Pco_2 > 50$, or cor pulmonale.
Modified from GOLD 2006 Executive Summary Table 2.

Smoking cessation above all requires that the patient want to quit; this is often not the case. Once the patient is ready to quit, techniques involve behavioral and medical therapies. Behavioral interventions include gradual reduction in smoking, habit substitution, lay support groups, clinician support at individual visits and group activities, and interventions such as acupuncture and hypnosis. Medical therapy uses nicotine replacement, buproprion, or varenicline. All of these interventions are effective in the short term, with quitting rates at 2–3 months often in the 75–90% range. Abstinence falls at 1 year, with typical continued abstinence in only 20–30% of initially successful quitters. Often, several attempts at quitting are necessary before the patient is finally tobacco free. Successful smoking cessation may be frustrated by weight gain, exacerbation of coexisting ulcerative colitis, and deteriorating cognitive function in patients with schizophrenia.

Medical therapy relies on bronchodilator therapy with SABA and LABA agents, ICS, systemic steroids, theophylline, and atropine analogs such as ipratropium and tiotropium. These drugs are described in greater detail in the **Medications for Airways Disease** section. Oxygen therapy plays a major role, particularly in Stages III and IV disease. Criteria for coverage of oxygen prescriptions under the US Medicare program are discussed in **Oxygen Therapy.** These criteria are based on scientific evidence and represent best practice. Some patients may benefit from chronic use of NIPPV for assisted nocturnal ventilation. Patients with severe, advanced COPD may be candidates for LVRS or lung transplantation, covered in the section on **Advanced Lung Disease.** In addition to palliation of symptoms and maintenance of functional status, medical therapy seeks to prolong the life of the patient. To date, only supplemental oxygen therapy in hypoxic patients has been shown conclusively to prolong life. Newer data regarding prognosis and ICS therapy are promising and will likely provoke further large-scale studies

(N Engl J Med 2007;356:775). Vaccination (influenza and
S. pneumoniae), mucolytics, and antitussives are adjuncts of
value. Vaccination in particular can be of great value. α-1-
antitrypsin replacement for α-1-antitrypsin deficiency-related
emphysema has been shown conclusively to raise α-1-antitrypsin
levels. Randomized, controlled clinical trials have not been performed that demonstrate that improved survival or better functional status. Observational studies do appear to show some
modest benefit to α-1-antitrypsin augmentation. Unlike asthma
guidelines, the step progression of treatment is not as rigid and/or
defined. The GOLD collaboration (Global initiative for
Obstructive Lung Disease) has offered an outline of management
outlined in Figure 4.2. Generally, patients should be initiated on
SABA therapy for intermittent symptoms. More severe symptoms are usually treated with a LABA and/or atropine analog.
Guidelines suggest adding ICS for Stage III or IV disease, but I
tend to add these agents relatively quickly. Guidelines state that
systemic steroids have no place in the chronic treatment of
COPD. However, I don't know a pulmonary doctor that doesn't
use them in his or her patients with advanced disease. My personal experience has been that the combination of ICS, LABA,
and tiotropium has markedly increased quality of life for patients
with advanced disease. Regular clinical assessment of the patient
should be performed so that changes in foundation therapy can
be made as the patient's condition changes. Supplemental
oxygen, NIPPV, LVRS, transplantation, and palliation are appropriate for advanced disease. With the exception of palliation,
which is a personal decision among the clinician, patient, and
family/partners, other advanced techniques are applied under
strict guidelines and protocols (see **Advanced Lung Disease**).
Treatment of secondary pulmonary hypertension is covered
separately.

Pulmonary rehabilitation is a multidisciplinary intervention
that provides supervised, graded exercise to maximize function,

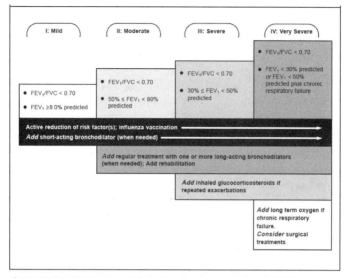

I: Mild	II: Moderate	III: Severe	IV: Very Severe
			• FEV₁/FVC < 0.70 • FEV₁ < 30% predicted or FEV₁ < 50% predicted plus chronic respiratory failure
		• FEV₁/FVC < 0.70 • 30% ≤ FEV₁ < 50% predicted	
• FEV₁/FVC < 0.70 • FEV₁ ≥80% predicted	• FEV₁/FVC < 0.70 • 50% ≤ FEV₁ < 80% predicted		

Active reduction of risk factor(s); influenza vaccination ⟶			
Add short-acting bronchodilator (when needed) ⟶			
	Add regular treatment with one or more long-acting bronchodilators (when needed); Add rehabilitation		
		Add inhaled glucocorticosteroids if repeated exacerbations	
			Add long term oxygen if chronic respiratory failure. *Consider* surgical treatments

*Postbronchodilator FEV₁ is recommended for the diagnosis and assessment of severity of COPD.

Figure 4.2 GOLD COPD treatment guidelines, by disease stage. From the Global Strategy for the Diagnosis, Management and Prevention of COPD, Global Initiative for Chronic Obstructive Lung Disease (GOLD) 2007. Available from: http://www.goldcopd.org. Used with permission.

nutritional counseling, extensive education, feedback as to the efficacy of self-assessment and self-management, and psychological support. There are no clinically proven exercises that improve FEV_1. Pulmonary rehabilitation seeks to maximize, optimize, and preserve the patient's remaining physical and emotional resources through education and exercise training. In this effort, most programs are quite successful, with studies showing that utilization of medical resources is reduced and patient quality of life is improved. Patients may benefit from pulmonary rehabilitation at any disease stage.

Patients should be reassessed on a regular basis. Symptom assessment and examination are usually sufficient. Patients should be queried as to their medical compliance, their ability to carry out common physical tasks, exacerbations since their last assessment, and symptoms such as cough, sputum, and dyspnea. I find it useful to seek aggressively evidence of uncontrolled comorbid conditions such as heart failure. As patients' disease progresses, repeat pulmonary function testing may help correlate symptoms with spirometric data. Arterial blood gas testing may also be helpful as dyspnea and exercise intolerance increase.

Prompt identification and treatment of exacerbations (acute exacerbation of COPD, AECOPD) are required to maintain the patient's functional status. Most patients develop a sense of what they can handle themselves, what needs a trip to a doctor's office, and what needs a trip to an emergency room. The educational component of pulmonary rehabilitation teaches these assessment and communication skills. Until the clinician and the patient have good communication, direct assessment (rather than telephone assessment) is appropriate. Patients should be considered for inpatient and/or hospital emergency room assessment and treatment when the symptoms are sudden and severe, there are significant comorbidities such as heart failure, there are new physical findings such as cyanosis or edema, there are new arrhythmias, or the patient is returning in the context of failed initial management. Advanced age and limited home care resources should also be considered in the overall assessment. Most AECOPD are caused by tracheobronchial infection and environmental changes such as air pollution. Cardiac decompensation may cause AECOPD and vice versa. The primary components of outpatient management are a pulse of systemic steroids, intensification of beta agonist therapy, and antibiotics if there is evidence of bacterial bronchitis. If a patient is not on steroids, I will usually pulse that patient with 30 mg prednisone for 3 days, 20 mg for 3 days, 10 mg for 3 days, and then stop. I will repeat this pulse once if the patient has a partial response. Patients who present to the emergency room require more careful evaluation as they are self-selecting to be sicker. Examination, chest X-ray, blood count, and blood gases are often indicated. Initial therapy usually consists of intensive nebulizer therapy and parenteral steroids (in our hospital usually methyprednisolone) with the dose usually reflecting the anxiety of the physician rather than following any particular protocol.

Antibiotics are also commonly used, generally similar to those used for CAP. Hospitalization is provided for patients who are severely ill, requiring aggressive nebulizer therapy, supplemental oxygen, treatment of comorbid conditions, intravenous therapy, and intensive nursing care. The latter cannot be overemphasized; bed rest and sleep are effective in this illness. Critical care unit admission is reserved for patients in shock or respiratory failure requiring intubation and mechanical ventilation. Depending upon the institution, patients requiring NIPPV may or may not be admitted to a CCU. My personal feeling on this is that if the patient is a potential candidate for intubation and ventilation, NIPPV should be supplied in a CCU setting. In both ward and ICU hospitalization scenarios, steroids and antibiotics as well as bronchodilators are continued at intensive levels until the patient starts to respond. The patient is then transitioned to the equivalent of outpatient therapy over the course of several more days. Discharge often includes home nursing services temporarily, permanent or temporary supplemental oxygen, a tapering course of steroids, and careful clinician reassessment.

All therapy should be undertaken with the understanding that COPD is a progressive illness that is often the cause of the patient's death, or at least a contributing factor. Early discussion of advance directives, palliation, attitude toward mechanical ventilation, and desire for aggressive care is extremely helpful to both the patient and the clinician. Discussion of these issues with the patient outside of an emergent or critical context gives the patient opportunity for reflection and permits development of communication and trust with the clinician so when patients reach the end of their lives, families and patients can trust and work with the clinician in this difficult time. Knowledge of state law, local resources regarding hospice availability, and execution of an advance directive make the transition to palliative care and end-of-life care easier for the patient. See **Palliative Care.**

4.3 Bronchiectasis

Bronchiectasis: N Engl J Med 2002;346:1383 excellent, recent general review.

Immotile cilia: Am J Med Sci 2001;321:3, Eur Respir J 1998;12:982

Cystic fibrosis: Cleve Clin J Med 2006;73:1065, Arch Dis Child 2001;85:62

Introduction: Bronchiectasis is a general term describing structural injury to the bronchial mucosa and airway wall causing permanent focal bronchial dilation, and a clinical syndrome manifested by chronic airway infection, cough, and often sputum production. The disease often follows infection but can also be a consequence of other forms of airway injury. Kartagener's syndrome and cystic fibrosis are systemic diseases that have very severe pulmonary complications.

Epidemiology: The prevalence of bronchiectasis is unknown. It is thought that there may be some clusters of high incidence of bronchiectasis in places with high rates of respiratory infection and poor access to health care. Bronchiectasis is associated with a number of illnesses. Although primarily of historical interest, pertussis has a very strong association with bronchiectasis. Many respiratory infections are connected with bronchiectasis, including viral infections, tuberculosis and atypical mycobacterial infections, and aspergillosis (allergic bronchopulmonary aspergillosis). Conditions that interfere with immune function such as congenital immunodeficiency syndromes, chemotherapy, and leukemia can lead to the condition. External agents such as foreign bodies leading to postobstructive pneumonia and chlorine gas exposure have been identified as etiologies as well. A number of congenital conditions cause the condition, including cystic fibrosis, immotile cilia syndrome, Marfan's, α-1-antitrypsin deficiency, and cartilage abnormalities. Several rheumatic illnesses including rheumatoid arthritis, Sjögren's syndrome, lupus, and relapsing polychondritis cause bronchiectasis. Finally, there are several miscellaneous conditions: yellow nail syndrome, inflammatory bowel disease, and Young's disease. Traction bronchiectasis from diffuse parenchymal lung disease can cause significant illness.

Pathophysiology: The most important component of the respiratory system's defense mechanism is effective mucociliary clearance. This requires an unobstructed airway, effective cough, normal mucus, and normal ciliary function. When the defense system is compromised, injurious agents such as bacteria, immune mediators, and host defense cells can stagnate and injure the bronchial wall. Failure of clearance can occur because of airway obstruction (such as foreign body), overwhelming infection, or because of impairment of mucociliary transport. One common form of localized bronchiectasis is right middle lobe syndrome. Anatomically, the right middle lobe bronchus is a long, thin tube (most bronchi are short, fat tubes) that is surrounded by lymph nodes at its orifice. When there is a right middle lobe pneumonia, compression of the already narrow airway can occur by enlarged lymph nodes, leading to right middle lobe bronchiectasis. Specific defects of mucus viscosity are seen in cystic fibrosis, and nonfunctional or dysfunctional cilia are seen in the immotile cilia syndromes. Structural injury takes place in the form of dilatation of airways. The abnormality can take the form of symmetric, cylindrical dilation (cylindrical or tubular form), alternating areas of constriction and dilation (varicose form), or actual cystic outpouchings from the airway (saccular form). In addition, these areas are scarred and either partially or completely denuded of ciliated cells. If the injury is from a localized process, such as a bad pneumonia, the bronchiectasis will be confined to a single area. More generalized illnesses will lead to diffuse bronchiectasis.

Once the structural injury has occurred, there is a repeating cycle of infection, host inability to clear infection, further host structural damage, with a result of more frequent and more serious infection. In many cases, particularly in patients with immotile cilia syndrome or CF (but can occur in anyone with extensive disease), patients will be colonized with resistant strains of *Pseudomonas aeruginosa*, *Burkholderia cepacia* (especially CF), and *S. aureus*. Chronic infection with *Haemophilus influenzae*, *Streptococcus pneumoniae*, and other respiratory pathogens is common.

Course/Prognosis/Complications: Hemoptysis is common and can be life threatening. Chronic bacterial antigen presentation can produce vasculitis. Patients with diffuse bronchiectasis have a high rate of hospitalization, often 1–2 hospitalizations per year, and have a higher death rate than age-matched controls. Pneumonia and parenchymal destruction are common, and respiratory failure can occur. Pulmonary hypertension and right heart failure can occur in advanced disease. Despite this, many patients become accustomed to the condition, develop good communication with their physicians, learn to assess and treat themselves, and handle the regimen, infection, sputum, and bleeding with surprising equanimity.

Laboratory: Indicators of chronic inflammation may be elevated, such as CRP and ESR. Culture of the sputum may provide direction for antibiotic therapy. Sweat chloride levels (CF), nasal ciliary biopsy (immotile cilia), and immune electropheresis may be appropriate. Pulmonary function testing usually shows obstruction. Many patients with advanced disease have parenchymal destruction as well and will demonstrate restriction on lung volumes.

Imaging: A conclusive diagnosis of bronchiectasis can be made from HRCT scanning of the chest. Plain chest X-rays can show so-called tram line bronchi, where the airway walls are parallel rather than tapering. Occasionally, cysts may be seen. HRCT, however, easily demonstrates the abnormalities of the disease. Tram lines and cysts can be easily identified. Airways can have irregular borders. The airway when seen in cross section should not be larger than the associated pulmonary vessels, and airways that are larger than their associated vascular structures indicate the presence of bronchiectasis. Of historical interest, bronchography was often used prior to the advent of CT scanning.

Diagnosis: Diagnosis requires identification of the condition and a search for the etiology. This is important in younger patients, where congenital, potentially treatable abnormalities sometimes may be missed until the patient is in his or her 20s or 30s. The classic presentation of bronchiectasis is purulent, copious sputum and unremitting cough, and it is easy to make a diagnosis in a patient producing sometimes literally one cup of layering sputum per day. The diagnosis may be more difficult in a patient with unremitting cough and some sputum but no obvious etiology such as COPD or asthma, a patient with many episodes of "bronchitis," and the patient with chronic cough and occasional hemoptysis. Patients who have bronchiectasis along with infertility (CF, immotile cilia), low BMI (CF), situs inversus (immotile cilia), or frequent nonpulmonary infections (hypogammaglobulinemia syndromes) should be evaluated for respective associated conditions. In the setting of localized bronchiectasis in an older individual, it is important to exclude airway obstruction (cancer, carcinoid, foreign body) and imaging and/or bronchoscopy may be indicated. Chest examination is often nonspecific, with rales, rhonchi, wheezing, and hyperinflation. Patients with severe bronchiectasis may have signs and symptoms of right heart failure, and the chronic infection may cause the patient to be catabolic to the point of malnourishment. An unusual complication (although I personally have had two patients with this) is a coexisting vasculitis from chronic *Pseudomonas* antigen presentation to the patient's immune system. Patients with palpable purpura, cough, and sputum may warrant careful evaluation for bronchiectasis (Chest 1997;112:1699). My unsubstantiated impression is that bronchiectasis is underdiagnosed and that a larger-than-recognized group of patients with chronic pulmonary disease has structural airway damage.

Treatment: My fellowship director, Dr. Roland Ingram, put it succinctly: "Ed, when you treat bronchiectasis you're just mowing the lawn. You aren't getting rid of the grass, you're just getting it down to where you can live with it again." It is next to impossible to return the bronchiectatic airway to a sterile state. Therapy is based on improving bronchial clearance, antibiotics, reducing inflammation, and occasionally resection of highly localized disease. A variety of chest physiotherapy devices and techniques (see **Chest Physiotherapy**) are used. Percussion and postural drainage and cough assist devices are essential elements of therapy. Mucolytics, such as dornase alfa (approved for CF only) and acetylcysteine, thin secretions. Only dornase alfa, however, has experimental evidence to support its use in improving endpoints. Ambulatory treatment of exacerbations with antibiotics should use a broad spectrum agent such as levofloxacin. Exacerbations requiring inpatient treatment should initiate therapy with a broad spectrum antibiotic, such as levofloxacin, and adjust antibiotics once there is identification of the offending organism(s). One article recommends therapy for 7–10 days, but my personal experience is that clinical results appear to be better with at least 2 weeks of treatment. A more difficult question is the suppression or reduction of chronic microbe load. It would make sense that reducing the *Pseudomonas* or *Haemophilus* would reduce the inflammatory mediator load. One large survey of the data suggests that there is a slight benefit to prolonged antibiotics, but that trials are so different that it is difficult to pool data (Cochrane Database Syst Rev 2003;CD001392). Specific protocols exist for the treatment of tuberculosis, atypical mycobacteria, and ABPA. These conditions differ from chronic bacterial infection and deserve aggressive treatment. Direct reduction in airways inflammation with inhaled corticosteroids and use of beta agonists also appears to be helpful. Erythromycin has been used with benefit to reduce inflammation in short trials. Indomethacin will reduce mediators of inflammation. Resection of localized bronchiectasis is reserved for patients failing more conservative measures, where there is associated airway obstruction, or there is recurrent life-threatening hemoptysis. A large survey of the data regarding surgical treatment of bronchiectasis performed in 2000 could not find controlled trials supporting surgical vs. nonsurgical care (Cochrane Database Syst Rev 2000;CD002180). Hemoptysis can also be treated with cannulation and embolization of the affected bronchial arteries. However, complications of this procedure can include infarction of the spinal cord, and should be attempted at major centers with experienced interventional radiologists. General supportive measures such as nutrition, good hydration, and supplemental oxygen are appropriate. Double lung transplant has been used with success in patients with immotile cilia and CF.

Chapter 5

Pulmonary Infectious Disease

5.1 Approach to the Patient with Suspected Pneumonia

Evaluation of the patient who is febrile and has pulmonary symptoms is a core competency for any clinician. Pneumonia, acute bronchitis, and acute exacerbations of chronic bronchitis are costly and associated with high morbidity and mortality. To improve outcomes and reduce cost, researchers have developed algorithms and tools to guide the management of common scenarios. When should such a pathway be used? Which one? When does a patient fall outside of a defined protocol? Once a patient is treated, how do we judge success or failure?

At the outset, it *is* reasonable to assume that a patient who is febrile and coughing, dyspneic, or producing sputum has a respiratory infection. It is the clinician's obligation to assess the patient, determine if it is reasonable to proceed with treatment for an infection, and choose the right therapy. Because morbidity and mortality can be so high in some populations, prompt presumptive treatment for pneumonia, in the absence of a firm diagnosis and isolation of an organism, is the usual approach. Indeed, it is frequent that an organism is never identified. Because therapy is so often empiric, treatment depends on predicting the organism(s) that would be expected in a given situation. Expected pathogens depend on host factors. For this reason, host assessment is the most important component of empiric treatment. Once the host has been assessed, the data are synthesized, the patient is placed in an appropriate treatment plan, and outcomes are assessed. This general algorithm is outlined in Figure 5.1.

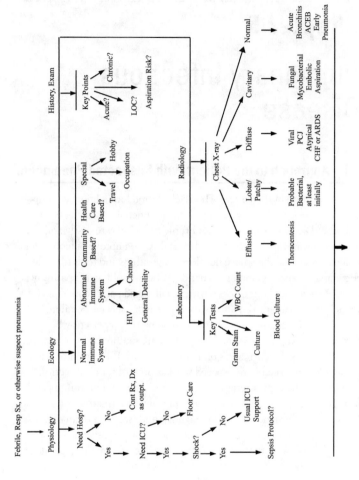

Febrile, Resp Sx, or otherwise suspect pneumonia

Figure 5.1 (Part 1) Pneumonia assessment algorithm.

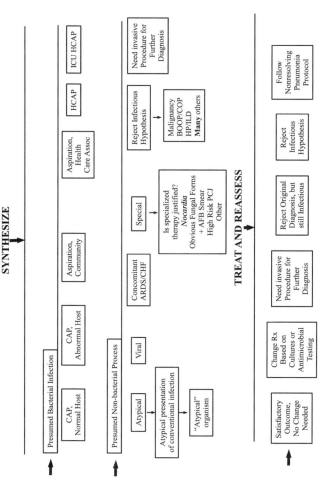

Figure 5.1 (Part 2) Pneumonia assessment algorithm.

When the patient presents, the approach that I use (and is similar to that used by most physicians) is to analyze five components of the patient's situation. First, we evaluate the overall physiologic status of the patient. The initial question is if the patient requires hospitalization and/or ICU care. In addition to clinical judgment, there are specific tools that can be used to assess the physiologic status of the patient and predict mortality (N Engl J Med 1997;336:243). Physiologic support (oxygen, ventilation, fluids, pressors, nursing care) buys time and creates an environment where antibiotics can function and the patient's immune system can activate. Many community-acquired pneumonia protocols include a formal physiologic assessment similar to that used in Tables 5.1a, b, and c; see **Community-Acquired Pneumonia**.

The patient's ecology (for want of a better term) is closely related to his or her immediate physiologic status but is more reflective of long-term health status. Does the patient have a normal immune system? Abnormalities, in addition to the obvious such as HIV infection and recent chemotherapy, include advanced age, alcoholism, anatomic abnormalities of the lung such as bronchiectasis, chronic malnutrition, and chronic steroid use. Does the patient live in the community, or has he or she recently been in contact with the healthcare system? Use of antibiotics, hospitalization, or institutional care within the last 60 days can alter host flora and requires different antibiotics. Finally, special circumstances should be sought. Travel will expose the patient to unusual flora. Occupations such as farmer (*Nocardia*) and hobbies such as spelunker (histoplasmosis) also change the patient's ecology. Homelessness, incarceration, and recent immigration also define the host. Assessment of risk for aspiration is the final component of patient ecology. Recent dental work, surgery, seizures, coma, advanced dementia, heavy use of sedatives/street drugs, and neuromuscular disease affecting the swallowing mechanism predispose the patient to aspiration. For patients in a healthcare setting, this is an important determinant of antibiotic choice. See Table 5.2 for a list of host conditions associated with specific pathogens.

Further assessment of the patient by physical examination and history is the next step. Much of the history is used to establish the patient's ecology. Additional information regarding specific symptoms such as hemoptysis, sputum production, pain, and chronicity helps complete the clinical picture. Other organ system involvement should also be sought. From a physical examination perspective, the "across the room gestalt" is probably the most important component of assessment: Is this patient at risk of dying or going into respiratory failure in the next 2 hours? Once acuity is established, vital signs, pulmonary exam, and other organ system examination will complete the initial data collection.

Chest imaging has great bearing on the next set of interventions. It is tempting in a busy practice or emergency room to get a chest X-ray, see an infiltrate, and give the patient antibiotics. Chest X-rays must be evaluated in the context of the patient's total clinical setting. Is it probable that the patient has pneumonia? Should we seek an alternative hypothesis? Should we deviate from the standard CAP protocol because of the patient's special circumstances? Review of the chest X-ray is the point at which these possibilities should be considered.

Figure 5.1 describes five major categories of abnormality. This list is neither exhaustive nor precise, and apologies to my colleagues who practice radiology. However, it is a useful first cut:

1. The patient may have a normal X-ray. This should raise considerations such as bronchitis, pulmonary embolism, very early pneumonia, or nonpulmonary etiology.
2. An effusion may be present. A patient who is acutely ill with what appears to be an infectious illness and has an effusion must have that effusion sampled and appropriately treated. (See **Empyema and Parapneumonic Effusion.**) This finding is in addition to any other X-ray findings that may be present.
3. The patient may have patchy or segmental/lobar infiltrates. Areas of consolidation that generally obey anatomic boundaries or follow the distribution of the bronchial tree often represent conventional bacterial infection, and this will often be

the most common scenario. However, hypersensitivity pneumonitis, BOOP/COP, exotic infections, and pulmonary infarction can have an identical appearance.

4. A cavity (or cavities) may be present. This should raise concerns for a variety of conditions, including mycobacterial infection, fungal infection, malignancy, and lung abscess. Many other noninfectious illnesses may also cause destruction of lung tissue, such as pulmonary infarction. The presence of a cavity *by definition* means that the patient does not have straightforward CAP and should be assessed carefully and individually.

5. Diffuse infiltrates are present. Diffuse parenchymal lung disease may be infectious, but it is often not. Many diffuse pulmonary processes may be seen in severely ill patients, such as ARDS, CHF, HP, BOOP/COP, and various other immunologic diseases such as SLE. Pulmonary infections may include viral pneumonia and atypical pneumonias. Diffuse infiltrates should prompt a careful search for alternative diagnoses to pneumonia. Also, remember that DPLD may obscure or hide a lobar or segmental infiltrate, and the X-ray should be reviewed carefully. Both congestive heart failure and ARDS are life-threatening complications of pneumonia and other infectious illnesses and must be treated aggressively.

Once these disparate pieces of data have been gathered, the data must be synthesized into a diagnosis and treatment plan. The treatment plan must include a feedback loop that monitors outcomes and adjusts the treatment plan as the patient's condition evolves. This process is outlined in Figure 5.1. If the patient has signs of pneumonia—fever, cough, sputum, relatively localized infiltrate, chest pain, elevated WBC count and/or elevation of band count (older patients in particular may have a left shift without an absolute elevation in white count), or abnormal sputum exam—it is reasonable to assume they have a bacterial pneumonia. Not all signs need to be present, and some clinical judgment must be applied in less clear-cut situations. Once the patient is felt to have a bacterial pneumonia, his or her ecology must be reviewed so that he or she can be further subcategorized. Risk factors, severity of illness, underlying health, and place of domicile direct the specific interventions. The treatment strategies are outlined in **Community-Acquired Pneumonia.**

If the patient is felt not to have a "standard" bacterial pneumonia, either by presentation, risks factors, or some combination of features, management becomes more complex. First, is this simply an atypical presentation of a conventional infection? Many competent physicians are aware of this possibility and will "cover" a patient for bacterial pneumonia even when that is not the primary diagnostic consideration. Stipulating that this decision is reassessed regularly as the patient's course unfolds, this is often a cautious and reasonable approach. The second so-called atypical presentation is that of the "atypical" organisms—mycoplasma, *Chlamydia*, *Legionella*. Depending upon the source and author, some specialists feel that these agents are consistently underdiagnosed. Because of this, CAP regimens include antibiotics that are active against these pathogens. The second diagnostic group is viral. Clues to this diagnostic group may include rash (varicella), epidemic (influenza), immunocompromised host (CMV), and outdoor activities with respiratory failure (Hantavirus). Infiltrates tend not to be localized, but diffuse. Care must be taken not to overlook bacterial superinfection, and purulent sputum or a superimposed localized infiltrate should prompt treatment with conventional antibiotics as well. The third diagnostic group is included to caution and remind readers that suffering from one disease does not offer immunity against a second or third. Severe pneumonia frequently can precipitate heart failure in the elderly, and ARDS may be the consequence of pneumonia. Conversely, a diffuse infiltrate and a fever do not necessarily mean the patient has pneumonia; diffuse infiltrates and a high fever in an elderly woman may be the consequence of ARDS in the setting of septic shock from a urinary tract infection, and a febrile diabetic patient's diffuse pulmonary infiltrates may be heart failure precipitated by a badly infected foot. The fourth situation is a true pulmonary infection not caused by conventional or "atypical" organisms. These situations are often difficult to recognize initially, and unfortunately at least some delay in diagnosis is common. Often, diagnosis will be prompted by a particular piece of information or specific clinical behavior of the patient. Some real-life examples: cavitary lesion in a homeless person (TB); diffuse alveolar infiltrates in an HIV-positive patient (PCJ); patchy, cavitating lesions in a farmer (*Nocardia*); patchy infiltrates and adenopathy in a spelunker (histoplasmosis); nonresolving dense pulmonary infiltrate in a patient with skin ulcers (blastomycosis). Prudence may again dictate "coverage" for conventional organisms while the clinical situation evolves. These cases will require individual review and literature review. Fifth, it is possible that the patient does not have an infectious illness. BOOP/COP, HP, and malignancy can all have the appearance of a conventional pneumonia, complete with infiltrate, cough, and fever. As in the previous situation, a noninfectious etiology begins to be considered as the patient does not respond to therapy. Finally, there is a small group of patients in whom the diagnosis is so unclear that treatment is withheld until there has been a biopsy or bronchoscopy or isolation/identification of an organism from the sputum. This is an uncommon situation. Scenarios might include a recurrent pneumonia, where antibiotic failure was questioned (and thus a need for specific culture-driven therapy); a severely immunocompromised patient where the likelihood of unusual infection was high (e.g., cavity in HIV+ patient); infectious vs. noninfectious etiologies are equally likely (e.g., patient with advanced lymphoma on aggressive chemotherapy with pulmonary infiltrates: drug vs. infection vs. lymphoma). In many cases, presumptive antibacterial therapy will be started immediately after a specimen is obtained.

Good outcome requires systematic assessment of therapy, the final component of pneumonia care. First, the patient may have a good outcome with the initial care plan. Second, the patient may be doing well, but culture and antibiotic sensitivity data indicate that a less expensive, narrower spectrum, or less toxic antibiotic is equally good. These changes when possible are good for the patient, the public health, and the healthcare system as a whole. Third, the patient's course may be unsatisfactory. Possibilities here include appropriate therapy but delayed response, incorrect diagnosis (but an infectious illness), or incorrect diagnosis (noninfectious illness). The clinician is faced with the choice of doing more testing (usually invasive), empiric change in therapy, or gritting one's teeth and pushing on. This is sometimes a difficult choice and is a function of local practice, confidence in the original diagnosis, availability of invasive evaluation, and severity of the patient's condition. Some clinicians declare treatment failure prematurely, and others may elect to "stay the course" to an excessive degree. Conventional bacterial infections can take 48–72 hours to respond, and frequent antibiotic changes will not make things better. Mycobacterial infections improve over weeks to months, and lung abscesses take days to weeks. X-ray findings *routinely* lag behind clinical improvement, and the patient's clinical condition, rather than the X-ray, should be the primary indicator of success or failure. Timing of invasive procedures, if contemplated, can be difficult. Unnecessary biopsy and bronchoscopy procedures can be avoided by making certain that a patient is truly not responding to therapy. However, the delay involved in developing that certainty may render the biopsy less safe or impossible. Once an unfavorable trend is established, intervention is appropriate. We favor bronchoscopic procedures for purulent pneumonias, and we favor surgical lung biopsy when there is a strong possibility of a noninfectious etiology. PCJ and evidence of viral infection can often be obtained from a bronchoscopy, and if these are the primary diagnoses, a bronchoscopy would be indicated as well. Patients in whom a surgical lung biopsy might be preferable would be patients who were rapidly deteriorating (can't wait the 2 days to do a bronchoscopy and get negative results), patients receiving chemotherapy (very broad differential diagnosis of infectious, neoplastic, and inflammatory conditions), and transplant patients (again, broad differential diagnosis). HIV+ patients have a clearly defined series of infections, most of which can be diagnosed from bronchial secretions or BAL, thus favoring bronchoscopy. Consultation in these situations is necessary. Finally, most authorities recommend successive chest X-rays after pneumonia to (1) assure that the appearance of the chest has returned to normal; (2) to document a new, scarred (but benign) appearance; or (3) to identify patients with a persistent pulmonary infiltrate that requires further evaluation (see **Nonresolving Pneumonia**).

5.2 Community-Acquired Pneumonia (CAP)

Clin Infect Dis 2007;44 Suppl 2:S27 is a comprehensive view of CAP, and is the gold standard reference.

Epidemiology: Lower respiratory tract infection is a common illness that results in a high rate of morbidity and mortality. By definition, *community acquired* means that the patient was living in a nonmedical, noninstitutional setting. It does not mean that the patient was previously well, nor does it imply that the patient did not have special risk factors. A wide spectrum of infectious agents can cause CAP, but from a practical standpoint the majority of infections arise from just a few organisms. Incidence is estimated in the population in the ~1% range. Most cases occur in the very young, very old, and impaired hosts. There appears to be an increase in pneumonia events in the wintertime.

Pathogenesis: Clinical lower respiratory tract infection is a product of the interaction between the pathogen and the host. The first line of defense of the lower respiratory tract is mechanical reduction and clearance of lower airway bacteria and viruses. Effective cough, functioning cilia, normal mucus production, structural airway integrity, and an ability of the upper airway to prevent contamination of the lower airway (cough in response to laryngeal contamination/irritation, prevention of aspiration) are the main components of pneumonia prevention and resolution. The second line of defense is the immune system itself. Depending upon the organism, humoral and/or cellular immune function may be required for resolution of the infection. A variety of processes can interfere with both layers of defense, including alterations in the level of consciousness, smoking, alcohol consumption (can also predispose to certain organisms), renal failure, malnutrition, malignancy, immunosuppressive agents, HIV infection, obstruction of a bronchus, advanced age, cystic fibrosis (both bronchiectasis and abnormal mucus production), bronchiectasis, COPD, cilial dysfunction syndromes, and immunodeficiency syndromes. Viral infection can predispose to superinfection with bacterial agents (influenza with subsequent staphylococcal pneumonia is the classic). Many bacteria and other pathogens have developed virulence factors (toxins, resistance to immunoglobulins, resistance to phagocytosis) that facilitate invasion and cause injury. An extended discussion of the mechanisms is beyond the scope of this book. Finally, the host must have sufficient physiologic reserve to withstand the effects of the infection. Pneumonia causes hypoxemia, increases the work of breathing, produces airway obstruction with mucus, can precipitate ARDS, and may initiate a SIRS picture with hypotension, shock, myocardial suppression, and renal failure. Infection of the pleural space and other forms of metastatic infection can complicate the primary infection and worsen the prognosis. Death, when it occurs, is usually the consequence of severe respiratory failure or SIRS. Hemorrhage and/or extensive destruction of parenchyma is a rare cause of death. The effect of comorbid conditions such as heart failure and malignancy as contributors to mortality should not be overlooked; pneumonia is often properly viewed as the final scene in a long play.

Symptoms/Signs: See **Approach to the Patient with Suspected Pneumonia.**

Course/Prognosis/Complications: Prognosis relates to the virulence of the organism and the robustness of the host; prognosis is predicted by the PSI. Complications include ARDS, SIRS, empyema (see **Empyema and Parapneumonic Effusion**), endocarditis, pericarditis, and meningitis as well as sepsis. Pleural effusion in the context of pulmonary infection is common; progression to empyema can often be controlled and effects minimized.

Imaging: See **Approach to the Patient with Suspected Pneumonia.**

Diagnosis: See **Approach to the Patient with Suspected Pneumonia.**
Definitive identification of an organism occurs in about 60–70% of cases of CAP. Conventional bacteria, when identified, are usually recovered from sputum or blood, occasionally from extrapulmonary sites such as the pleural space. There is growing interest in urinary antigen testing for some conventional bacteria such as *S. pneumoniae*. Viral illness is usually identified serologically, although there are direct nasal swab tests for influenza. *Legionella* is difficult to grow, and identification techniques have focused on serological means such as urinary antigen testing. Mycobacterial diseases, depending upon local resources, potentially may be rapidly identified despite their slow growth. This is dependent upon the equipment and local expertise available in any given area. Rickettsial and chlamydial illnesses will depend upon serological testing. PCJ usually is identified by recognition of organisms in sputum, BAL fluid, or biopsy material. *Nocardia* and fungal illnesses also are recovered from the sputum or blood. In a substantial number of cases no organism will be identified, and recovery (reduced white count, reduced left shift, improving gas exchange, improving imaging, improving sense of well-being) temporally associated with antibiotic administration will be the best indication that an infection was present. Finally, it should be remembered that even in immunocompromised hosts, common things happen commonly; the diagnosis will usually be a common organism and only less frequently something interesting and exotic.

Treatment: See **Approach to the Patient with Suspected Pneumonia** as an adjunct to this discussion. We recommend assessment of the patient's physiologic status first and categorization of host ecology second, although in practice these are done simultaneously. There have been numerous attempts to develop some metric for the severity of a patient's respiratory infection. One widely used tool is the pneumonia severity index (PSI) (N Engl J Med 1997;336:243), which has been validated and is part of many hospitals' pneumonia protocols. This is shown in Tables 5.1a, b, and c. The patient is first matched against a series of criteria (Step 1) that determine if the patient has a potential for a morbid outcome. If a possible bad outcome is predicted, a weighted multicomponent tool is used to develop a PSI score (Step 2). This PSI score in turn assigns the patient to a risk category (I–V) (Step 3). Most authorities agree that patients who fall in risk categories I and II can be safely cared for in the outpatient setting. Patients who are category III are often but not always admitted to inpatient units. Some authorities advocate an overnight observation stay in these patients to get a better sense of the patient's response to the illness and treatment. There is full

Table 5.1a   Pneumonia Severity Index, Step 1

Age of patient >50 years
Active neoplasm
CHF
Chronic renal insufficiency
Chronic liver disease
Altered mental status
Pulse ≥125
Respiratory rate ≥30
Systolic BP <90 mmHg
Temp <35 or ≥40 (Celsius)

If the patient has none of the properties listed, he or she is risk Class I.

Table 5.1b   Pneumonia Severity Index, PSI Step 2
Calculate the sum of points. Sum is the pneumonia severity score (PSI).

Risk Factors	Points
Age, men	Age, in years
Age, women	Age in years − 10
Nursing home resident	Age in years + 10
Active neoplasia	+30
Chronic liver disease	+20
Congestive heart failure	+10
Cerebrovascular disease	+10
Chronic renal disease	+10
Altered mental status	+20
Respiratory rate ≥30	+20
Systolic BP <90 mmHg	+20
Temperature <35 or ≥40°C	+15
Pulse ≥125	+10
Arterial pH <7.35	+30
BUN ≥30	+20
Sodium <130	+20
Glucose ≥250	+10
Hematocrit <30	+10
Pao_2 <60 or O_2 saturation <90%	+10
Presence of pleural effusion	+10

Table 5.1c   Pneumonia Severity Index, PSI Step 3
Determine class and mortality using PSI.

Class	Point Sum	Probability of Mortality, %
I	0	0.1
II	<70	0.6
III	71–90	2.8
IV	91–130	8.2
V	>130	29.2

Table 5.2   Host Conditions Associated with Specific Pathogens

Condition	Related Pathogens
Alcoholism	*S. pneumoniae,* anaerobes, gram-negative bacilli, tuberculosis
COPD/smoker	*S. pneumoniae, H. influenzae, Moraxella catarrhalis, Legionella* sp.
Nursing home resident	*S. pneumoniae,* gram-negative bacilli, *H. influenzae, S. aureus,* anaerobes, *Chlamydia pneumoniae,* TB, MRSA
Poor dental hygiene	Anaerobes
Epidemic Legionnaire's	*Legionella* sp.
Bat exposure	*Histoplasma capsulatum*
Bird exposure	*Chlamydia psittaci, Cryptococcus neoformans, Histoplasma* sp.
Rabbit exposure	*Francisella tularensis* (tularemia)
Travel SW United States	Coccidioidomycosis
Farm animal, parturient cats	*Coxiella burnetti* (Q fever)
Epidemic influenza in community	Influenza, *S. pneumoniae, S. aureus, H. influenzae*
Aspiration	Anaerobes, chemical pneumonitis, obstruction
Bronchiectasis, CF, other structural lung disease	*Pseudomonas aeruginosa, P. cepacia, S. aureus* (incl MRSA)
IVDU	*S. aureus,* anaerobes, TB, PCJ
Endobronchial obstruction	Anaerobes
Recent antibiotic Rx	DRSP, *P. aeruginosa,* MRSA

Modified from Am. J. Resp Crit Care Med 2001: Vol 163, p. 1738 and updated.

agreement that patients in categories IV and V require hospitalization; a category V patient should be admitted to a critical care setting if aggressive care is globally appropriate for the patient. The placement of category IV patients probably depends upon individual patient circumstances and the resources of the institution providing the care. Selection of initial antibiotic therapy depends on the classification of the patient's host status and severity of illness. Table 5.3 identifies the host categories and initial recommended therapies. These tables use data from recommendations made in the ATS/IDSA 2007 CAP treatment

Table 5.3   Initial Treatment of Community-Acquired Pneumonia Based on Host Status

Risk Group	Organism	Antibiotic
OUTPT, healthy, No risk for DRSP	*S. pneumoniae, M. pneumoniae Chlamydia pneumoniae Haemophilus influenzae* Respiratory viruses *Legionella* sp., *M. tuberculosis* Local endemic fungi	Macrolide (azithromycin, clarithromycin, erythromycin) Doxycycline
OUTPT, + comorbidities (chronic heart or lung disease, DM, alcoholism, active neoplasm, asplenia, immunosuppressed [disease or drugs], use of AB within preceding 3 months, other risks for DRSP)	*S. pneumoniae, M. pneumoniae Chlamydia pneumoniae* Mixed infection (bact. + other pathogen) *Haemophilus influenzae* Enteric gram-neg. Respiratory viruses, *Legionella* sp. *Moraxella catarrhalis* Mixed aspiration (anaerobic) *M. tuberculosis* Local endemic fungi	Respiratory fluoroquinolone (moxifloxacin, gemifloxacin, levofloxacin @ 750 mg) β-lactam **AND** macrolide (β-lactam as high-dose amoxicillin @ 1g. tid **OR** amox/clav. Alternatives incl. ceftriaxone, cefpodoxime, cefuroxime). Could also use doxycycline instead of macrolide.
OUTPT, High-risk DRSP	Drug-resistant strep. Pneumo.	Macrolide plus cephalosporin listed above rather than amox. or amox/clav
Influenza	Influenza A + B	Oseltamivir or zanamivir
INPT, non-ICU	*S. pneumoniae Haemophilus influenzae M. pneumoniae Chlamydia pneumoniae* Mixed infection (bact. + other pathogen) Enteric gram-neg. Respiratory viruses Mixed aspiration (anaerobic)	Respiratory fluoroquinolone (moxifloxacin, gemifloxacin, levofloxacin @ 750 mg) **OR** β-lactam **AND** macrolide (β-lactam as high-dose amoxicillin @ 1g. tid or amox/clav. Alternatives incl. ceftriaxone, cefpodoxime, cefuroxime). Could also use doxycycline.

Table 5.3

Risk Group	Organism	Antibiotic
	Legionella sp., *Moraxella catarrhalis* *M. tuberculosis*, local fungi	instead of macrolide; may consider ertapenem for some pts. Fluoroquinolone for **PCN allergic pts.**
INPT, ICU (general)	*Strep. pneumoniae,* *Legionella* sp. *Haemophilus influenzae,* Enteric gram neg. *Staph. aureus,* *M. pneumoniae* Respiratory viruses *M. tuberculosis,* local fungi	β-lactam (cefotaxime, ceftriax-one, or amp/sulbactam) **AND** azithromycin **OR** resp. fluoroquinolone Use azithromycin + resp. fluoro-quinolone for **PCN allergic pts.**
INPT, ICU w/ *Pseudomonas* risk	Same as gen. + *Pseudomonas*	Anti-pseudomonal β-lactam (pip/taz, cefipime, imipenem, meropenem) **AND** ciprofloxacin **or** levofloxacin **OR** Anti-pseudomonal β-lactam **AND** aminoglycoside **AND** azithromycin **OR** Anti-pseudomonal β-lactam **PLUS** aminoglycoside **AND** respiratory fluoroquinolone Use aztreonam for **PCN allergic pts.**
INPT, ICU w/ community-acq. MRSA	Same as gen + community-acq MRSA	As in INPT, ICU (general) **AND** vancomycin **OR** linezolid

Note: Capitalized, bolded conjunctions are used as logical operators.
Data from Mandell, 2007.

consensus statement (Clin Infect Dis 2007;44 Suppl 2:S27). Individual choice of antibiotics suggested in the tables should be based on (in no particular order) the patient's allergy/sensitivity profile, renal and hepatic function, comorbid conditions, potential drug interactions, knowledge of local microbial environment, and local formulary policy. Although there is lingering debate on the subject as to the value of the recommendation, most authorities recommend prompt administration of empiric antibiotics (in the emergency ward) and within 4 hours of presentation to the point of care. Patients usually should start to respond to therapy within 24–48 hours. The antibiotics recommended will treat the common causes of pneumonia. Failure to respond to therapy, recent previous antibiotic therapy, and/or a prolonged illness prior to medical attention raise concern for an unusual or resistant organism. These patients should be followed carefully. In severely ill patients, SIRS may take on a life of its own, and infection may be easily controlled while the resultant inflammation runs rampant. Finally, the role of prevention must be emphasized. Influenza vaccination (see **Influenza**) and *Strep. pneumoniae* vaccination in appropriate populations reduce morbidity and mortality. Smoking cessation also reduces propensity to pneumonia and should be encouraged.

5.3 Healthcare-Related Pneumonia (HCRP)

Pneumonia that develops while a patient is in a healthcare-related setting is a frequent and serious problem, often associated with high rates of morbidity and mortality. Patients in healthcare setting are vulnerable to infection. They are sick. They have underlying illnesses that predispose them to infection, such as malignancy or other chronic illnesses. We as clinicians have done things to these patients. We have bypassed their upper respiratory tract with intubation. We've given them chemotherapy. We've made them unconscious. We've given them antibiotics. We have changed their flora, often changing the balance between saprophytic and pathogenic organisms, and we have applied selective pressure for antibiotic-resistant organisms to survive. We have cared for these vulnerable patients in hospitals and nursing homes and clinics. We have clustered these patients where their exotic (and not so exotic) organisms can be passed from patient to patient by poor handwashing, crowding, and contaminated equipment. These factors combine to create a different series of requirements for diagnosis and treatment of patients in this category.

Patients are further subdivided into three subcategories with differing needs and prognoses. Ventilator-associated pneumonia (VAP) is pneumonia that develops more than 48–72 hours after intubation. Hospital-acquired pneumonia (HAP) is pneumonia that develops 48–72 hours after admission to the hospital, assuming that the disease was not incubating at the time of admission. (These patients may be intubated, but that would be different from VAP). Finally healthcare-associated pneumonia (HCAP) extends the concept of healthcare-related pneumonia to patients who reside in nursing homes, have received intravenous antibiotics, chemotherapy, or wound care within the last 30 days, have had a >48 hour hospitalization in an acute care hospital within the last 90 days, or have attended a hospital clinic or hemodialysis unit within the last 30 days. The concept of HCAP recognizes the extended effect of contact with the healthcare system on both bacterial flora and host vulnerability.

While general principles of pneumonia care still apply (prompt empiric treatment, physiologic support, etc.; see **Approach to the Patient with Suspected Pneumonia**), additional factors should be considered. First, particularly for VAP, there are specific strategies that can be applied to lessen the likelihood of pneumonia. Second, although common pathogens such as S. *pneumoniae* may occur, there is a high likelihood of gram-negative infections and resistant staphylococcal infections. This changes empiric therapy. Third, diagnosis of pneumonia may be difficult (fever from other sources, pneumonic infiltrate "hiding" in preexisting congestive heart failure, purulent secretions from endotracheal colonization), and the clinician may have difficulty deciding when to treat. Fourth, because of the fragility of the patients and the desire to prevent further change in patient and institution ecology, there is much greater impetus to identify the offending organism, narrow treatment, and/or stop treatment if the hypothesis of pneumonia is disproved. Finally, the clinician needs knowledge of the ecology of the healthcare entity in question; *Serratia* species may be a problem at one hospital, but across town just a mile or two away staph is the culprit.

The American Thoracic Society and Infectious Disease Society of America issued a joint statement in 2005 regarding management of these pneumonias (http://thoracic.org/sections/publications/statements /pages/mtpi/guide1-29.html 2004;2007). Prevention is paramount. Appropriate isolation techniques and handwashing reduce spread of infection. Some highly contagious agents, such as TB, require negative pressure rooms. Patients on mechanical ventilation present special problems since the protection afforded by the upper airway is bypassed, and these patients are often partially or completely sedated. Many institutions have developed a ventilator "order bundle" to assure that patients receive uniform care to minimize complications. Good respiratory therapy technique minimizes or eliminates opening the closed breathing circuit. This includes suction catheters that are integrated into the circuit. Circuit tubing is not changed automatically every 2 days, but as soiled and once a week. Other simple and effective interventions include treating the patient in the semirecumbent position, subglottic continuous suction, decontamination of the gut, and maintenance of normal gastric pH. Authors of the IDSA/ATS document recognize that the last recommendation is difficult to follow, and recommend stress ulcer prophylaxis with H2 blockers rather than PPIs as a compromise. All interventions to minimize the length of intubation, and to use NIPPV when possible, are appropriate.

Patients with suspected pneumonia are at risk for multiply drug-resistant pathogens. Risk factors for MDR bacteria include antimicrobial therapy in the last 90 days, current hospitalization of 5 days or more, high frequency of MDR in the community or hospital unit, and immunosuppression. In the case of HCAP, risk factors have already been defined. Patients with suspected HCRP should have every effort made to obtain a microbiological sample from the lower respiratory tract. This should be balanced against the need for prompt empiric therapy. Most authorities recommend the use of quantitative or semi-quantitative cultures for intubated patients. The reason for culture is twofold: first, to identify a pathogen and permit antimicrobial testing, and second to confirm or deny the hypothesis of pneumonia. Leukocytosis (or leukopenia), infiltrate on chest X-ray (new or progressive), and purulent secretions should trigger a concern for pneumonia. Quantitative cultures use either protected specimen brush (PSB) or BAL bronchoscopic collection techniques. Most authorities consider a PSB culture positive at 10^3 CFU/ml, and BAL culture positive at 10^4 CFU/ml.

Table 5.4   Initial Empiric Antibiotic Therapy for Hospital-Acquired Pneumonia or Ventilator-Associated Pneumonia in Patients with No Known Risk Factors for Multidrug-Resistant Pathogens, Early Onset, and Any Disease Severity

Potential Pathogen	Recommended Antibiotic*
Streptococcus pneumoniae†	Ceftriaxone
Haemophilus influenzae	*or*
Methicillin-sensitive *Staphylococcus aureus*	Levofloxacin, moxifloxacin, or
Antibiotic-sensitive enteric gram-negative bacilli	ciprofloxacin
Escherichia coli	*or*
Klebsiella pneumoniae	Ampicillin/sulbactam
Enterobacter species	*or*
Proteus species	Ertapenem
Serratia marcescens	

*See Table 5.6 for proper initial doses of antibiotics.

†The frequency of penicillin-resistant *S. pneumoniae* and multidrug-resistant *S. pneumoniae* is increasing; levofloxacin or moxifloxacin are preferred to ciprofloxacin and the role of other new quinolones, such as gatifloxacin, has not been established.

Neiderman, Craven, et al. 2005. ATS/IDSA Guidelines for the management of adults with hospital acquired, ventilator associate, and healthcare associated pneumonia. American Journal of Respiratory and Critical Care Medicine 171; p 388-416. Official Journal of the American Thoracic Society. © American Thoracic Society.

If pneumonia is suspected, empiric therapy is indicated. Initial therapy is guided by risk for MDR pathogens. If the risk is low, the low-risk protocol (see Table 5.4) should be used. If high risk, the protocol outlined in Table 5.5 should be used. Initial antibiotic doses for these drugs are outlined in Table 5.6.

Table 5.5   Initial Empiric Therapy for Hospital-Acquired Pneumonia, Ventilator-Associated Pneumonia, and Healthcare-Associated Pneumonia in Patients with Late-Onset Disease or Risk Factors for Multidrug-Resistant Pathogens and All Disease Severity

Potential Pathogens	Combination Antibiotic Therapy*

Pathogens listed in Table 5.3 and MDR pathogens
Pseudomonas aeruginosa
Klebsiella pneumoniae (ESBL+)†
Acinetobacter species†
Methicillin-resistant
  Staphylococcus aureus (MRSA)
Legionella pneumophila†
Methicillin-resistant
	Antipseudomonal cephalosporin
	  (cefepime, ceftazidime)
	  or
	Antipseudomonal carbapenem
	  (imipenem or meropenem)
	  or
	β-Lactam/β-lactamase inhibitor
	(piperacillin–tazobactam)
	  plus
	Antipseudomonal fluoroquinolone†
	  (ciprofloxacin or levofloxacin)
	  or
	Aminoglycoside
	  (amikacin, gentamicin, or tobramycin)
	  plus
	Linezolid or vancomycin‡

*See Table 5.6 for adequate initial dosing of antibiotics. Initial antibiotic therapy should be adjusted or streamlined on the basis of microbiologic data and clinical response to therapy.

†If an ESBL+ strain, such as *K. pneumoniae,* or an *Acinetobacter* species is suspected, a carbapanem is a reliable choice. If *L. pneumophila* is suspected, the combination antibiotic regimen should include a macrolide (e.g., azithromycin) or a fluoroquinolone (e.g., ciprofloxacin or levofloxacin) should be used rather than an aminoglycoside.

‡If MRSA risk factors are present or there is a high incidence locally.

Neiderman, Craven, et al. 2005. ATS/IDSA Guidelines for the management of adults with hospital acquired, ventilator associate, and healthcare associated pneumonia. American Journal of Respiratory and Critical Care Medicine 171; p 388-416. Official Journal of the American Thoracic Society. © American Thoracic Society.

Table 5.6 Initial Intravenous, Adult Doses of Antibiotics for Empiric Therapy of Hospital-Acquired Pneumonia, Including Ventilator-Associated Pneumonia, and Healthcare-Associated Pneumonia in Patients with Late-Onset Disease or Risk Factors for Multidrug-Resistant Pathogens

Antibiotic	Dosage*
Antipseudomonal cephalosporin	
Cefepime	1–2 g every 8–12 h
Ceftazidime	2 g every 8 h
Carbapenems	
Imipenem	500 mg every 6 h or 1g every 8 h
Meropenem	1 g every 8 h
β-Lactam/β-lactamase inhibitor	
Piperacillin–tazobactam	4.5 g every 6 h
Aminoglycosides	
Gentamicin	7 mg/kg per d†
Tobramycin	7 mg/kg per d†
Amikacin	20 mg/kg per d†
Antipseudomonal quinolones	
Levofloxacin	750 mg every d
Ciprofloxacin	400 mg every 8 h
Vancomycin	15 mg/kg every 12 h‡
Linezolid	600 mg every 12 h

*Dosages are based on normal renal and hepatic function.
†Trough levels for gentamicin and tobramycin should be less than 1 μg/ml, and for amikacin they should be less than 4–5 μg/ml.
‡Trough levels for vancomycin should be 15–20 μg/ml.
Neiderman, Craven, et al. 2005. ATS/IDSA Guidelines for the management of adults with hospital acquired, ventilator associate, and healthcare associated pneumonia. American Journal of Respiratory and Critical Care Medicine 171; p 388-416. Official Journal of the American Thoracic Society. © American Thoracic Society.

A general approach to subsequent management is outlined in Figure 5.2. The emphasis of this management algorithm is on deescalation of therapy when appropriate (clinical clearing if 48–72 hours with sterile cultures; stop antibiotics), shortened treatment duration (7–8 days), and directed therapy (narrow spectrum antibiotics after identification of an organism).

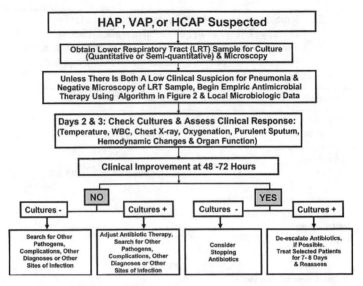

Figure 5.2 Algorithm for treatment of HAP and VAP. Summary of the management strategies for a patient with suspected hospital-acquired pneumonia (HAP), ventilator-associated pneumonia (VAP), or healthcare-associated pneumonia (HCAP). The decision about antibiotic discontinuation may differ depending on the type of sample collected (PSB, BAL, or endotracheal aspirate), and whether the results are reported in quantitative or semiquantitative terms (see text for details). Niederman, Craven, et al. 2005. ATS/IDSA guidelines for the management of adults with hospital-acquired, ventilator associate, and healthcare-associated pneumonia. American Journal of Respiratory and Critical Care Medicine 171; p 388-416. Official Journal of the American Thoracic Society. © American Thoracic Society.

Nonresolution or clinical deterioration must be judged in light of the known clinical course of pneumonia in the seriously ill patient. A trial of initial therapy of 48–72 hours is appropriate, and clinical indicators (favorable WBC changes, reduction in temperature, better oxygenation, resolution of hypotension, patient reporting improved sense of well-being) are far more reliable than radiographic changes (see

Table 5.7   Possible Causes of Failed Treatment of Healthcare-Related Pneumonia

Failure of Therapy Related to Infection	Noninfectious Causes of Failed Therapy
Antibiotics correct, organism ID correct, patient's immune system cannot respond	Congestive heart failure
	Progression of underlying disease
Inadequate dose of antibiotics	Adult respiratory distress
Incorrect antibiotics, organism ID OK	syndrome
Incorrect identification of organism	Atelectasis
Multiple organisms	Pulmonary embolism
Inherently resistant organism	Neoplasm
(mycobacteria,viral, fungal)	Pulmonary hemorrhage
Complications (empyema, *C. difficile* colitis)	

Nonresolving Pneumonia). If a patient is judged to be failing therapy, reasons for failure can be classified as unsuccessful treatment of the infection or that a noninfectious hypothesis must be considered. These possibilities are outlined in Table 5.7. Overlap among these possibilities must be considered as well. At this juncture, consultation with pulmonary and/or infectious disease physicians is appropriate.

5.4   Pneumonia in Immunocompromised Hosts

N Engl J Med 1998;338:1741, Clin Chest Med 1990;11:55, N Engl J Med 2004;350:1339, Infect Dis Clin North Am 1998;12:781

Patients who are immunocompromised present an additional layer of problems and concerns for respiratory infections. A general approach to infections has already been outlined in other articles. Because of the unique issues faced by HIV+ patients, pulmonary manifestations of that illness are discussed separately (see **HIV and the Lung**). Besides HIV infection, patients may have impaired systemic immune function from an underlying illness (common variable immune deficiency, SLE), use of steroids (probably the most common source of immunosuppression), chemotherapy, and organ transplantation. More subtle abnormalities may be identified in patients with diabetes, abnormal gastric pH, and malnutrition. The approach to these patients should follow that followed for any patient with a suspected pneumonia. The observations below are a reflection of my experience supplemented by literature-based recommendations.

1. Common things happen commonly. Immunosuppression will render the patient susceptible to all forms of exotic infections. However, pneumonia with *S. pneumoniae* will still be more common than *Aspergillus*.

2. Despite observation #1, the incidence of less common infection is high. The clinician must remain vigilant and have a low threshold for looking for less common pathogens.

3. Aggressive attempts to achieve a conclusive diagnosis are appropriate. Because of the compromised status of the patient and the high degree of uncertainty in presumptive diagnosis, minimally invasive and highly invasive (bronchoscopy, surgical lung biopsy) diagnostic procedures may be lifesaving (Am J Respir Crit Care Med 2000;161:723). Early consultation is appropriate.

4. The clinician should maintain a high suspicion for a noninfectious etiology. Many of the diseases prompting immunosuppression and the immunosuppressive agents themselves (chemotherapeutic agents, radiation) may cause pulmonary infiltrates, fever, and hypoxia. Failure to respond to antibiotics promptly (48–72 hours) should prompt a reevaluation of the diagnosis.

5. Many specialty services (e.g., oncology) have specific protocols in place for problems such as neutropenic fever. These should be followed. If these protocols are not in place, they should be developed, as there is a large body of data to support this approach (Clin Infect Dis 2002;34:730).

6. Radiographic abnormalities may be subtle. Review images yourself, and, if possible, compare to older studies.

7. Multiple pathologic states may exist simultaneously.
8. The risk of fungal infection, particularly aspergillosis, is high and rising. Nodular and/or cavitating lesions should immediately raise concern for this organism.

5.5 Acute Bronchitis

N Engl J Med 2006;355:2125

Epidemiology: Acute bronchitis is a common illness in the community. Although a source of misery, the condition carries little risk of morbidity and almost none of mortality. Acute bronchitis should be differentiated from acute exacerbations of COPD.

Pathophysiology: Acute bronchitis is by definition an infectious inflammation of the airways without parenchymal involvement. By convention, the term *acute bronchitis* also implies that the host was previously healthy and that there is no underlying lung disease present. Generally, bronchitis is caused by a virus, such as RSV, coronavirus, rhinovirus, influenza, or parainfluenza. There is little evidence that there is such a disease as acute bacterial bronchitis. Although bacteria do play a role in airways infection, it is in the setting of underlying lung disease. Irritation of the bronchial mucosa leads to cough and sputum production. The illness may last between 5 and 15 days ($\pm$).

Symptoms: Cough, occasionally paroxysmal. Severe coughing may lead to syncope and/or emesis. Sputum production is common.

Course/Prognosis/Complications: In the great majority of cases, acute bronchitis is a benign, self-limited illness. Injury to the tracheal and bronchial mucosa may lead to superinfection and pneumonia. There is some evidence that an episode of acute bronchitis may trigger clinical manifestations of asthma in patients predisposed to that illness.

Imaging: Nonspecific. Usually normal. The primary role of imaging (when required at all) is to exclude pneumonia. Some patients may have some accentuation of bronchial markings (peri-bronchial cuffing) as an indication of inflammation.

Diagnosis: This benign condition should be differentiated from other processes. Pertussis and mycoplasma may cause profound degrees of coughing. Identification of pertussis (see **Pertussis**) is particularly important from a public health standpoint. Pneumonia may be difficult to distinguish from bronchitis on clinical grounds, especially in the elderly. However, fever, tachycardia, and tachypnea are not seen with uncomplicated bronchitis. Repetitive episodes of "bronchitis" may be manifestations of asthma or postnasal drip, and acute bronchitis must be differentiated from acute exacerbations of chronic bronchitis (AECB) seen in patients with COPD. Chest X-rays are indicated if physical exam is abnormal (rales, rhonchi, evidence of consolidation) or the patient has abnormal vital signs.

Treatment: The literature does not support the use of antibiotics for this condition, and acute bronchitis is responsible for wholesale misuse of outpatient antibiotics (Ann Intern Med 2001;134:518). Routine use of bronchodilators such as β agonists or inhaled (or systemic) corticosteroids does not appear to be supported by adequate controlled trials.

5.6 Atypical Pneumonia

Atypical pneumonia is an archaic term used to describe pneumonias that do not fit into the "typical" patterns of bacterial pneumonia. There are a number of different agents that can cause a febrile illness with infiltrate and cough, and where causative bacteria cannot be identified using conventional culture techniques. This article reviews two prototypic organisms: mycoplasma and chlamydia. These agents, although biologically and morphologically different, share obligate use of host cellular mechanisms for metabolism and reproduction. This renders them refractory to culture by conventional microbiological techniques. Additionally, these agents share the ability to infect normal hosts and are highly contagious (Infect Dis Clin North Am 1991;5:585). Legionella is often referred to as an atypical pneumonia, but personally I think this is a misnomer, and the organism is covered with other organisms in **Bacterial Pneumonia.**

Mycoplasma pneumoniae

This agent is a common cause of CAP, and tends to occur in younger patients. It is spread by droplet infection. The spectrum of illness is wide, ranging from asymptomatic to life threatening. Outbreaks in closed populations (military recruits, college campuses) occur regularly. Typical pulmonary disease begins as headache, general malaise, and fever. Rigors are uncommon. Cough is a prominent symptom, and may persist for many weeks. There can be a disconnect between patient complaints and physical findings, with a benign respiratory exam even in the face of considerable patient misery. Upper respiratory tract disease such as pharyngitis and myringitis may be seen as well. Immunologic consequences of infection are common and cause several extrapulmonary manifestations of disease including skin rash, joint complaints, and hemolytic anemia. Exacerbation (and some think precipitation) of asthma is described as well. Conclusive diagnosis in real time is difficult. Fifty percent of patients will have positive cold agglutinin titers, and many patients will have a low-grade hemolytic anemia. Serologies are accurate but provide a diagnosis only after the fact. Antigen identification and PCR techniques are primarily investigational. Radiologic patterns include bronchopneumonia, platelike atelectasis, lymphadenopathy, and nodular infiltrates. In common practice, the disease is often suspected in the context of a young, otherwise healthy individual presenting with cough, low-grade pneumonia, and patchy infiltrates, although other patient groups may be affected. Treatment with macrolides, doxycycline, and fluoroquinolones is effective. This organism will be adequately treated by use of CAP protocols (Clin Chest Med 1991; 12:237, Clin Infect Dis 1993;17 Suppl 1:S32).

Chlamydia

Our taxonomist friends have recently changed the name to *Chlamydophila*. *C. pneumoniae* is a common illness, seen typically in older patients (in contrast to mycoplasma). Clinical and radiographic presentation are indistinguishable from other atypical and typical pathogens. It is likely that true incidence of *C. pneumoniae* is underestimated because there is no reliable real-time means of diagnosis. As with mycoplasma, treatment with a macrolide is effective, as is a quinolone. However, if (somehow) there is a conclusive diagnosis of *C. pneumoniae*, doxycycline is the preferred drug. There is an interesting sidebar to *C. pneumoniae*, with a number of investigators questioning the role of the organism in asthma, atherosclerosis, and Alzheimer's dementia (Clin Microbiol Rev 1995;8:451). In contrast, *C. psittaci* is an unusual zoonosis, with psittacine birds the primary reservoir. However, domestic fowl may also pose a risk. Contact with infected birds is required. Infection with *C. psittaci*, psittacosis, can be a severe illness and cause death. Patients may have high fever, cough, and purulent/bloody sputum. Extrapulmonary manifestations are also seen, with cardiac and CNS involvement possible. The organism responds to the same agents as *C. pneumoniae*. Diagnosis may be difficult, as there are no real-time conclusive diagnostic tests. Contact with fowl or birds in the parrot family should raise suspicion for this agent (Br Med Bull 1983;39:163).

5.7   Bacterial Pneumonia

Bacterial pneumonia is a common illness and frequent cause of hospitalization. A wide variety of conventional bacterial organisms cause pneumonia, but most clinicians implicitly are referring to a relatively small group of organisms that cause the bulk of inpatient and outpatient pneumonia. Some of these are so-called atypical pneumonias (see **Atypical Pneumonia**). This article is a brief overview of conventional gram-positive and gram-negative organisms.

Pneumonias share a common etiology in that the majority of pulmonary infections are caused by micro-aspiration or inhalation. A small number of bacterial pulmonary infections are the result of hematogenous spread (e.g., septic embolism). Many individuals' nares are colonized with potential respiratory pathogens; *S. pneumoniae* and *S. aureus* are common colonizers. Patients (and sometimes care practitioners) who spend time in healthcare institutions may be colonized by bacteria that have multiple antibiotic resistances and different species from the general population. Antibiotic recommendations, even when there is conclusive identification of an organism, should be driven by antibiotic sensitivity testing and local patterns of susceptibility and resistance.

Once the organism(s) have been inhaled, there is an interaction between host defenses (mechanical defenses such as cough, effective cilial function, intact mucosal barrier and immune function) and the bacteria. Some organisms (*S. pneumoniae*, *H. influenzae*) will cause an intense inflammatory response with pulmonary hyperemia and pus formation in the alveoli, but the host will be left with essentially normal lung tissue if they survive the illness. Other organisms (*P. aeruginosa*, *K. pneumoniae*, *S. aureus*) destroy lung tissue, and the host may be left with scarring and loss of pulmonary function.

Streptococcus pneumoniae

Streptococcus pneumoniae is the archetypal organism causing pneumonia. When organisms are isolated from patients, particularly in patients ill enough to warrant inpatient care, *S. pneumoniae* is the most common isolate in most series. This gram-positive diplococcus has a capsule that affords it some protection from the host's immune system. The disease typically causes a lobar or segmental pneumonia; the classic presentation is a mild upper respiratory infection punctuated by an abrupt rigor, high fever, and blood streaked sputum. The illness is seen in all ecological settings. The infection tends to be most dangerous in the very young and very old, and some of my older professors (trained in the 1920s and 1930s) referred to pneumococcus (the old name for the bug) as the old man's friend. My personal experience, and that of some of my colleagues, is that there is a subset of patients in whom the disease is overwhelming despite prompt treatment of a sensitive organism and good physiologic support. I have seen this most frequently in alcoholics. This has been recognized for decades (Ann Intern Med 1964;60:4). Complications of the infection include empyema, hematogenous spread, meningitis, and pericarditis. S. pneumoniae has become increasingly resistant to therapy (in the late 1970s patients were treated with 600,000 units of procaine penicillin intramuscularly twice daily for a couple of days) and in some communities highly penicillin-resistant and/or moderately penicillin-resistant organisms constitute over 20% of isolates. Pneumococcal vaccine reduces invasive infection in high-risk patients and should be given to all patients over 65 and younger high-risk patients. However, immunity conferred on the vaccinated population is neither uniform nor complete (Chest 1995;107:457, Medicine [Baltimore] 2005;84: 147, Am J Med 1999;107:12S, J Gen Intern Med 2000;15:638, Clin Infect Dis 2004;38:222, Semin Respir Infect 1999;14:227, Clin Infect Dis 2006;43:1004).

Haemophilus influenzae and *Moraxella catarrhalis*

H. influenzae and M. catarrhalis are gram-negative coccobacillary organisms that are also frequently seen in clinical practice. Although gram negative, they tend to behave in a similar fashion to S. pneumoniae in that they can cause a severe, lobar, nonnecrotizing pneumonia. Although these organisms can be seen in normal hosts, they seem to be more common in patients with underlying pulmonary problems such as smokers and patients with COPD. They are also both common causes of AECB. H. influenzae strains seen in adults with pneumonia are nontypable, different from the invasive organisms associated with pediatric meningitis. Pediatric immunization against H. flu does not confer protection against the nontypeable strains. Although these organisms used to be sensitive to amoxicillin, they now require at least a second-generation cephalosporin, modern macrolide (clarithromycin, azithromycin), or respiratory fluoro-quinolone. Complications are similar to those seen in *S. pneumoniae* infection (Curr Opin Infect Dis 2003;16:129, Clin Microbiol Rev 2002;15:125).

Group A Streptococcal Infection

This is a serious infection with gram-positive cocci. It is often fulminant, even in previously healthy young patients. This is thought to occur by hematogenous spread from a skin site that can be so small as to be overlooked. Early empyema formation and tissue destruction are very common. Mortality rate is high, near 40% in one series (Chest 2006;130:1679). The organism should be considered when there is rapid progression of pneumonia and cardiovascular collapse with rapid development of a large effusion. If group A strep is recovered from the patient, many clinicians feel that combination β-lactam and clindamycin therapy is appropriate because clindamycin (although bacterio*static* rather than bacteri*cidal*) interferes with protein (and therefore toxin) synthesis (Arch Intern Med 2003;163:467).

Staphylococcus aureus

S. aureus infection is a major problem for inpatient clinicians. A clustering gram-positive coccus, *S. aureus* pneumonia was classically described as an infection occurring postinfluenza. The organism is often seen infecting patients with abnormal airways or who are immune incompetent. The organism has several characteristics that enhance virulence, and the patient is usually severely ill. Unlike *S. pneumoniae*, the X-ray appearance can be that of a patchy pneumonia following bronchial outlines (bronchopneumonia). Staph pneumonia may be associated with extensive tissue destruction if the patient survives (CJEM 2007;9:300). Within the last 10 years, there has been widespread dissemination of methicillin-resistant *S. aureus* (MRSA) strains requiring treatment with vancomycin, linezolid, or tigecycline (or similar agents). These strains appear to be particularly virulent as well, and are associated with high mortality; this is in part why so many arms of the HCAP initial treatment algorithm include vancomycin. Cavitating staph infection in the lung should prompt a search for an endovascular source (heart valve, prosthesis, catheter-related sepsis) as this typically occurs as a consequence of septic embolization (Emerg Infect Dis 2006;12:894, MMWR Morb Mortal Wkly Rep 2007;56:325).

Pseudomonas aeruginosa

P. aeruginosa is a gram-negative bacillus commonly associated with nosocomial pneumonia. It has a relatively nonspecific X-ray pattern (lobar vs. bronchopneumonia) but can be associated with cavitation, particularly later in the course. *P. aeruginosa* infection often occurs in association with respiratory equipment and mechanical ventilation. The organism has a variety of virulence factors that cause severe illness with sepsis syndrome. Additionally, the organism is often highly antibiotic resistant, requiring treatment with specific β-lactams, cephalosporins, fluoroquinolones, carbapenems, and/or aminoglycosides. Because the organism can develop resistance quickly, many authorities recommend treatment with two drugs that have dissimilar mechanisms of action. In contrast, at least one group feels that monotherapy may be adequate when directed by antimicrobial testing. Pseudomonal ventilator-associated pneumonia has, in some series, mortality in excess of 50%. Pseudomonas is also seen in outpatients with bronchiectasis (see **Bronchiectasis**). These patients can become chronically infected/colonized (sometimes it's hard to tell the difference), and when they flare they can develop a pseudomonas bronchopneumonia. Treatment of pseudomonas infection may be prolonged, often 2 weeks or more (Antimicrob Agents Chemother 2003; 47:2756).

Enteric Organisms

Enteric organisms is an umbrella term for gram-negative bacilli associated with the human gut (*E. coli, K. pneumonia, P. mirabilis, E. cloacae*, etc.). These organisms are typically a cause of HCAP.

Antibiotic sensitivities can vary, but initial treatment with a broad spectrum penicillin derivative is usually effective. The X-ray picture can also vary, including bronchopneumonia, lobar pneumonia, and cavitation. Associated mortality is high. Because these gram-negative organisms produce endotoxin, shock and SIRS are frequent (Chest 1991;100:439).

Anaerobic Lung Infections

These infections are the result of aspiration of oral or nasal contents. These are complex infections with anaerobic, aerobic, and facultative anaerobic organisms present. The major risk factor for these infections is depressed consciousness (anesthesia, drug overdose, alcohol intoxication, seizures) leading to loss of control of upper airway defense mechanisms. Patients with esophageal dysfunction and abnormal swallowing mechanisms from neuromuscular disease are also at risk. Poor dental hygiene with periodontal disease increases the potential organism load and increases risk of infection if aspiration occurs. Dental work itself also increases the risk of aspiration. These infections may be more indolent than other bacterial pneumonias, and days or weeks of symptoms may be seen. Tissue necrosis is more common with anaerobic infections than other conventional bacterial infections, and abscess formation and empyema are seen frequently. Anaerobic infections are also seen in pneumonias forming behind bronchial obstructions (postobstructive pneumonia) and with superinfection of bullae. Interestingly, the synergistic effect of these mixed infections is also their Achilles heel; antibiotic therapy need not be effective against all species present. If the synergism can be interrupted by destroying some fraction of the bacteria in the infection with antibiotics, the immune system can often control the remainder of the organisms present. Usually, clindamycin or ampicillin/sulbactam is used. Surgical or minimally invasive drainage of lung abscesses is generally unnecessary; failure of a lung abscess to respond to therapy should prompt bronchoscopy to evaluate the airway for a foreign body or obstruction (Clin Chest Med 1991;12:269, Clin Infect

Dis 1993;16 Suppl 4:S248, Chest 2005;127:1276, Curr Infect Dis Rep 2000;2:238).

Legionella

Legionella species are a relatively common etiology of pneumonia in both immune-competent and immunosuppressed patients. Active smokers, patients with COPD, and immunosuppressed patients appear to be particularly susceptible. Often grouped with the "atypical" pneumonias, implying a pattern of diffuse infiltrates, this is a widely held misconception: *Legionella* respiratory infection has a pattern of bronchopneumonia or lobar pneumonia in the immune-competent patient and can have a somewhat more unusual pattern of peripheral (pleural-based) opacities in immunosuppressed patients. Patients with *Legionella* infection often have gastrointestinal symptoms and headache in addition to cough and sputum (sometimes blood streaked). Hyponatremia, high fever, and mental status changes (confusion) are common. Sputum exam does not show organisms, and this fastidious organism is difficult to grow in culture. Diagnosis is made (when made at all) *ex post facto* through serological testing or through newer methods such as urinary antigen testing. Azithromycin and fluoroquinolones such as levofloxacin are the cornerstones of therapy. β-*lactams do not work*, and coverage for *Legionella* is the major reason for basing empiric therapy CAP protocols (and some HCAP protocols) on azithromycin- and/or fluoroquinolone-containing regimens. Recovery is slow, and, because many patients often have underlying lung disease, risk of mortality or respiratory failure can be high (N Engl J Med 1997;337:682).

5.8 Pertussis

Ann Intern Med 2005;142:832, N Engl J Med 2005;352:1215, J Clin Microbiol 1997;35:2435

Epidemiology: Until the 1940s when a vaccine was developed, pertussis was a severe childhood illness. It was (and is) highly contagious and had a high rate of complication among infants. In the adult population, particularly in the era of vaccination, the illness is probably underrecognized, and presentation may not be typical. Between 10,000 and 15,000 cases of pertussis are reported annually in the United States. A larger number of cases are seen worldwide, particularly in developing countries. Some authors have reported serologic evidence of recent infection with pertussis in 10–15% of patients with prolonged course of acute onset cough. Overall, the literature suggests that true adult incidence and prevalence figures may be difficult to obtain because of difficulty recognizing the illness.

PULMONARY INFECTIOUS DISEASE

Pathophysiology: Whooping cough is caused by *Bordetella pertussis*, a gram-negative coccobacillus. It is highly infectious, spread by droplet infection, with same-household attack rates of 50–100%. The organism has multiple virulence factors and produces toxins that paralyze cilia and are cytotoxic to the respiratory epithelium. Invasion beyond the bronchial epithelium is uncommon. Pertussis pneumonia, when it occurs, comes about by direct spread down the airway rather than through the airway walls. The patient is the most contagious during the initial (catarrhal and early paroxysmal) phases of the illness.

Symptoms: Whooping cough often starts as a "catarrhal phase" that is indistinguishable from a common cold. This lasts ~7 days and then the patient enters the "paroxysmal phase" during which the hallmark whooping cough (although not required for disease diagnosis) is heard. Severe, unremitting coughing associated with rib fractures, emesis, and lumbar strain are typical. This phase can last anywhere between 1 and 10 weeks. The "convalescent phase" can last another 2 months, where the cough persists but at less intensity. Adult patients may have an altered, less severe course.

Course/Prognosis/Complications: This is a difficult illness for the patient with a prolonged period of severe coughing that can lead to rib fractures, syncope, vomiting, pneumomediastinum, pneumothorax, and secondary infection. Pertussis may also lead to bronchiectasis, and was a common etiology of bronchiectasis in the prevaccination, preantibiotic era. The patient also presents a public health hazard, and pertussis is a reportable illness in every jurisdiction in the United States.

Imaging: Nonspecific, often normal. Some peribronchial cuffing may be present.

Laboratory: Pertussis infection is unusual in that lymphocytosis (often high) rather than neutrophilia is the cause of leukocytosis, and should raise the concern for pertussis in a patient with a severe coughing illness.

Diagnosis: Pertussis can escape detection unless clinical suspicion is high. Clinicians will be more alert during outbreaks, but sporadic cases may be difficult to detect. The CDC uses a clinical diagnosis (during outbreaks) that consists of 2 weeks of cough plus at least one of the following: posttussive vomiting, paroxysms of cough, and/or inspiratory whoop. Differentiation from asthma, protracted exacerbation of COPD, viral infections, GERD, tuberculosis, mycoplasma, and airway abnormality such as foreign body or tumor should be considered. Laboratory diagnostic methods include culture early in the illness; PCR methods and DFA methods may also be used for real-time diagnosis. After-the-fact diagnosis may be possible with serologic methods.

Treatment: Erythromycin is the "official" drug for treatment. Newer macrolides such as azithromycin and clarithromycin appear to be as effective, better tolerated, and require a shorter course of therapy (and hence a greater probability of compliance). Trimethoprim-sulfa is the preferred agent for macrolide intolerant/allergic patients. Most authorities recommend treatment even if there is a significant delay in diagnosis (up to 4–6 weeks into the illness). Newer vaccines present almost no risk to the recipient, and aggressive vaccination for this illness is appropriate.

5.9 Tuberculosis (TB)

The CDC has a terrific Web site that offers authoritative information and guidelines for diagnosis and treatment. See http://www.cdc.gov/tb/pubs/mmwr/Maj_guide/default.htm. The June 2005 issue of *Clinics in Chest Medicine* is devoted entirely to tuberculosis and is also an excellent reference.

Epidemiology: Epidemiology of TB in the United States over the last 30 years has been reflective of other societal and health trends. In the 1970s and 1980s, effective chemotherapy and effective case identification (as well as downward trends in TB rates) suggested that eradication of the disease in the United States would be a feasible goal. Several external forces combined to increase the incidence of TB and rendered it more difficult to control. First, appearance of HIV/AIDS created a population of potential patients unusually susceptible to the disease. Second, large increases in infected immigrant populations from Asia and Latin America increased incidence and prevalence. These immigrants, along with increasing numbers of patients with TB who were noncompliant with medications, created a reservoir of TB organisms resistant to first-line and some second-line agents. Today, TB is overrepresented among the poor, the homeless, and the incarcerated. These individuals have limited resources for the extended course of treatment necessary for cure. Intermittent and/or no compliance lead to development of resistant strains and persistent sources of contagion. The crowding of penal institutions and homeless shelters amplifies the risk of spread. Extralegal immigration bypasses the screening process designed to diagnose and treat TB in legal immigrants. Furthermore, extralegal immigrants have limited access to medical care and are afraid that a TB diagnosis will result in deportation, prompting active avoidance of treatment. HIV disease impairs cellular immunity functions necessary to prevent reactivation TB, and reactivation rates among HIV-positive, PPD-positive patients may be as high as 7–10% per year. TB also tends to occur in the subgroup of HIV+ patients from lower socioeconomic groups, further compounding risk. Other risk groups include patients on steroids, with certain forms of malignancy, and patients receiving tumor necrosis factor (TNF) antagonists.

Pathogenesis: The pathogenesis of TB has been well understood for decades. Tubercle bacilli are inhaled and lodge in the alveoli. Often, these organisms are immediately destroyed, with no further immunologic or pathologic sequelae. If the organisms are not destroyed, they reproduce and injure and destroy surrounding alveolar tissue. This in turn produces cytokines and chemotactic factors that attract macrophages, neutrophils, and monocytes. Usually, growth of the organisms will be checked once there is adequate cellular immunity response (cellular-mediated immunity, CMI), which occurs in 2–6 weeks. The cells and bacteria form a nodule, a granuloma containing TB bacilli, referred to as a tubercle. At this point, depending upon host factors and the virulence of the strain, several different endpoints may be reached. First, if there is no more growth, the tubercle may be the only site of disease, and the organisms are maintained in a latent stage. Second, if there is further growth, bacilli may enter lymphatics and infect hilar lymph nodes, causing lymphadenopathy. Both the tubercle and the lymph nodes may have calcification as a long-term consequence of the scarring and containment process. The combination of a peripheral tubercle and a calcified, enlarged hilar lymph node is termed a Ghon complex. The majority of infections that progress to this point are generally held in check, creating latent infection. A small minority of patients may go on to have progressive primary disease in the lung, and an even smaller number of patients (often immunosuppressed through one mechanism or another) go on to have hematogenous spread, with production of innumerable tubercles throughout the body. This is termed miliary tuberculosis and is associated with a very high mortality. Patients who have a successful CMI response will reflect immunological memory of the infection with a positive Mantoux test. This consists of intradermal injection sterile TB protein and observing for signs of immune response, induration of the injection site 48–72 hours after injection. The Mantoux test is the mainstay of exposure testing, covered in greater detail in the Treatment and Prevention section below. Latent infection does not always remain latent. Approximately 10% of patients will reactivate their latent infection within the first 3 years after infection, going on to have a necrotizing, destructive infection with prominent constitutional symptoms. The tissue destruction appears to be the effect of both the organism and the host immune response. An additional group of patients will go on later in life to reactivate decades after exposure, as age, medication, or intercurrent disease changes the balance between host and organism.

Symptoms: Initial, controlled infections are usually asymptomatic. Progressive, primary disease may include fever, vague chest pain, and shortness of breath. Reactivation TB, the most common manifestation seen in the United States, generally has a chronic course with weeks to months of low-grade fever, cough, sputum, and weight loss. Occasionally, reactivation TB may be associated with pneumothorax and/or tuberculous empyema, which may cause dyspnea. Hemoptysis may occur when there is destruction of pulmonary or bronchial blood vessels. Miliary tuberculosis may be difficult to diagnose, with fevers, malaise, and more of an "FUO" (fever of unknown origin) flavor than a respiratory disease. Patients with HIV and TB have a higher incidence of extrapulmonary disease and have a higher organism load.

Course/Prognosis/Complications: TB incites an immune response causing significant tissue destruction. Even successful treatment of TB will often leave permanent areas of scarring and fibrosis. Untreated TB can progress to tuberculous empyema and fibrothorax. Cavities may on occasion not close, permitting formation of a mycetoma (see **Aspergillosis**). Damage to bronchial and pulmonary blood vessels may cause hemoptysis, which can be fatal. Active TB is a wasting illness that causes weight loss, fevers, and loss of appetite; the course can be indistinguishable from malignancy.

Imaging: Latent tuberculosis may manifest as a calcified nodule in the lung periphery. The Ghon complex described above consists of a calcified hilar lymph node and a calcified pulmonary nodule. Primary tuberculosis may occur in any lung field, and commonly may be seen in lower lung fields. A pleural effusion is common, occurring in ~25% or more of patients with primary TB. Reactivation TB imaging reflects the aerobic character of the organism, with higher partial pressures of oxygen in the upper lung zones, and a preponderance of infiltrates in the upper lung zones. Typically, a poorly marginated nodular and reticular infiltrate can be seen. The infiltrate may have a central cavity; one of the characteristics that raises suspicion for TB is a ragged interior cavity wall. However, reactivation TB is not confined to the upper lung zones, and as many as 10% of cases may have lower lobe manifestations. Imaging of patients with HIV and TB may be untypical, and TB should be a consideration in HIV+ patients with chronic lung infection, irrespective of X-ray appearance.

Laboratory: Blood testing is nonspecific. An elevated ESR and/or CRP is common. Most laboratory testing revolves around recovery of conclusive evidence for TB bacilli in the patient. This may include visual identification of acid-fast bacilli (characteristic of mycobacteria) in sputum or tissue, detection of M. tuberculosis DNA, or successful culture of the organism. Laboratory methods for decades have been hampered by the slow growth of the organism. However, use of molecular genetic methods combined with culture to amplify early growth has reduced positive ID intervals from weeks and months to days from specimen collection. Laboratory methods are highly specific, but sensitivity can be a problem. Patients without cavitary disease (where there is a high organism load and the organisms are in communication with the airway) may have few organisms in sputum even when ill from the disease. In these cases, sputum induction with inhalation of hypertonic saline may improve yield. Most authorities recommend three morning sputum collections as the compromise between best sensitivity and diminishing returns with larger numbers of specimens. Invasive procedures such as bronchoscopy are best left for patients who simply cannot produce any sputum, or where an alternative diagnosis, more amenable to bronchoscopic diagnosis, is under consideration.

Skin Testing (Mantoux): Stimulation of the anamnestic CMI response with intradermal M. *tuberculosis* protein (tuberculin) is evidence only of prior infection. It does not provide any information regarding active disease. Older methodology (prior to ~1990) used a single criterion for a positive test, namely 10 mm or greater of induration at the site of the injection. Current testing uses multiple criteria based on pretest probability of exposure and infection; the higher the risk, the less robust a reaction is needed for a positive result. This is outlined in Table 5.8. Up to ~25% of patients who have had TB infection may have a negative Mantoux test. Some reasons for a negative test are outlined in Table 5.9. Skin testing should be used for evaluation of latent infection. Although a negative skin test in a healthy, nonanergic patient is strong evidence against active TB, a negative skin test in a chronically ill, immunosuppressed patient provides no information. Similarly, a positive skin test does not provide assurance that the cavity seen on X-ray is tuberculosis. A patient may have a true positive Mantoux but an initially negative skin test. A second skin test, administered in 1–3 weeks may be positive. This is termed *booster phenomenon*, and two-stage testing is appropriate in initially screening individuals who will then go on to have

Table 5.8   Interpretation of Mantoux Testing Based on Risk of Infection

Induration	>5 mm	>10 mm	>15 mm
Risk group	• HIV+ • Recent contacts of TB patient • Fibrotic changes on CXR c/w old TB • Immunosuppressed pts (= to >15 mg prednisone/day)	• Recent arrival from high-prevalence country • IV drug users • Residents and employees of jails, prisons, nursing homes, healthcare facilities, AIDS residential setting, home-less shelter • Specific clinical conditions: silicosis, DM, renal failure, leukemia/lymphoma, ca. of head/neck/lung, gastrec-tomy, jejunoileal bypass, wt. loss >10% body weight • Children <4 yrs; infants, children, adolescents ex-posed to high-risk adults	• All others

regular testing in the future (healthcare workers, prison inmates, nursing home residents, etc.).

Diagnosis: The diagnosis of TB is primarily clinical. Scenarios that should raise a concern for TB include: a patient with a nonre-solving pneumonia; patients with pulmonary infiltrates in high-risk groups who do not have obvious bacterial pneumonia; pulmonary infiltrates in anyone associated with a chronic or sub-

Table 5.9   Reasons for False-Negative Mantoux Testing

Malnutrition
Anergy (HIV+, malignancy)
Severe TB
Simultaneous immunosuppressive disorder
Concurrent viral infection
Steroid therapy

acute course and constitutional symptoms; upper lobe cavitary disease, regardless of chronicity; exudative pleural effusion of unknown etiology (often seen with primary tuberculosis); any wasting illness with pulmonary infiltrates.

Treatment and Prevention: *Prevention* of TB in the United States depends upon multiple strategies. First, prompt identification of the patient with active TB, isolation of that individual, and rendering the patient noncontagious as rapidly as possible minimizes spread. Second, contacts of that patient are screened for skin test conversion, identifying individuals who have new latent infection. Third, screening programs are conducted periodically in high-risk populations to identify individuals who have developed latent infection since the last screening. Additionally, screening may be applied to patients when they enter a high-risk group (e.g., receive a prison sentence or convert their HIV status). Chemoprophylaxis is provided to converters to reduce the risk of reactivation TB in the future. Chemoprophylaxis for appropriate candidates can reduce the risk of reactivation from a lifetime risk of 10–15% to approximately 1%, with minimal side effects and risk. Programs are in place to physically reduce spread of unidentified or identified disease with interventions such as isolation and high-efficiency respiratory masks for healthcare workers. *Treatment* of TB is constrained by the long course of therapy required to achieve cure and the relative toxicity of some of the antibiotics. Successive iterations of therapy protocols have shortened the course of treatment, improving compliance and reducing the incidence of failed treatment (which results in clinical deterioration, continued capacity for infection, and development of drug resistance). Use of directly observed therapy (literally, watch the patient put the pills in his or her mouth and swallow them) in select high-risk populations has also reduced treatment failure. From a medical standpoint, duration and intensity of therapy is driven by the patient's HIV status, and protocols differ on whether a patient is HIV+ or HIV−.

Treatment of multidrug-resistant tuberculosis requires special expertise and should not be attempted without the assistance of an experienced TB physician. At all points in the prevention and treatment chain, local public health officials should be apprised of patients with a new diagnosis of TB and treatment status so that case-contact finding may be conducted, and therapy appropriately supervised. The decision to initiate treatment is based on multiple factor, and can be complicated by delay in getting a culture or DNA-based conclusive positive or negative result. A compelling clinical picture plus AFB on sputum smear should prompt immediate treatment. A patient who is systemically ill and has a convincing clinical presentation without a positive smear also should probably start therapy while cultures are pending. As the likelihood of disease lessens, the indications to initiate therapy in the absence of conclusive microbiological evidence become successively less clear. Consultation is recommended. The following tables and figures provide the basic framework of therapy for TB that is *not* drug resistant. Figure 5.3 is an overall treatment algorithm for culture-proven disease. Figure 5.4 is a treatment algorithm when the patient is treated pending culture results. Table 5.10 provides the specific treatment recommendations for first-line drugs. Patients who are HIV+ and are receiving antiretroviral agents are at high risk for drug interactions and also require consultation and careful monitoring. General monitoring includes clinical evaluation, monitoring of the chest X-ray, monitoring of drug side effects (e.g., liver function studies, eye exams), and successive sputum cultures to document sterilization of the sputum. Treatment of latent tuberculosis should go forward only after active TB has been excluded. Once active TB has been excluded, high-risk patients who have positive skin tests should be treated. Table 5.11 delineates current drug regimens for treatment of latent tuberculosis. Tables 5.12 and 5.13 review relative risk for development of TB and incidence of TB infection in patients with a positive tuberculin skin test.

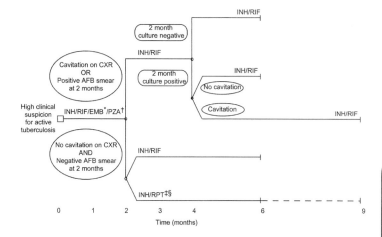

Patients in whom tuberculosis is proved or strongly suspected should have treatment initiated with isoniazid, rifampin, pyrazinamide, and ethambutol for the initial 2 months. A repeat smear and culture should be performed when 2 months of treatment has been completed. If cavities were seen on the initial chest radiograph or the acid-fast smear is positive at completion of 2 months of treatment, the continuation phase of treatment should consist of isoniazid and rifampin daily or twice weekly for 4 months to complete a total of 6 months of treatment. If cavitation was present on the initial chest radiograph and the culture at the time of completion of 2 months of therapy is positive, the continuation phase should be lengthened to 7 months (total of 9 months of treatment). If the patient has HIV infection and the CD4+ cell count is <100/μl, the continuation phase should consist of daily or three times weekly isoniazid and rifampin. In HIV-uninfected patients having no cavitation on chest radiograph and negative acid-fast smears at completion of 2 months of treatment, the continuation phase may consist of either once weekly isoniazid and rifapentine, or daily or twice weekly isoniazid and rifampin, to complete a total of 6 months (bottom). Patients receiving isoniazid and rifapentine, and whose 2-month cultures are positive, should have treatment extended by an additional 3 months (total of 9 months).

* EMB may be discontinued when results of drug susceptibility testing indicate no drug resistance.
†PZA may be discontinued after it has been taken for 2 months (56 doses).
‡RPT should not be used in HIV-infected patients with tuberculosis or in patients with extrapulmonary tuberculosis.
§ Therapy should be extended to 9 months if 2-month culture is positive.
CXR = chest radiograph; EMB = ethambutol; INH = isoniazid; PZA = pyrazinamide; RIF = rifampin; RPT = rifapentine.

Figure 5.3   Treatment algorithm for tuberculosis. From ATS/IDSA/CDC Recommendations for the Treatment of Tuberculosis, 2003. Used with thanks.

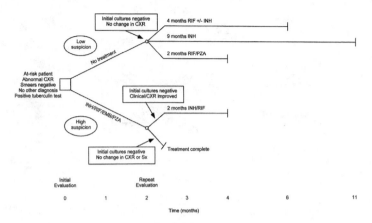

The decision to begin treatment for a patient with sputum smears that are negative depends on the degree of suspicion that the patient has tuberculosis. The considerations in choosing among the treatment options are discussed in the text. If the clinical suspicion is high (bottom), then multidrug therapy should be initiated before acid-fast smear and culture results are known. If the diagnosis is confirmed by a positive culture, treatment can be continued to complete a standard course of therapy (see Figure 1). If initial cultures remain negative and treatment has consisted of multiple drugs for 2 months, then there are two options depending on repeat evaluation at 2 months (bottom): (1) if the patient demonstrates symptomatic or radiographic improvement without another apparent diagnosis, then a diagnosis of culture-negative tuberculosis can be inferred. Treatment should be continued with isoniazed and rifampin alone for an additional 2 months; (2) if the patient demonstrates neither symptomatic nor radiographic improvement, then prior tuberculosis is unlikely and treatment is complete once treatment including at least 2 months of rifampin and pyrazinamide has been administered. In low-suspicion patients not initially receiving treatment (top), if cultures remain negative, the patient has no symptoms, and

the chest radiograph is unchanged at 2–3 months, there are three treatment options: these are (1) isoniazid for 9 months, (2) rifampin with or without isoniazid for 4 months, or (3) rifampin and pyrazinamide for 2 months. CXR = chest X-ray; EMB = ethambutol; INH = isoniazid; PZA = pyrazinamide; RIF = rifampin; Sx = signs/symptoms. (It should be noted that the RIF/PZA 2-month regimen should be used only for patients who

Figure 5.4 Algorithm for treatment of culture-negative and inactive TB. From ATS/IDSA/CDC Recommendations for the Treatment of Tuberculosis, 2003. Used with thanks.

Table 5.10 Drug Regimens for Treatment of Susceptible, Culture Positive TB

	Initial Phase			Continuation Phase			Range of Total Doses (minimal duration)	Rating (evidence)	
Regimen	Drugs	Interval and Doses‡ (minimal duration)	Regimen	Drugs	Interval and Doses‡§ (minimal duration)			HIV−	HIV+
1	INH RIF PZA EMB	7 days per week for 56 doses(8 wk) or 5 d/wk for 40 doses (8 wk)¶	1a	INH/RIF	7 days per week for 126 doses (18 wk) or 5 d/wk for 90 doses (18 wk)¶		182–130 (26 wk)	A (I)	A(II)
			1b	INH/RIF	Twice weekly for 36 doses (18 wk)		92–76 (26 wk)	A (I)	A (II)#
			1c**	INH/RPT	Once weekly for 18 doses (18 wk)		74–58 (26 wk)	B (I)	E (I)
2	INH RIF PZA EMB	7 days per week for 14 doses (2 wk), then twice weekly for 12 doses (6 wk) or 5 d/wk for 10 doses (2 wk)¶ then twice weekly for 12 doses (6 wk)	2a	INH/RIF	Twice weekly for 36 doses (18 wk)		62–58 (26 wk)	A (II) B (I)	B (II)# E (I)
			2b**	INH/RPT	Once weekly for 18 doses (18 wk)		44–40 (26 wk)	B(I)	E(I)

(continues)

Table 5.10 (continued)

3	INH RIF PZA EMB	Three times weekly for 24 doses (8 wk)	3a	INH/RIF	Three times weekly for 54 doses (18 wk)	78 (26 wk)	B (I)	B(II)
4	INH RIF EMB	7 days per week for 56 doses (8 wk) or 5 d/wk for 40 doses (8 wk)¶	4a	INH/RIF	7 days per week for 217 doses (31 wk) or 5 d/wk for 155 doses (31 wk)¶	273–195 (39 wk)	C (I)	C (II)
			4b	INH/RIF		118–102 (39 wk)	C (I)	C (III)

Definition of abbreviations: EMB = ethambutol; INH = isoniazid; PZA = pyrazinamide; RIF = rifampin; RPT = rifapentine.

*Definitions of evidence ratings: A = preferred; B = acceptable alternative; C = offer when A and B cannot be given; E = should never be given.

†Definition of evidence ratings: I = randomized clinical trial; II = data from clinical trials that were not randomized or were conducted in other populations; III = expert opinion.

‡When DOT is used, drugs may be given 5 days/week and the necessary number of doses adjusted accordingly. Although there are no studies that compare five with seven daily doses, extensive experience indicates this would be an effective practice.

§Patients with cavitation on initial chest radiograph and positive cultures at completion of 2 months of therapy should receive a 7-month (31 week; either 217 doses [daily] or 62 doses [twice weekly]) continuation phase.

¶5-day-a-week administration is always given by DOT. Rating for 5 day/week regimens is AIII.

#Not recommended for HIV-infected patients with CD4+ cell counts <100 cells/μl.

**Options 1c and 2b should be used only in HIV-negative patients who have negative sputum smears at the time of completion of 2 months of therapy and who do not have cavitation on initial chest radiograph (see text). For patients started on this regimen and found to have a positive culture from the 2-month specimen, treatment should be extended an extra 3 months.

From ATS/IDSA/CDC Recommendations for the Treatment of Tuberculosis, 2003. Used with thanks.

Table 5.11   Treatment Regimens for Latent TB Infection

Drug/Dose	Frequency/Duration	Rating* (Evidence)† HIV negative	Rating* (Evidence)† HIV positive
Preferred Regimen Isoniazid Adult: 5 mg/kg Children: 10–20 mg/kg Maximum dose 300 mg	Daily × 9 months	A (II)	A (II)
Alternate Regimens Isoniazid Adult: 15 mg/kg Children: 20–40 mg/kg Maximum dose 900 mg	Twice weekly × 9 months§	B (II)	B (II)
Isoniazid Adults: 5 mg/kg Maximum dose 300 mg	Daily × 6 months	B (I)	C (I)
Isoniazid Adults: 15 mg/kg Maximum dose 900 mg	Twice weekly × 6 months§	B (II)	C (I)
Rifampin Adults: 10 mg/kg Children: 10–20 mg/kg Maximum dose 600 mg	Daily × 4 months	B (II)	B (II)

Note: *Strength of the recommendation: A = preferred regimen; B = acceptable alternative; C = offer when A and B cannot be given

†Quality of the supporting evidence: I = randomized clinical trials data; II = data from clinical trials not randomized or from other population

§A regimen of rifampin and pyrazinamide for the treatment of LTBI should generally not be offered due to risk of severe adverse events. In situations in which rifampin cannot be used (e.g., HIV infected persons receiving protease inhibitors), rifabutin may be substituted. Intermittent regimen must be provided via directly observed therapy (DOT), i.e., health care worker observes the ingestion of medication

From CDC Guide for Primary Health Care Providers: Targeted TB Testing and Treatment of Latent Tuberculosis, 2005. Used with thanks.

PULMONARY INFECTIOUS DISEASE

Table 5.12   Incidence of Active TB in Patients with Positive Skin Test, by Condition

Risk Factor	TB Cases/1000 person-years
Recent TB infection	
Infection <1 year past	12.9*
Infection 1–7 year past	1.6
Human immunodeficiency virus (HIV) infection	35.0–162
Injection drug use	
HIV seropositive	76.0
HIV seronegative or unknown	10.0
Silicosis	68
Radiographic findings consistent with prior TB	2.0–13.6
Weight deviation from standard	
Underweight by 15%	2.6
Underweight by 10–14%	2.0
Underweight by 5–9%	2.2
Weight within 5% of standard	1.1
Overweight by 5%	0.7

From ATS/CDC. Targeted tuberculin testing and treatment of latent tuberculosis infection, 2000. Used with thanks.

Table 5.13   Relative Risk* for Developing Active Tuberculosis (TB), by Selected Clinical Conditions

Clinical Condition	Relative Risk
Silicosis	30
Diabetes mellitus	2.0–4.1
Chronic renal failure/hemodialysis	10.0–25.3
Gastrectomy	2–5
Jejunoileal bypass	27–63
Solid organ transplantation	
Renal	37
Cardiac	20–74
Carcinoma of head or neck	16

*Relative to control population; independent of tuberculin test status.
From ATS/CDC. Targeted tuberculin testing and treatment of latent tuberculosis infection, 2000. Used with thanks.

5.10 Nontuberculous Mycobacteria (NTM)— Avium–Intracellulare

This is the most useful reference: Am J Respir Crit Care Med 2007; 175:367 . Other references include N Engl J Med 1989;321:863, Lancet Infect Dis 2004;4:557, Clin Chest Med 1989;10:13.

Introduction: In addition to M. *tuberculosis*, there are approximately 100 other species of mycobacterium, some of which are capable of causing human disease. Some species, such as M. *bovis*, are considered to be in the M. *tb* family and cause disease (and are treated) in a manner indistinguishable from M. *tb*. A number of other organisms such as M. *fortuitum*, M. *chelonae*, and M. *kansasii* are capable of causing human disease but are encountered uncommonly in the practice of respiratory medicine. In the United States, the most common NTM infections are caused by the avium-intracellulare group (MAC), which are not distinguished in testing. Infections caused by this group of agents will be reviewed. References above can provide detailed information on the clinical syndromes and treatment of the organisms not covered here.

Epidemiology: Prior to the AIDS era, three groups of patients developed MAC infections. First, patients with bronchiectasis would develop pulmonary infiltrates and exacerbations of their underlying lung disease. Second, older male patients with underlying COPD could develop a syndrome that was virtually indistinguishable from tuberculosis. Finally (and the group I have personally encountered most frequently) were older (>60) women who had cough and progressive apical nodular infiltrates. With the advent of AIDS, MAC was also recognized to cause a form of disseminated infection associated with low CD4+ counts with little pulmonary involvement. MAC has been identified as the antigen responsible for an unusual HP, "hot tub lung" (Environ Health

Perspect 2007;115:262). Since NTM infection is not a reportable disease, precise incidence is unknown; some authorities suggest incidence at 1–2/100,000. The risk of MAC infection in patients with AIDS and low CD4+ count is high, in the range of 20%.

Pathogenesis: As with other mycobacterial infections, tissue injury is a consequence of both direct bacterial injury and host response. It is unclear if infection represents reactivation or acquisition of new infection. Patients with progressive disease may have destruction of lung tissue by cavitation or progressive fibrosis. Loss of lung tissue may lead to dyspnea and respiratory failure.

Symptoms: There is no hallmark symptom of this infection. Cough, sputum, low-grade hemoptysis, and fever are common. Lymphadenitis and lymphadenopathy may also occur. Patients with HIV/MAC will be quite ill systemically, with unremitting fevers and further wasting. Diarrhea and lymphadenopathy may also be seen.

Course/Prognosis/Complications: Progressive destruction of lung tissue may lead to respiratory failure. Many patients, particularly the older female subgroup, find the cough to be disabling and socially paralyzing. My personal experience has been that 30–50% of geriatric patients cannot tolerate the drug regimen. Patients with HIV/MAC by definition have advanced disease and have a poor prognosis.

Imaging: As with symptoms, X-ray and HRCT findings may be nonspecific. Cavitation and nonspecific infiltrates in the area of known bronchiectasis may be the imaging findings. Older women may have a pattern of upper lung zone fibrotic and nodular changes. The presence of micronodules and bronchiectasis on HRCT should raise the possibility of MAC infection. HIV/MAC patients may have few CXR findings.

Laboratory: Skin testing is not performed routinely for the diagnosis of this condition. The role of the laboratory in MAC infection is to grow and isolate the organism. Specimens may include sputum, bronchial washings/BAL, or tissue. In HIV/MAC patients, organism burden may be so high that blood cultures may be positive for organisms.

Diagnosis: Requires a plausible clinical scenario, as outlined above, *and* microbiological and/or histological evidence of infection. Positive sputum cultures for MAC, particularly in patients with underlying lung disease, may represent colonization rather than infection. Conversely, many of the clinical scenarios described above are consistent with M. *tb* infection, fungal infection, or bacterial infection; these must be excluded. HIV− patients diagnosed with MAC infection have persistent cough, nonspecific pulmonary infiltrates, and often have underlying lung disease. The clinician has made multiple efforts to treat symptoms with conventional antibiotics and/or bronchodilators unsuccessfully. Sputum cultures and/or bronchoscopic specimens grow MAC, and the decision must be made as to whether or not to treat the patient. The ATS and IDSA have issued detailed criteria for diagnosis and treatment of NTM; it is strongly recommended that this document be reviewed before embarking upon treatment for MAC or any other NTM.

Treatment: Treatment is expensive, prolonged, and often poorly tolerated in the elderly. Table 5.14 outlines 2007 recommendations for therapy. Care should be taken to reduce dosage when necessary for body weight and creatinine clearance, and regular monitoring of hematologic, hepatic, neurologic, and visual function is warranted. Therapy should be continued for 1 year after sterilization of the sputum. Treatment of HIV/MAC patients is complicated by drug interactions and higher organism burdens and is beyond the scope of this book.

Table 5.13   Treatment Regimens for MAC

Disease Type	Fibronodular/Bronchiectatic	Fibrocavitary (or Severe Fibronodular)
Regimen	Clarithromycin 1000 mg **OR** Azithromycin 500 mg **AND** Rifampin 600 mg **AND** Ethambutol (25 mg/kg)	Clarithromycin 500 mg or 1000 mg **OR** Azithromycin 250 mg **AND** Rifampin 600 mg **OR** Rifabutin 150–300 mg **AND** Ethambutol 15 mg/kg
Frequency	Thrice weekly	Daily

Note: Some authorities recommend addition of streptomycin or amikacin (both 10–15 mg/kg) thrice weekly for first 8 weeks. Reduce to 6–8 mg/kg in pts >50 y.o., <50 kg, or who require prolonged therapy. Some older patients may require reduction in clarithromycin dose to 500 mg (as in far-right column) to prevent excessive drug levels. Capitalized, bolded conjunctions are treated as logical operators.

5.11 Pulmonary Viral Infections

Numerous viruses may cause pulmonary infections. As with other classes of pathogens, host status defines susceptibility and severity of illness. The most common viral pulmonary infection is influenza and is seen in immune-competent and -incompetent individuals. Respiratory syncitial virus is being recognized with increasing frequency in adults. Varicella pneumonia, although uncommon can cause severe disease in adults and can be seen in healthy adults. Cytomegalovirus and herpesvirus are prototypical agents seen in immunocompromised patients. SARS and hantavirus are seen in normal individuals. They are capable of causing severe disease and are highly contagious. Because of these properties, they require different public health and therapeutic interventions.

Influenza

The human form of influenza has two types, A and B. Type A in particular has a remarkable ability to change its antigenic appearance. Depending upon previous exposure to influenza antigen and the similarity between the current strain and previously experienced strains, the host may have minimal or effective immunity. Major changes in antigenic appearance, termed antigenic *shifts*, are associated with pandemics and high rates of morbidity and mortality because of widespread lack of immunity in the populations at risk. Minor changes, called antigenic *drifts*, have less drastic effects on populations. Influenza will enter a community or region and reach maximal levels of infectivity in 2 or 3 weeks. The prevalence will then start to drop in 2 or 3 months. Highest levels of morbidity and mortality are seen in the elderly and the chronically ill. Transmission is by droplet.

Clinical manifestations include abrupt high fever, myalgias, cough, and sore throat. Uncomplicated influenza will resolve usually in a few days (~3–5). Patients with complicated courses may develop pneumonia. Neurological manifestations and rhabdomyolysis are uncommon but severe complications. Pneumonia may be primary, due to the effect of the virus itself, secondary (an opportunistic bacterial infection that takes advantage of cilial dysfunction and injured bronchial mucosa), or both. Staphylococcal infection is the "classic" secondary pneumonia. Both primary and secondary pneumonias have a high rate of morbidity and mortality, particularly in the elderly and chronically ill.

Diagnosis is often presumptive. A patient with typical symptoms at the right time of year (November to March in North America) has influenza until proven otherwise. Nasal swabs may provide rapid diagnostic information but do not have perfect sensitivity and/or specificity. Many practitioners, myself included, will perform rapid testing until it is clear that the infection is in the community; the diagnosis is then clinical. Serological testing and viral culture may also be used, but these are more epidemiologic than clinical tools.

Treatment and prevention are inseparable. US vaccine manufacturers try to anticipate the correct antigenic strain(s) that will be prevalent by monitoring influenza activity in other parts of the world. The better the prediction, the more effective the vaccine. Vaccination has been demonstrated to be highly effective in immune-competent nonelderly adults; it is less so in the elderly where only modest reductions in mortality have been noted. Nonetheless, vaccination is still recommended in many population subgroups; one goal of widespread vaccination is to create "herd immunity" where contagion in the population at risk is reduced by causing fewer individuals to be susceptible to infection. This protects high-risk populations such as the elderly indirectly but effectively. Preparations include an injected split virus vaccine and a live attenuated intranasal vaccine. Current treatment regimens are based on the neuraminidase inhibitors zanamivir and oseltamivir. The former is inhaled and the latter is ingested. Both will shorten length of illness by 1–3 days if taken within the first 24 hours of illness; efficacy drops rapidly after that interval. Severity of the infection is also reduced if the drug is started promptly. Amantidine and rimantidine are M2 inhibitors that have been used in the past. High levels of viral resistance to these agents caused the CDC to issue warnings against their use for the 2005–6 and 2006–7 seasons. The CDC Web site should be queried for current recommendations. Interestingly, there is little information on the efficacy of any of these agents for severe disease.

No discussion of influenza is complete without reference to zoonotic influenza. Avian and swine influenza strains have the potential to mutate to forms which have greater human virulence. At the time of this writing, the greater concern is for avian strains hopping to human hosts. Human infection is most prevalent in China and southeast Asia where animals and humans live in close proximity. However, human-to-human transmission is very rare. Human and zoonotic influenza is a rapidly changing subject, and the CDC Web site should be consulted for current threat assessment (Geriatrics 2002;57:56, Arch Intern Med 2000;160:3243, JAMA 2000;284:1655, Ann Intern

Med 1995;123:518, CMAJ 2003;168:49). Perusal of the CDC Web site and archives of MMWR may also be very helpful.

Respiratory Syncytial Virus (RSV)

RSV in the past has been associated with pediatric and infant infections, but there has been an increasing recognition that RSV infections occur repeatedly throughout life. A significant proportion of infections attributed to influenza may in fact be due to RSV. The disease is particularly dangerous in the elderly and chronically ill. Ribavirin inhaled (contraindicated in pregnancy) may be of value. In both children and adults RSV infection can be associated with bronchiolitis and reactive airways (Clin Microbiol Rev 2000; 13:371).

Varicella Pneumonia

Varicella (chickenpox) is a common infection in childhood, although the incidence may decrease in the future as immunization becomes more common. Varicella is a relatively benign illness in children, but can be a serious infection in adults who did not experience the virus as a child and become infected as adults. Varicella is highly contagious, and an adult who has never had the illness and comes in contact with an infected child has a high likelihood of infection. It is unlikely that the pneumonia will precede the rash, and, as such, the infection should be readily identified. Fever, cough, and respiratory distress are common, and if the patient needs to be intubated, mortality can be in the 30–50% range. Treatment with steroids and acyclovir has been shown to reduce mortality and morbidity. Patients who recover from varicella pneumonia have a signature X-ray appearance of a profusion of tiny calcified nodules throughout the lung; these have no clinical meaning. Varicella pneumonia can be severe in immunocompromised patients (Arch Intern Med 1988;148:1630, Chest 1998;114:426).

Cytomegalovirus

Cytomegalovirus is a common infection, acquired through sexual or other forms of close contact. Most individuals who are immuno-competent will have no respiratory symptoms or signs at the time of initial infection. CMV does not clear after acute infection and remains latent. Severe changes in the patient's immune status, such as acquisition of HIV infection or organ transplant, can activate the virus. CMV can be recovered from BAL fluid collected from both HIV and transplant patients. There is controversy as to whether HIV patients who shed CMV actually have a pneumonitis, and if treat-ment is necessary. On the other hand, CMV pneumonitis is an accepted complication of transplantation, and in the case of lung transplantation is thought to contribute to rejection syndromes. Patients with CMV infection have cough, low-grade fever, dyspnea, and pulmonary function abnormalities. X-ray appearance can be vari-able, but may include pleural effusions, perihilar infiltrates, diffuse pulmonary infiltrates, or even focal consolidations. Often, the differ-ential diagnosis is between CMV infection and rejection; CMV infection usually occurs between 2 weeks and 2 months after trans-plantation, whereas acute rejection will occur earlier. Treatment is usually with ganciclovir. Many transplant protocols include some form of prophylaxis, which may include both ganciclovir and immune glob-ulin. Additionally, efforts are made (when possible) to transplant seronegative recipients with organs from seronegative donors. Diagnosis is through transbronchial lung biopsy or BAL with culture; PCR or histology is used for identification of the organism. This is a dangerous disease that requires infectious disease consultation (J Clin Virol 2002;25 Suppl 2:S1, Semin Respir Infect 1999;14:353).

Herpesvirus

Reactivation of herpesvirus presents a problem for organ trans-plant recipients, where reactivation of HSV-1 can run as high as 70%. Although pulmonary involvement is uncommon, it can manifest as an erosive tracheobronchitis or a diffuse pneumonitis. Treatment is with acyclovir, as is prophylaxis. The latter has decreased all forms of herpes reactivation illness (Postgrad Med J 2000;107:67).

Hantavirus

Hantavirus is the umbrella term for a number of related virus species that cause a severe, progressive respiratory illness in previously healthy individuals. The illness is acquired from contact with rodents (bites are not required), and mortality can range from 10–70%, depending upon the strain. The clinical picture is that of noncardiogenic pulmonary edema. There is no effective antiviral treatment for this condition, and supportive care is necessary. Early treatment with vasopressors appears to improve survival (N Engl J Med 1994;330:949).

SARS

Severe acute respiratory syndrome is a newly recognized coronavirus syndrome. It was first seen in China and Southeast Asia in 2002. High rates of person-to-person transmission were seen, and case mortality was approximately 10% even in previously healthy individuals. An initial prodrome of fever and myalgias suggested a nonspecific viral illness, but progressed in patients to respiratory failure requiring intubation and mechanical ventilation. An ARDS-like picture was the most common X-ray finding. *Ex post facto* diagnosis by serologic means is possible, but there are no real-time tests currently available. The only treatment is supportive.

Because of the high virulence of both Hanta and SARS infections, protection of healthcare workers is mandatory. The prodrome of a relatively mild illness with SARS allowed inadvertent spread of the illness until it was realized that quarantine and interdiction of travel were key elements of controlling the outbreak in 2003. It is anticipated that this would be part of future strategies as well (Clin Infect Dis 2004;38:1420).

5.12 *Nocardia,* Actinomycosis, and *Rhodococcus*

Eur Respir J 2003;21:545, Clin Microbiol Rev 1991;4:20, J Clin Microbiol 2003;41:4497

Introduction: *Nocardia,* actinomycosis, and *Rhodococcus* species are members of the family Mycobacteria, sharing genetics and cell wall fatty acids with agents such as M. *Tb. Nocardia* and *Rhodococcus* are both found in the environment and can frequently be isolated from soil samples. Actinomycosis is harbored by humans. All three agents share a propensity for infection in immunocompromised hosts but can also affect immune-competent hosts. All are unusual infections with delay in diagnosis frequent (see **Nonresolving Pneumonia**).

Epidemiology: All three are infrequent infections, with *Nocardia* species the most common of the three. Approximately one third of *Nocardia* infections occur in immune-competent hosts, as do one fifth of *Rhodococcus* infections. The majority of actinomycosis cases are reported in immune-competent individuals. *Nocardia* and *Rhodococcus* are frequently seen in patients with exposure to farms or soil. *Rhodococcus* has a strong association with domesticated herbivores such as horses. Actinomycosis organisms are carried in the mouth and periodontal area of humans, and pulmonary disease results from aspiration. Actinomycosis is frequently a mixed infection since it is a consequence of aspiration. Risk for *Nocardia* infection is high in patients with pulmonary alveolar proteinosis and lupus.

Pathophysiology: All three agents destroy pulmonary tissue producing cavitation, hemoptysis, and chest pain. Extension to and involvement of the pleural space is common. Actinomycosis is distinguished from the other two organisms by its disregard for anatomic boundaries and its propensity for sinus tract formation. Actinomycosis is aspirated; *Nocardia* and *Rhodococcus* are inhaled.

Course/Prognosis/Complications: Soft tissue invasion and pleural disease occur with all three organisms; *Nocardia* and *Rhodococcus* have a predilection for neural tissue, and CNS infection is the worst complication. A diligent search for CNS disease is necessary. *Rhodococcus* may spread to bone or cause renal disease or a hepatic abscess. *Nocardia* may spread to bone or kidneys, and may cause endocarditis. Actinomycosis may form sinus tracts and empyemas, requiring surgical intervention. Actinomycosis may also disseminate. Cure and mortality depend on extent of disease, length of delay in diagnosis, and immune status for all three organisms. Pulmonary nocardiosis is associated with mortality of 30–50%.

Diagnosis: Presentation of all three organisms is a chronic to subacute course with fever, weight loss, malaise, cough, and sputum. Frequently there is a delay in diagnosis as the patient is treated for a conventional pneumonia but there is persistence of symptoms and abnormal X-ray. Alternative diagnoses include tuberculosis and atypical mycobacteria, fungal infections, lung abscesses, and malignancy. Diagnosis is made when clinical suspicion is high (pneumonia not resolved, bronchoscopy negative for malignancy, immune status, etc.), and these organisms are sought specifically. Sputum may be diagnostic, but bronchoscopy or TTNB may be necessary. Laboratory values will reflect chronic infection; there are no specific findings. Suspicion for actinomycosis should be high in patients with cervical/facial infection, poor dentition, and a pulmonary cavity. *Rhodococcus* may be associated with gastrointestinal disease. *Nocardia* may have cutaneous manifestations, and patients with SLE and PAP appear to be susceptible to *Nocardia* infection. *Nocardia* and actinomycosis are weakly acid fast and appear on Gram's stain as gram-positive branching rods. *Rhodococcus* is a gram-positive coccobacillary rod. Farm or soil contact is not a prerequisite for contraction of *Rhodococcus* or *Nocardia*. Actinomycosis is described as having "sulfur granules" (i.e., little yellow clumps) in the sputum or pus. Conclusive diagnosis is made by culture.

Imaging: Lobar/segmental infiltrates that are persistent; fluffy nodules, cavities, and cavitating nodules. Actinomycosis may cross anatomic barriers such as the pleura and invade the chest wall directly. Pleural effusions may be seen with all three infections.

Treatment: Actinomycosis: High-dose penicillin or amoxicillin are the drugs of choice and are usually a successful treatment. Penicillin V is used at 2–4 grams/day, amoxicillin at 500 mg tid. Macrolides are also successful. *Nocardia* is difficult to treat, requiring months of therapy. High-dose trimethoprim-sulfa is the drug of choice; amikacin, minocycline, imipenem, and linezolid are alternatives. Speciation and antimicrobial testing is very important, as a significant number of *Nocardia* isolates are not *N. asteroides* sensitive to sulfa. Duration of therapy is at least 6 months for immune-competent individuals, and at least 12 months for immune-incompetent patients or those with CNS infection (see below). TMP-SMX is used at 15mg/kg/day; amikacin 7.5 mg/kg/day to start; if CNS infection is present ceftriaxone should be used instead of amikacin at 2 gm/day. *Rhodococcus* is treated with a macrolide (azithromycin 250mg/day), quinolone (levofloxacin 500 mg/day), rifampin, vancomycin, or imipenem. Multiple agents used simultaneously for a prolonged period are required in the immunocompromised patient. Prophylaxis for recurrence may be indicated for immunocompromised patients once apparently disease free. HIV patients with *Rhodococcus* are at risk for drug interactions if on antivirals and at risk for relapse/recurrence. Infectious disease consultation is recommended for all three infections, irrespective of patient's immune status.

5.13 *Pneumocystis jiroveci* Pneumonia (PCJ)

Mayo Clin Proc 1996;71:5, N Engl J Med 2004;350:2487

Epidemiology: *Pneumocystis jiroveci* is the current name for an organism that has been variously classified as a bacteria, protozoan, and fungus. The most recent classification, based on DNA analysis, suggests that this organism is most closely related to the fungus family. Previously named *Pneumocystis carinii*, the organism causes severe, potentially life-threatening infections in patients who are immunocompromised. The organism was first identified in malnourished, premature infants in post–World War II Europe. Up until the AIDS era, infection was seen most commonly in patients undergoing aggressive treatment for hematologic malignancy or who were solid organ transplant recipients. The common factor appeared to be treatments that included corticosteroids and suppression of T-cell immunity. Other conditions treated with long courses of corticosteroids, such as inflammatory and rheumatologic conditions, also produce appropriate conditions for PCJ infection. In the era of HIV/AIDS, this rare infection became quite common. The infection also took on considerable prognostic importance as an AIDS-defining illness. As treatment of HIV/AIDS entered the HAART era, the frequency of infection has dropped, but it is still the most common opportunistic infection in AIDS patients. PCJ has two distinct clinical presentations, depending upon the patient's HIV status.

The mode of transmission is uncertain. Frequency of infection in HIV+ patients increases as the CD4 count drops, with the illness becoming more common as the CD4 count drops below 200. In the pre-HAART era, frequency of infection in the low CD4 count population was as high as 8%, and, conversely, over 95% of patients with PCJ had CD4 counts below 200. HAART and prophylaxis have reduced the frequency of PCJ both as the AIDS-defining illness and as a complication of HIV infection. PCJ remains an unusual infection in patients without HIV infection (Emerg Infect Dis 2004;10:1713).

Pathophysiology: Infection is confined to pneumonitis. There can be destruction of lung tissue, or more frequently there is alveolar filling with organisms and inflammatory exudates. Diffuse untreated infection can cause hypoxic respiratory failure and death.

Symptoms: In the non-HIV patient, PCJ infection is a fulminant illness with abrupt onset of fever, cough, and dyspnea. Presentation often occurs in the context of the patient's steroid requirement dropping, presumably permitting an inflammatory response to the presence of the organisms. In the HIV+ patient, the presentation is often slower, with gradual onset of symptoms over weeks to months. Fevers, cough, and dyspnea are present, but the time course is so different between HIV+ and HIV− patients that clinically the two presentations appear to be different illnesses.

Course/Prognosis/Complications: PCJ pneumonia is a serious illness with a high death rate. Patients who are HIV+ and who require mechanical ventilation for PCJ pneumonia have a 60% mortality—high enough to warrant great concern, but enough to warrant a period of intensive care (N Engl J Med 2006;355:173). HIV+ patients who survive the illness may have pneumatoceles and other structural lung damage. In both HIV+ and HIV− patients undergoing treatment for PCJ pneumonia, the large number of concomitant medications can lead to drug interactions between maintenance medications and the anti-infectives.

Imaging: The common presentation in both HIV+ and HIV− patients is that of diffuse parenchymal lung disease. The lungs have a ground glass or nodular appearance, and there is no lung zone predominance. In patients who are HIV+, patients can present with lobar infiltrates, pneumothorax, pneumatoceles, nodules, and even pleural effusions.

Laboratory: A variety of laboratory tests have been evaluated and recommended in patients with possible PCJ disease. Indirect tests such as pulmonary functions and serum LDH have been evaluated, but definitive testing rests upon identification of the organism in tissue or alveolar fluid. Organisms are identified with the use of silver stain, immunofluorescent staining, or Giemsa. Organisms can be identified in sputum (~50%), BAL fluid (~95+%) or transbronchial lung biopsy (~95+%). Organism load tends to be high in HIV+ patients, making induced sputum samples a feasible initial test. Arterial blood gas testing is used prognostically in patients with HIV/PCJ and helps define indications for concomitant steroid therapy.

Diagnosis: PCJ is one of many infections and inflammatory conditions seen in immunocompromised patients. The articles on **HIV and the Lung** and **Pneumonia in Immunocompromised Hosts** review the differential diagnosis more completely. Presumptive diagnosis and therapy (with the exception of obvious bacterial pneumonia) may lead to delayed treatment and unfavorable outcomes in these patients.

Treatment and Prophylaxis: In HIV− patients, therapy usually consists of trimethoprim/sulfamethoxazole as 15/75 to 20/100 per kg per 24 hours divided into four doses. This can be given orally or intravenously. TMP/SMX is usually well tolerated in HIV-negative patients. Alternatives include pentamidine and the alternatives used in HIV+ patients. Duration of therapy is usually 14 days. In my experience, and that of other practitioners, recovery is dependent upon reconstitution of the patient's immune system. Corticosteroids are used in severe cases. Prophylaxis in HIV− patients is warranted in patients with long-term high-dose steroids and is accomplished with low-dose TMP/SMX (1 double-strength tablet 3 days/week). Inhaled pentamidine does not work as well as other regimens and is not optimum. Patients who are HIV+ require 21 days of therapy and may worsen during initial treatment. They are often intolerant of TMP/SMX. Patients who have a Po_2 <70 on room air or an A-a gradient of >35 should be considered for steroid therapy. One regimen is 40 mg prednisone bid × 5 d; 40 mg q day × 5 d; 20 mg po q day × 11 d. TMP/SMX is administered as 2 double-strength tablets every 8 hours. Hepatotoxicity, fever, rash, and hyperkalemia are all possible and can be severe enough to require cessation of therapy. TMP-dapsone, atovaquone, and primaquine-clindamycin are alternatives, and dosing should be reviewed at the time of initiation of therapy. If the patient is sufficiently ill to warrant intravenous therapy, TMP/SMX is the drug of choice, and other regimens can also be given IV. If the patient has developed PCJ on TMP/SMX prophylaxis, an alternative regimen (atovaquone or clindamycin-primaquine) is appropriate. Prophylaxis in HIV+ patients is usually with TMP/SMX and should be provided in patients with CD4 <200, with prior PCJ infection, or who have oral candidiasis. Dapsone is the second choice. Inhaled pentamidine is well tolerated but less effective. TMP/SMX doses are similar to those for non-HIV patients. Prophylaxis is effective, greatly reducing the rate of PCJ pneumonia. Prophylaxis may be stopped when immune reconstitution occurs such that the CD4 count is >200 (Treat Respir Med 2004;3:381).

5.14 Fungal Infections

Fungi That Affect the Normal Host

Blastomycosis

Fraser and Pare 1999;3:3076, 899–902, Clin Infect Dis 2000;30:679, N Engl J Med 2007;356:1456

Epidemiology: This is an uncommon illness caused by *Blastomyces dermatitidis*, a fungus endemic to much of the eastern half of the United States and the St. Lawrence valley in the United States and Canada. The disease has been seen in Africa. Central

America and South America as well as India have also reported cases. In Wisconsin, where the disease is reportable, incidence is <1.5/100,000. The organism tends to be found in wooded areas, although patients have been infected in other venues.

Pathophysiology: The disease is most often acquired by inhaling the conidial (spore) form. The fungus is dimorphic, having a yeast form at 37°C and a mycelial phase at room temperature. The yeast cell wall is thick and has surface proteins that resist phago-cytosis. The organism is a primary pathogen and does not have a propensity for immunocompromised individuals, although the disease, when it does occur in this population, tends to be more serious. Severe infection is thought to be caused by inhalation of a large number of spores that overwhelm host immune defenses.

Symptoms: The disease has a variety of manifestations, ranging from a mild illness indistinguishable from a viral illness to a progressive multiorgan disease leading to respiratory failure and death. The lungs are involved in the majority of cases. Skin lesions and geni-tourinary tract disease are also common. Skin lesions can be ulcerating nodules, subcutaneous nodules, or papulopustular lesions. Lesions tend to be pyogenic and provide material for microbiological analysis. Arthralgias and myalgias often accom-pany the disease, and bone involvement is common.

Course/Prognosis/Complications: Patients with progressive, severe disease may go on to have CNS disease or ARDS. Patients treated with amphotericin B or itraconazole have an 80–90% cure rate if they are compliant with therapy. If respiratory failure occurs, mortality can be 50% or greater.

Imaging: Nonspecific, usually that of an acute, dense pulmonary infiltrate.

Diagnosis: This disease should be suspected when there is a presenta-tion of pulmonary infiltrates and skin nodules; the presence of GU disease as well should raise the suspicion. Another common scenario is that of what appears to be a "typical" pneumonia that is not responding to therapy. Residence or travel in an endemic area is necessary. Differential diagnosis includes other primary pathogen fungi and the *Nocardia*, actinomycosis, and *Rhodococcus* family. If the disease is limited to the lungs, resistant pyogenic bacteria may cause a similar picture. Diagnosis is made from identification of the organism in sputum or skin lesions, either on smear or culture.

Laboratory: Nonspecific. Yeast forms may be seen in the sputum, urine, or skin lesions. WBC count will be elevated. Skin testing is of little or no value. Definitive diagnosis is made from culture (at room temperature, to encourage the mycelial form which is easier to grow and identify).

Treatment: Some cases are self-limited (the mild, viral syndromelike variant) and require no treatment. More serious cases require therapy with an azole (itraconazole is favored, 200–400 mg/day for at least 2 months). Patients with CNS infection, who are immunocompromised, or who have life-threatening illness should be treated with amphotericin B with a cumulative dose of 1.5–2.5 grams.

Coccidioidomycosis

J Clin Microbiol 2007;45:26, N Engl J Med 1995;332:1077, Clin Infect Dis 2005;41:1217

Epidemiology: This fungus lives in the soil of the southwest United States and northern Mexico (Sonoran Plateau). Some authors feel that geographic distribution of the illness may be more widespread. Probability of infection is ~3%/year with residence in an endemic area.

Pathogenesis: Inhalation of fungus leads to replication of the organism(s) with primary infection. A large number of patients do not become sufficiently ill to require medical care. Early illness ("Valley Fever") may last 2–8 weeks with fever, arthralgias, and cough. There appears to be a prominent immune response, with some patients having erythema nodosum. Most patients resolve this illness without difficulty. A small percentage will have persistent pulmonary abnormalities such as nodules and thin-walled cavities, which may require evaluation. Some thin-walled cavities may go on to rupture and create a bronchopleural fistula, but most resolve within 2 years. Other patients will go on to have fibrocavitary disease, which requires treatment. Patients who are immune compromised or pregnant may go on to have disseminated disease both in the lung and in extrapulmonary sites such as lymph nodes, skin, and CNS.

Symptoms: Valley Fever is a mild subacute illness with fevers, cough, and arthritis. This is a self-limited illness. Residual nodules are generally asymptomatic. Patients with thin-walled cysts are also asymptomatic. Rupture into a pleural space will produce signs and symptoms typical of a pneumothorax. Chronic fibrocavitary disease is typical of chronic granulomatous infection with fever, cough, weight loss, and constitutional symptoms. Patients with disseminated disease may be ill with a disseminated reticulonodular pneumonia with an X-ray appearance similar to PCJ. Skin lesions, adenopathy, and meningitis may also be seen.

Course/Prognosis/Complications: Prognosis of primary disease and pulmonary sequelae in normal hosts is good. Fibrocavitary disease responds satisfactorily to treatment. The feared complication is dissemination, which carries a high mortality.

Imaging: Valley Fever may have no findings or nonspecific areas of consolidation. Pulmonary nodules are large, close to the pleural surface, and often single. Thin-walled cavities may have very thin walls, often are single, and also are close to the pleural surface. Fibrocavitary disease is a mixture of infiltrate, scarring, and cavitation. The appearance may be similar to TB. Disseminated pulmonary coccidioidomycosis will have a reticulonodular pattern that is indistinguishable from PCJ.

Laboratory: Conclusive diagnosis depends upon identification of the organism by culture, identification in tissues, or use of serologic means. Some patients may have an associated eosinophilia.

Diagnosis: Suspicion for coccidioidomycosis will be present in endemic areas. Southern California clinicians will recognize Valley Fever readily. Patients from endemic areas with thin-walled cysts, nodules, or fibrocavitary disease should raise suspicion for this illness. Malignancy and tuberculosis may be among the alternative diagnoses. For Valley Fever, typical pneumonia is an alternative diagnosis. Immunocompromised patients may be more difficult to diagnose, and the close clinical appearance of disseminated pulmonary coccidioidomycosis and PCJ pneumonia is reason not to provide empiric PCJ therapy to patients with AIDS. Definitive diagnosis relies on laboratory methods described below.

Treatment: Valley Fever generally does not need treatment, and thin-walled cysts also do not require treatment. Nodules require diagnosis and observation to distinguish from malignancy; use the solitary pulmonary nodule algorithm (see **Solitary Pulmonary Nodule**) including old chest films and CT/PET/biopsy/excision when appropriate. Bronchopulmonary fistula may require excision of the cyst to achieve closure of the fistula. Treatment of fibrocavitary disease, severely symptomatic Valley Fever, and disseminated disease is usually accomplished with a member of the azole family. Treatment of fibrocavitary disease is generally for 1 year. Fluconazole appears to be favored.

Histoplasmosis

Semin Respir Crit Care Med 2004;25:129, Am Rev Respir Dis 1978;117:929, Medicine (Baltimore), 1988;67:295, Medicine (Baltimore) 2007;86:162

Epidemiology: Histoplasmosis is distributed worldwide. There is a pattern of geographic distribution in the United States with large number of cases in the Ohio River valley and the Midwest. There is also a band of activity that corresponds with the St. Lawrence valley in the United States and Canada. Internationally, the disease is seen in South and Central America. It is estimated that over 50,000,000 persons in the United States have been infected, and that approximately half a million new cases accumulate each year. Certain occupations, such as chicken farming, and hobbies, such as caving, carry a high risk of exposure.

Pathogenesis: Infection is caused by inhalation of fungus *Histoplasma capsulatum*. In cases of low inoculum, infection may be clinically inapparent as the organism disseminates throughout the body. As cellular immunity develops in 10–14 days after exposure, the organism is contained. The patient may appear as though they have a somewhat atypical URI. Immune-competent patients who inhale a large organism load may become acutely ill with abnormal chest X-rays, dyspnea, and even respiratory failure. Progressive histoplasmosis is uncommon in immune-competent patients, generally described as occurring in <5% of exposed individuals. In patients with underlying lung disease, the patient may develop chronic histoplasmosis with chronic infiltrates and cavitation. Inflammation of mediastinal lymph nodes is common and can lead to serious complications. Patients who lack T-cell immunity, such as patients who are HIV+, have undergone transplant, are on corticosteroids, or are receiving anti-TNF therapies, can rapidly disseminate the infection with pulmonary, hepatic, splenic, and CNS disease as well as skin disease. Some patients may progress to respiratory failure and death. Severe illness may occur either immediately after infection or may be delayed for months or years.

Symptoms: Symptoms associated with low-inoculum disease may be nonspecific and include headache, malaise, anorexia, and cough. Patients with large-inoculum disease may have severe dyspnea and may progress to respiratory failure. Chronic illness in otherwise immune-competent hosts may have a clinical course indistinguishable from tuberculosis with chronic cough, inanition, hemoptysis, and progressive respiratory compromise. Patients may have mediastinal disease, pericarditis, and arthritic complaints as well. Immunocompromised patients with disseminated histoplasmosis can have pancytopenia, hepatosplenomegaly, and skin and oral lesions. A subgroup of patients may progress to a SIRS-like picture with respiratory failure, shock, and death despite antifungal treatment.

Course/Prognosis/Complications: Acute disease in healthy patients carries an excellent prognosis. Mortality of 50% or greater can be seen in patients with disseminated disease who are not treated (Rx reduces mortality to 25%). In addition to destruction of pulmonary tissue, a significant complication of histoplasmosis is mediastinal disease. Mediastinal granuloma denotes a condition of multiple enlarged lymph nodes with caseous breakdown; symptoms occur from compression of surrounding mediastinal structures. Fibrosing mediastinitis describes the progressive fibrosis of mediastinal structures with constriction and obstruction of blood vessels, airways, and esophagus as well as pericarditis. Fibrosing mediastinitis is a difficult condition to treat with a poor prognosis.

Imaging: May vary from nonspecific infiltrates to cavities to miliary pattern. Patients may also have pleural effusions. Mediastinal and hilar lymphadenopathy is a prominent finding.

Lab Findings: Skin testing, similar in execution to Mantoux testing, has value primarily as an epidemiologic tool. A positive skin test does not predict active disease. Recovery of organisms (either through culture or tissue staining) of biopsy material is considered diagnostic. Positive serology, such as complement fixation or immunodiffusion, is also considered diagnostic. Antigen detection in urine, blood, or BAL/airway secretions has some value as well.

Diagnosis: Histoplasmosis should be considered in patients in endemic regions when they have a clinical appearance similar to that of reactivation TB (chronic upper lobe cavitation) but negative skin testing; in patients with pulmonary infiltrates and hilar/mediastinal adenopathy; sarcoid-like picture (one of the reasons for not making a presumptive diagnosis of sarcoidosis and for staining tissue for fungi at biopsy). If there is heavy mediastinal involvement, the patient may have severe dyspnea, superior vena cava syndrome, or esophageal stricture. Conclusive diagnosis is laboratory based, as described below.

Treatment: Patients with low-inoculum disease do not need treatment, and fewer than 5% go on to chronic illness. Patients with heavy-inoculum disease will often clear their infection, but be miserable. These patients are usually treated. Chronic illness should be treated, and disseminated disease must be treated urgently. Patients capable of oral intake may be treated with itraconazole; higher initial serum levels may be achieved with IV itraconazole. Severely ill patients should be treated with amphotericin or one of its lipid derivatives. Acute disease should be treated for 6–12 weeks. Chronic disease should be treated for 18–24 months. Experts recommend that disseminated disease be treated for 6–12 months. There may be a role for chronic suppressive therapy in patients who do not reconstitute their immune system (Clin Infect Dis 2007;45:807).

Opportunistic Fungal Infections

Introduction: Although not as common as bacterial infections, fungal infections are a serious consequence of immune incompetence. Many fungi may cause severe, invasive infections in patients with compromised immune status. Four representative organisms are presented. Primary candidal pneumonia is uncommon but can be associated with systemic candidiasis. Mucormycosis is an aggressive illness with high mortality. *Aspergillus* is an interesting infection in that three clinical presentations may be seen: invasive aspergillosis, mycetoma, and allergic bronchopulmonary aspergillosis. While many persons are exposed to *Cryptococcus*, the illness is rarely serious in immune-competent patients. In immunocompromised patients, however, the disease may be life threatening and difficult to eradicate.

Candida

Several different species of *Candida* cause human infection, including C. *albicans*, C. *glabrata*, and C. *tropicalis*. Blood-borne infections are seen in patients receiving parenteral nutrition and who are immunocompromised from malignancy, chemotherapy, or other forms of immunosuppression. Concomitant use of antibiotics increases risk of candidal infection, as do large open wounds such as burns. Patients with suppression of cellular immunity are prone to these infections, and invasive candidal esophagitis is an AIDS-defining illness in HIV+ patients. Catheter-related sepsis is commonly associated with candidal species. The diagnosis of candidal *infection* as opposed to *colonization* can be difficult. Candidal species are resident in the oropharynx and in the lower airway of intubated patients, as well as skin, wounds, and urinary catheters in patients with severe systemic illness. Use of antibacterial antibiotics increases the risk of candidal colonization. Thus, recovery of *Candida*, from sputum or bronchial aspirates is not *prima facie* evidence of pneumonia, and most infectious disease authorities feel that *Candida*, must be isolated from at least two body sites with appropriate supporting evidence of an infectious illness; the single exception is recovery of *Candida*, from the bloodstream. Conclusive diagnosis of candidal pneumonia is thus difficult in the absence of a tissue specimen showing invasive infection. As stated in the introduction, primary candidal pneumonia is rare. Pulmonary involvement as a component of systemic infection is more common. X-ray appearance is nonspecific. *Candida*, like other fungal infections, may create a halo sign on CT with an area of ground glass attenuation surrounding a denser infiltrate. Treatment of candidal disease has become complex as resistant strains of candidal species emerge. Fluconazole, the old standby, has become less effective, and newer agents, such as the echinocandins and other azoles (such as voriconazole and posoconazole), are used as first-line agents with greater frequency. Amphotericin and its lipid derivatives remain effective. Sensitivity patterns vary among medical centers. Knowledge of local ecology is necessary for good antifungal choices. Overall, systemic candidiasis is associated with a high mortality. As with other infections in immunocompromised hosts, cure and survival depends most on reconstitution of the patient's immunocompetence. High-risk populations, such as solid organ transplant recipients, may receive prophylactic antifungal therapy (Medicine [Baltimore] 1993;72:137, Clin Infect Dis 2002;34:400, Clin Infect Dis 2004;38:161).

Mucormycosis

Mucormycosis is an aggressive, invasive infection seen in patients with immune compromise. Patients with iron overload or receiving desferoxamine are also at high risk. The organisms are ubiquitous in the environment, and spores are constantly inhaled. When the patient's immune system fails, this rapidly growing organism causes tissue infarction by vascular invasion. The most aggressive infection is rhinocerebral infection, which has a high mortality. Patients who develop pulmonary infection have tissue destruction, infarction, and invasion of mediastinal structures by the infection. Diagnosis may be difficult because mucor infection will not be the clinician's first thought when presented with an aggressive pneumonia, and the organism does not have a signature X-ray pattern. Recovery of characteristic hyphae from bronchial specimens is inconsistent. Therapy *requires* debridement, and amphotericin is felt to be adjunctive at best (Arch Intern Med 1999;159:1301).

Aspergillosis

This organism is widely distributed in the environment and is not a problem for immune-competent individuals. However, any failure of the immune system may increase the risk of infection. Unlike the previous two fungi, failure of the immune system may include structural abnormalities of the lung and/or mucosal abnormalities of the airways. *Invasive aspergillosis* is the most feared complication with tissue invasion and infarction. This is often seen in the context of severe neutropenia such as that seen in the treatment of hematopoeitic malignancy and transplantation. The patient is severely ill with *Aspergillus* recoverable from bronchial secretions. X-ray appearance can include dense pneumonia with cavitation. Rarely, tracheobronchial ulceration may occur. Pulmonary aspergillosis can be seen in the context of disseminated aspergillosis with hematogenous spread of disease in the liver, spleen, brain, and kidneys. The mortality for this illness is high, with rates of 50–70% mortality even without disseminated disease. Most authorities recommend treatment with amphotericin or one of its lipid derivatives (e.g., liposomal preparations) although some of the newer azoles such as voriconazole or itraconazole also have activity against invasive disease. Recovery is contingent upon reconstitution of the patient's immune system. Some patients at high risk for infection, such as lung transplant recipients, may receive prophylaxis with itraconazole (Am J Respir Crit Care Med 2006;173:707). *Mycetoma* or alternatively *aspergilloma* refers to a ball of *Aspergillus* that resides in an otherwise sterile cavity from old tuberculosis or sarcoid. Other etiologies of chronic cavities may also be colonized. The fungus ball is not invasive but may erode the walls of the cavity causing hemoptysis, occasionally massive. An exposed pulmonary artery in an old TB cavity (Rasmussen's aneurysm) is particularly vulnerable. When visible on chest X-ray or CT scan, there is a "crescent moon" sign with a filling defect within a cavity, the remaining cavity forming the crescent. If the patient's position is changed, the ball may roll within the cavity. There can be focal areas of invasion as well within the cavity wall. Treatment is undertaken for recurrent large-scale hemoptysis. This usually consists of surgical resection of the cavity. Some authorities have used itraconazole or intracavitary amphotericin B with varying degrees of success (Kekkaku 1997;72:557, Arch Intern Med 1983;143:303, Ann Thorac Surg

1992;54:1159). *Allergic bronchopulmonary aspergillosis* is a condition where there is chronic colonization of abnormal airways with *Aspergillus*. This occurs in patients with bronchiectasis, cystic fibrosis, and asthma. Here, the pathology is one of inciting an allergic inflammatory response rather than aggressive tissue invasion. These patients present with increasingly refractory reactive airways disease and may cough up brown "cigar plugs," Chest X-ray may show proximal bronchial plugging and atelectasis. Laboratory abnormalities include positive prick or skin tests for *Aspergillus*, the presence of *Aspergillus* precipitins, blood eosinophilia, and an elevated IgE level. Treatment has been directed at interrupting the allergic response with steroids, and this works well. More recent therapy includes attempts to suppress the *Aspergillus* organism load with an oral antifungal such as itraconazole (fluconazole has no activity against *Aspergillus*) (Mayo Clin Proc 2001;76:930, N Engl J Med 2000;342:756).

Cryptococcus

Cryptococcal exposure is common with a majority of children demonstrating evidence of exposure. The lung is the portal of entry for the organism, and the infection is quickly controlled in the vast majority of immune-competent individuals. In a minority of patients, symptomatic cryptococcal infection may be seen, with the X-ray appearance usually that of noncalcified nodules. Organisms may be recovered from tissue (although not necessarily on culture) or from BAL fluid. Unless there is evidence of systemic spread, some authorities elect not to treat these patients as it is often a self-limited illness. When treatment is required, usually because of symptoms (cough, sputum, chest pain, hemoptysis, constitutional symptoms), fluconazole is safe and effective. Cryptococcal disease is more aggressive in immunocompromised patients and may be associated with CNS involvement, notoriously in HIV+ patients. There appears to be a difference in presentation between patients who are immunocompromised from HIV disease and those who have malignancy or transplantation. The non-HIV group has symptoms similar to those seen in the immune-competent group, while the HIV+ group is acutely ill with high fever, hypoxia, and diffuse pulmonary infiltrates. Concomitant CNS illness is the rule rather than the exception. Diagnosis may be from tissue samples, BAL fluid, or cryptococcal antigen detected in the blood and/or CNS. When treating the patient with possible cryptococcosis who is HIV+, there should also be evaluation for the presence of concomitant opportunistic infections. Treatment is complex with initial use of amphotericin and flucytosine, followed by long-term (some say indefinite) fluconazole first at treatment then at maintenance doses (Scand J Infect Dis 2006;38:788, Rev Infect Dis 1991; 13:64, Clin Infect Dis 2000;30:710).

5.15 HIV and the Lung

Thorax 2003;58:721; J Thorac Imaging 1998;13:247; Curr Opin Pulm Med 2005;11:203; Curr Opin Pulm Med 2005;11:208; Am J Respir Crit Care Med 1997;155:72

Epidemiology: The lung is a common target of infectious and noninfectious complications of HIV/AIDS. Pulmonary illnesses that occur in HIV-infected patients depend upon the degree of immune deficiency, use of HAART, geographic location, socioeconomic status, and use of prophylactic regimens for various specific illnesses. All of these factors should be taken into account when evaluating the patient. HAART has changed the presentation of illness and has made empiric therapy unreliable because as it has changed the course of the illness, it has changed the frequency of some opportunistic infections at a given stage of disease. It is unlikely that a patient will have disseminated blastomycosis, histoplasmosis, or coccidioidomycosis unless they live in an endemic area. TB is much more prevalent in African patients with AIDS. Patients with early-, intermediate-, advanced-, and late-stage illness have susceptibilities to different infections; PCJ is uncommon in patients with a CD4 count >200. Patients who have been in prison or homeless shelters have a higher incidence of tuberculosis, and patients who have taken inhaled pentamidine for PCJ prophylaxis may have an unusual X-ray presentation of PCJ disease.

Pathophysiology: Manifestations of disease are an interaction between host inflammatory response and the infection, tumor, etc. Alterations in immune response will cause atypical or severe presentations of common illnesses, and permit pathogens with limited virulence in the presence of a normal immune system to thrive in the HIV-infected patient. The surveillance function of the immune system is compromised. Proliferating lines of potentially malignant cells are not destroyed, and high rates of malignancy are seen in these patients. As natural balances between components of the host's immune system are disrupted, some inflammatory states may progress unimpeded.

Symptoms: There are no special symptoms associated with pulmonary illness in this population. Cough, fever, sputum, and dyspnea are the presenting complaints. Chest pain can occur with pleural inflammation. Hemoptysis can occur with tissue/vessel destruction. Constitutional symptoms are common. Adenopathy may be present depending on the illness. Skin lesions may be seen with various fungal and viral illnesses. Duration of illness may help predict etiology as well. Ocular findings may be present with some fungal infections.

Course/Prognosis/Complications: See individual disease articles. Reconstitution of the immune system with HAART can cause a temporary worsening (sometimes severe) of the patient's condition as the inflammatory response becomes more appropriate (immune reconstitution syndrome).

Imaging: A variety of X-ray and CT abnormalities are possible. See differential diagnosis.

Laboratory: A variety of laboratory abnormalities are possible. See differential diagnosis. The first step for etiologic diagnosis is an attempt to obtain a sputum or bronchoscopic specimen. PCJ can be identified in induced, expectorated sputum ~50% with low sensitivity and high specificity. PCJ can be identified in BAL fluid ~95% or greater, and TBLB is rarely needed for this diagnosis. Viral and bacterial illnesses often can be diagnosed from BAL fluid as well. Some noninfectious etiologies can be identified with minimally invasive techniques (bronchoscopy, TTNB) but may require surgical lung biopsy. Antigen testing is of limited value except for histoplasmosis and *Cryptococcus*. Older studies discuss the usefulness of elevated LDH levels associated with PCJ, blood gas abnormalities, and pulmonary function abnormalities. These are probably less relevant as the diagnostic issues have become better defined.

Diagnosis: Three concepts govern the initial treatment of HIV+ patients with pulmonary disease:

1. Empiric therapy for opportunistic infection, except in unusual circumstances, is not appropriate. (This does not apply to obvious bacterial pneumonia.) In the pre-HAART era in the United States, PCJ was so much more common relative to other illnesses that empiric therapy for PCJ was justified in the patient presenting with acute or subacute diffuse infiltrates. In the present, HAART has caused an equalization of disease incidence, and any number of HIV/AIDS infections may be possible and have similar clinical and X-ray appearances. Additionally, the first diagnosis of PCJ is an AIDS-defining illness and changes prognosis and treatment. In light of the impact of the illness, the patient should have a definite, not presumed, diagnosis.

2. Chest X-ray changes, even in the absence of symptoms, warrant vigorous evaluation.

3. New infiltrates should be considered infectious until proven otherwise.

Bacterial bronchitis and pneumonia commonly occur at all stages of HIV/AIDS disease. X-ray appearance is that of a single area or multiple consolidated areas. Common pathogens include

S. pneumoniae, H. influenzae, S. aureus, K. pneumoniae, and *P. aeruginosa.* Most authorities recommend that HCAP, rather CAP guidelines should be followed for empiric treatment. Less common, but significant pathogens include *Nocardia* species and *Rhodococcus.* These patients will have prostration, fever, cough, sputum, dyspnea, and sometimes chest pain. Presentation is usually abrupt.

As referenced earlier, PCJ is a common infection. "Typical" presentation is that of a fine nodular, almost granular appearing chest X-ray in association with dyspnea, dry cough, and fever over weeks. Alternative scenarios are possible with nodules, cysts, and upper lung zone predominant diffuse parenchymal disease possible (the latter especially with inhaled pentamidine prophylaxis). Approximately 25% of patients may have a normal X-ray but an abnormal CT scan.

Tuberculosis and atypical mycobacteria have a variety of presentations. Areas of consolidation and/or cavitation may be seen. "Typical" reactivation TB pattern on X-ray is many times not seen and the suspicion for TB must remain high even when this pattern is absent. Mantoux testing may be unreliable because of immune deficits. In the appropriate populations (homeless, prisoners, IVDU, Africans in Africa) this diagnosis must be actively excluded to prevent contagion and prevention of MDRTB.

A variety of viral illnesses are encountered in this population, including influenza, CMV, and *Herpes* (simplex and zoster). Chest X-ray will demonstrate diffuse interstitial changes.

Fungal illnesses include *Cryptococcus,* histoplasmosis, *Aspergillus,* blastomycosis, and coccidioidomycosis. Cavitating (or noncavitating) infiltrates and nodules are all seen. Diffuse parenchymal lung disease is also possible. These patients may have a variety of presenting complaints.

Parasitic infections include toxoplasmosis, leishmaniasis, and strongyloides.

Noninfectious problems include malignancy, inflammatory states, and structural parenchymal changes. Lung cancer and non-Hodgkin's lymphoma are frequent and lymphoma may present as a pulmonary infiltrate. Kaposi's sarcoma, a herpesvirus-related malignancy, may present as nodules. At bronchoscopy, typical sarcoma lesions may be seen in the airway. Both lymphocytic interstitial pneumonitis, a rare condition in normal hosts, and COP/BOOP can be seen in HIV/AIDS patients. Cyst formation as a consequence of infection and primary emphysematous changes in the lung has been identified.

Pleural disease is usually associated with a primary pulmonary problem such as pneumonia or TB. Body cavity lymphoma, an unusual AIDS-related lymphoma, can be seen primarily in the pleural space. Pneumothorax as a consequence of PCJ has been recognized.

Therapy is based on accurate diagnosis, which in turn often requires a minimally invasive or invasive procedure. The precise approach to lung sampling is a technical decision that rests upon the opinions and competencies of the pulmonary physicians, infectious disease physicians, surgeons, and radiologists. Primary clinicians will play an important role providing context for these discussions and coordinating the overall direction and intensity of care. Empiric treatment should be avoided unless the patient is felt to have an acute bacterial pneumonia. In that case, the ATS/IDSA guidelines for pneumonia in the abnormal host should be followed. A sputum sample should still be pursued. If there is greater concern for an opportunistic infection, the patient should undergo bronchoscopy with BAL, with or without TBLB. The incremental yield of TBLB probably will be limited. Rapid mycobacterial, PCJ, and fungal stains are available, and a cytologist can identify viral "footprints" readily. Nodules and dense consolidations lend themselves to TTNA with cytologic and microbiological analysis. If no diagnosis is forthcoming, or the patient is worsening despite therapy, surgical lung biopsy may be indicated. Both VATS and OLB procedures are safe, with VATS having a shorter recovery time. Pleural effusions should be sampled (and drained if possible) and analyzed so as to further diagnostic yield, determine need for drainage of empyema, and to define extent of disease.

Treatment: See individual disease articles. Treatment is also based on reconstitution of the immune system (with HAART) if feasible.

5.16 Parasitic Lung Disease

Higher complexity organisms can infect the lung. These include helminths and complex single-cell organisms such as amoebae and malaria. These infections are uncommon in North America. However, immigrants, travelers, and returning military personnel may present with parasitic infections and the practitioner must be alert to unusual infections, especially in these risk groups.

Injury to the host occurs from direct attack by the parasite or by immune response, often a Type I (IgE-mediated) hypersensitivity. A general overview of tropical lung disease (including parasitic lung disease) is in the June 2002 issue of *Clinics in Chest Medicine* and in Curr Opin Pulm Med 2006;12:212. Tropical pulmonary eosinophilia and Loeffler's syndrome are reviewed in **Eosinophilic Lung Disease.**

Roundworm

Includes *Ascaris* and *Toxocara* species, found worldwide. These worms have a complex life cycle, part of which includes residence in the lungs. Eosinophilia, fever, cough, and pulmonary infiltrates are the most common pulmonary manifestations. The presence of eosinophilia and pulmonary infiltrates is the indicator to assess the patient for these infestations. These are benign conditions that are usually self-limited. The patient is treated to prevent nonpulmonary complications (N Engl J Med 1972;286:965).

Hookworm

Strongyloides stercoralis is the prototypical agent for this group, and distribution is worldwide in tropical and subtropical regions. It can be seen in the southeastern United States. Cough, fever, and pulmonary infiltrates in the presence of eosinophilia suggest hookworm infection. Disseminated disease with autoinfection may produce a syndrome of hyperinfection resulting in a SIRS-like picture. Immune-incompetent patients are at risk for this complication (Chest 1990;97:1475). Current therapy for this condition is ivermectin.

Microfilaria

See **Eosinophilic Lung Disease.**

Trematodes

Schistosomiasis and paragonimiasis are the two major offenders in this category. Schistosomiasis does not affect the lung until there is a heavy portal circulation burden of disease. In this setting, eggs may lodge in the pulmonary arterioles and form pulmonary endarteritis with pulmonary hypertension. Dyspnea is the primary manifestation, and a fine, miliary pattern of nodules may be seen on X-ray. Physiologic changes are usually irreversible. There may also be involvement of the lung in Katayama syndrome, a form of acute schistosomiasis. Some authors feel that pulmonary involvement in schistosomiasis has been underemphasized and/or underrecognized in the past (Lancet Infect Dis 2007;7:218, Clin Chest Med 2002;23:433). Paragonimiasis is a chronic trematode infection that may be clinically indistinguishable from tuberculosis. Cough, hemoptysis, fever associated with pleural disease, cavitary disease, and infiltrative/nodular disease is described. Diagnosis depends upon an appropriate level of suspicion for the infection (travel history) and the identification of eggs in feces or sputum. Praziquantel is an effective treatment (Clin Chest Med 2002;23:421, Clin Chest Med 2002;23:409).

Echinococcus

Echinococcus granulosus is a primarily tropical/subtropical tapeworm with humans representing an anomalous host. This species is responsible for hydatid cyst disease, where the larvae form cysts in the lungs and liver. Symptoms may be caused by direct destruction of tissue by cyst expansion, or by cyst rupture with a severe hypersensitivity reaction, which can be fatal. Treatment is surgical removal, with care exercised not to rupture the cyst(s) during removal from the host. *Echinococcus multilocularis* is seen in temperate climates. Humans are accidental hosts. The multilocularis organism forms masses of fibrous inflammatory tissue containing larvae. On X-ray, evidence of calcification is prominent. These masses are often asymptomatic until growth of the mass causes organ dysfunction. Treatment is surgical, and an aggressive, "cancer surgery" approach to excision is recommended (Clin Chest Med 2002;23:397).

Amebiasis

Entamoeba histolytica is a common illness responsible for a large number of deaths globally. Infection is from ingestion of contaminated food or water. Invasive intestinal disease leads to systemic disease with hematogenous spread to the lungs an uncommon source of pulmonary involvement. A more common source of pulmonary involvement occurs when a liver abscess ruptures into the pleural space. This can lead to parenchymal lung involvement and formation of bronchial-pleural-biliary fistulas. The "classic" clinical finding in this illness is "anchovy sauce" sputum. Metronidazole is the treatment of choice (Clin Chest Med 2002;23:479).

Malaria

The biology, diagnosis, and treatment of malaria are well beyond the scope of this article. Pulmonary malaria is very rare. However, noncardiogenic pulmonary edema in severe and complicated falciparum disease may reach the 10–30% range. Supportive treatment for ARDS and aggressive treatment of the underlying malarial infection are required for survival (Clin Chest Med 2002;23:457).

Chapter 6
Pulmonary Malignancy

6.1 Bronchogenic Carcinoma

Chest, September 2007 Supplement: Diagnosis and Management of Lung Cancer: ACCP Evidence-Based Clinical Practice Guidelines (2nd ed.) is highly recommended.

Epidemiology: Lung cancer, like COPD, is a largely preventable illness and is one of the medical tragedies of the last 50 years. Epidemiologic trends in lung cancer have changed over the last several decades as tobacco marketing and smoking cessation programs have had their impact. Smoking cessation and prevention programs have been successful in middle-class white men; incidence of lung cancer and COPD has dropped sharply in this group. Lung cancer, which used to be a disease of middle-aged, middle-class white men, has become more of an equal opportunity killer as targeted minority marketing and marketing to women has leveled the playing field. Blue collar and lower-class sectors of society continue to have greater cultural tolerance for smoking than do middle-class and upper-class groups. Tobacco use in developing countries occurs at a very high rate. As these populations age, chronic lung disease and lung cancer will become severe public health problems. In the United States (2003 figures) respiratory tract cancer incidence was 73/100,000 for whites and 79/100,000 for blacks. Rates for Native Americans, Asians, and Hispanic populations were approximately half that rate. Overall US incidence was 73/100,000. Death rate was very high (indicating a highly lethal disease) of 56/100,000 and 64/100,000 respectively for whites and blacks (http://apps. nccd.cdc.gov/uscs/Table.aspx?Group=TableAll&Year= 2003&Display=n 2003;2007). Although female breast cancer remains the most common invasive malignancy (excluding skin cancers), lung cancer is the most lethal. Lung cancer in the United States is seen almost exclusively in smokers or ex-smokers. A small portion of patients may trace the etiology of their cancer to other carcinogenic exposures such as radon, environmental tobacco smoke, and uranium mining. Asbestos exposure also leads to increased risk for lung cancer and is a synergistic risk factor when coupled with smoking. Diseases that cause pulmonary fibrosis, such as scleroderma, are also associated with higher risks of lung cancer.

Pathogenesis: The interplay of host and environmental factors that cause chromosomal deletion and inactivation of tumor suppressor genes is at the first stages of investigation. Murray and Nadel, 2005, p. 1311 offer a good introduction to the biology of lung cancer. Common lung cancers include adenocarcinoma, squamous cell carcinoma, large cell undifferentiated carcinoma, and small cell carcinoma. At present, adenocarcinoma is the most common histopathology, accounting for 30–40% of lesions. Squamous cell cancer used to be most common, but has been overtaken by adenocarcinoma. Large cell undifferentiated is a large cell histology that cannot be differentiated as to squamous or glandular origin. Small cell cancer arises from neuroendocrine cell lines and has a faster growth rate. It is much more aggressive with a poorer prognosis. In current treatment planning, there is less emphasis placed upon distinguishing between squamous, adenocarcinoma, and large cell varieties; the primary distinction is between small cell or nonsmall cell. As a lung cancer grows, it can have a variety of symptoms and effects depending upon the location and biology of the tumor:

1. Behave as a space-occupying lesion. Injury to the host occurs by compression of normal structures, e.g., superior vena cava syndrome or compression of the recurrent laryngeal nerve resulting in hoarseness.
2. Invade normal tissue, causing direct tissue damage such as erosion of bones, and blood vessels, producing pain and bleeding. Invasion of the pleura or pericardium can cause pleural or pericardial effusions respectively.
3. Block airways, causing pneumonia, cough, and respiratory distress.
4. Produce biologically active chemicals producing paraneo-plastic syndromes such as SIADH, hypertrophic pulmonary osteoarthropathy, and hypercalcemia. Lung cancer also causes a wasting illness with weight loss and fatigue. The mechanism of this effect is not known.
5. Metastasize, causing damage in remote locations. Liver, adrenals, brain, and bone are common sites of extratho-racic disease.

Lung cancer starts as a small focus of abnormal cells; occasionally there may be two or more synchronous tumors. Tumors have a prolonged quiescent or slow growth phase. Patients may be asymptomatic from the cancer during that period. As the tumor enters a rapid growth phase, symptoms occur (with specific symptoms depending upon anatomic site of disease). Often, by the time symptoms are recognized by the patient, the tumor has grown and/or spread to such a degree that cure is difficult or impossible.

Symptoms: The most common symptom is cough, often associated with sputum. Hemoptysis and dyspnea are also common. Unilateral wheezing is less common, but is a potential indicator of bronchial obstruction. Patients when questioned may report loss of energy, fatigue, and weight loss. Patients with cancer may have an initial appearance similar to pneumonia; lung cancer is one of the major points of differential diagnosis for nonresolving pneumonia (see **Nonresolving Pneumonia**). Chest pain or arm pain, as a result of chest wall invasion, pleural invasion, or brachial plexus invasion is less common, but must be investigated. Hoarseness may occur as a consequence of recurrent laryngeal nerve injury. Clubbing and joint pain (hypertrophic pulmonary osteoarthropathy) are unreliable findings but can be dramatic when present. Occasionally, patients may have their cancer detected because of extrapulmonary manifestations of metastasis. In my experience, severe bone pain and neurologic changes of brain metastasis are most common in this category. Superior vena cava syndrome with edema and venous prominence of the face, neck, and arm(s) is a radiation oncology emergency and requires prompt confirmation and intervention. Rarely, patients may present with a neurologic or metabolic abnormality such as a myasthenia gravis type picture (Eaton-Lambert syndrome), hyponatremia (syndrome of inappropriate ADH, SIADH), or hypercalcemia. Findings on examination span the spectrum of a healthy-appearing patient with a normal exam, shocked to hear the diagnosis to a haggard, worn-out dyspneic patient coughing up blood. Most patients are somewhere in between. Patients who present for evaluation because of symptoms may have weight loss (ask about changes in fit of clothes, taking in a notch on a belt, etc.) and may complain of feeling run down. Even in this setting, examination may be normal. Subtle areas of bronchial breath sounds or reduced breath sounds, unilateral wheezing, and dullness to percussion are inconsistently present, even in the presence of significant X-ray abnormalities. Identification of cervical and supraclavicular adenopathy can define extent of disease and a biopsy target. I have found that asking a patient to do a Valsalva maneuver while examining for supraclavicular adenopathy can enhance the detection of small lymph nodes. Normal examination and absence of symptoms provide no reassurance in the face of an abnormal, worrisome chest X-ray. Most curable lung cancers have no symptoms and are detected as the result of an incidental finding on chest X-ray done for other reasons. Don't "follow" these patients just because they feel well.

Course and Prognosis: This is a dismal, difficult disease. Most patients present with stage III or stage IV disease. These patients have a prognosis measured in months to a couple of years. A small percentage (~5–20%) of these patients may go on to have a prolonged complete remission that probably represents cure. The biology of these tumors varies widely, and a minority of patients can have measurable disease with a good quality of life for many years; my personal observation is that this occurs more commonly in the elderly. Patients with stage II disease will have cure rates of ~30%. Patients with Ib disease have a slightly higher cure rate. Patients with Ia disease have cure rates frequently in excess of ~60–70%. It is worth restating that this is, in large part, a preventable disease.

Imaging: X-ray findings associated with bronchogenic carcinoma are diverse. The most common finding is a mass: an area of increased radio-opacity without any lung markings. Borders are usually well circumscribed, or may be stellate or spiculated. Atelectasis and pneumonia-like infiltrate are also common. Bronchoalveolar carcinoma may have a pneumonia-like appearance or circumscribed area of interstitial abnormality. Pleural effusions, cavities, and mediastinal widening can be seen on plain films. Radio-dense single abnormalities surrounded completely by the pulmonary parenchyma are termed *solitary pulmonary nodules* and permit application of an algorithm (see **Solitary Pulmonary Nodule**). CT scanning will confirm the presence of the abnormality, permit precise location and presence of invasion of surrounding structures, determine the presence or absence of subtle abnormalities such as calcification and/or microcavitation, and identify additional abnormalities beyond the resolution of the plain film. Radioactive glucose (FDG) scanning (PET scanning) is discussed in sections below. Many different X-ray and CT appearances can suggest malignancy. It is the responsibility of the clinician to recognize the risk, evaluate the patient, and accept or reject the hypothesis of cancer as an integrated clinical decision. Lung cancer in the presence of a *normal* (i.e., *completely normal*) X-ray is uncommon. Screening is discussed below. Increasing reliance on high-tech imaging procedures has reduced reliance on old baseline films. Comparison of current imaging to previous films is a powerful tool both to reassure and to promote further evaluation. It is worth 20 or 30 minutes with a radiologist and a stack of X-rays to avoid a procedure. The transition in many radiology departments to digital imaging can make it more difficult to compare digital images to older film images. The latter often are now off-site or in a remote part of the organization, requiring "retrieval." Inconvenience notwithstanding, these old studies must be obtained and compared to current films.

Laboratory: There is no test for lung cancer. Several areas of research are evaluating exhaled organic compounds as cancer markers, but no methods are ready for clinical use. Conclusive diagnosis depends upon histopathology or cytology examination of a specimen retrieved from the patient. Lung origin of a mass or nodule can sometimes be an issue, and immunochemical evaluation of the biopsy material can help determine derivation. Common routine laboratory abnormalities associated with lung cancer include anemia, hyponatremia, elevated platelet count, elevated markers of inflammation (ferritin, CRP), and hypercalcemia.

Diagnosis: The diagnosis of lung cancer rests upon the identification of malignant cells retrieved from the patient that are plausibly of lung origin. (Occasionally, this rule may be violated in the very elderly or infirm.) Accurate, rapid diagnosis must be weighed against the risks and costs of imaging and invasive diagnostic and therapeutic procedures. Diagnosis is achieved by manipulating seven basic tools: plain chest X-ray, CT scan, PET scan, bronchoscopy, transthoracic needle biopsy, surgical lung biopsy, and time. Extrathoracic biopsy may sometimes be valuable (obvious liver metastases or extrathoracic adenopathy). Indications for extrathoracic biopsy will usually be self-evident and will not be reviewed here. Patients are stratified into groups based on pretest probability of malignancy. Patients with a high (>50%) pretest probability undergo invasive biopsy promptly, and negative results are presumed to be false negative until proven otherwise. In this group, diagnostic planning primarily addresses technical aspects of specimen procurement and the overall utility of a diagnostic evaluation (see **Treatment,** below). Patients with moderate risk (10–50%) are subjected to maneuvers designed to push the patient into a high-risk category and prompt biopsy or to lower the likelihood of malignancy (e.g., PET scanning, observation of an X-ray abnormality over time). Patients who stratify to a low-risk category (<10%) are reassured. Some of these patients may be subjected to long-term monitoring, usually in the context of the SPN algorithm described in Table 6.1.

With the exception of the solitary pulmonary nodule, there are few formal guidelines to direct risk stratification. Table 6.2 outlines some common clinical scenarios that fall into the three risk groups. This table is not definitive, but tries to give the flavor of various clinical problems. Because solitary pulmonary nodules are common, algorithms have been developed to guide management. See Table 6.1. All decisions regarding invasive procedures should be taken in the context of the patient's suitability for surgery, discussed below in the treatment section. The decision regarding which procedure (bronchoscopy, TTNB, surgical lung biopsy) to use for which patient is usually a joint decision among the pulmonary physician, surgeon, and radiologist. Primary clinicians and patients provide input as to the patient's overall health and philosophy of care.

The clinical problem of lung cancer diagnosis boils down to how much testing to do before doing a biopsy. Much of the decision is still art and based on local skills and preferences. The

Table 6.1   Evaluation and Management of SPN Based on Risk Stratification

Risk	Criteria	Action
Nil	Benign calcification pattern; present on previous images ≥2 years	No further testing, reassure patient
Low	Diameter <1.5 cm Pt age <45 Nonsmoker OR quit >7 years ago Smooth border to lesion	Serial followup CT at 3, 6, 9, 12, 18, 24 months; if change noted proceed to VATS/DS
Intermediate	Diameter 1.5–2.2 cm Pt age 45–60 Smoker (<1 ppd) OR quit <7 yrs ago Scalloped border	Add'l testing: PET, TTNB (if peripheral), bronchoscopy (if air bronchus sign), contrast enhanced hi-res. CT scan. If positive proceed to VATS/DS; if negative serial follow-up CT
High	Diameter ≥2.3 cm Age >60 Current smoker (≥1 ppd) Spiculated border	VATS/DS. TTNB or bronchoscopy if patient not a surgical candidate and diagnosis is still desirable

Note: VATS/DS denotes video-assisted thoracoscopic surgery followed by frozen section and definitive surgery if indicated. Approach to the patient with mixed criteria (e.g., diameter ≥2.3 cm but age <60) is not defined but prudence would dictate defaulting to the higher risk category. Testing suggested in intermediate action plan can be tailored to the needs of the patient and institution. Not all tests need be done. Data from Istm 2003.

capabilities of the local cytology laboratory, pulmonary physician, surgeon, and radiologist have an effect on the outlined recommendations. The division between diagnosis and treatment for bronchogenic carcinoma is arbitrary. Treatment planning is an integral part of diagnosis and will be discussed below.

Screening for lung cancer has been a topic of debate for decades. Recent articles, such as N Engl J Med 2006;355:1763, suggest that a screening strategy using low-dose CT scanning in a high-risk population is effective. This has been challenged by other authors, and, at present, there is no professional society or

Table 6.2 Scenarios of High, Medium, and Low Risk for Pulmonary Malignancy

High Risk	Intermediate Risk	Low Risk
Hemoptysis with abnormal CXR	Hemoptysis with normal CXR	Hemoptysis previously evaluated, in context of hemoptysis-prone illness (e.g., bronchiectasis)
Subacute or chronic cough with infiltrate	Cough w/infiltrate in context of infectious illness (covers most pneumonias)	Cough with normal CXR in context of cough prone illness (e.g., asthma)
Pleural effusion with parenchymal mass and/or wasting illness	Parapneumonic effusion	Waxing and waning pleural effusion in context of CHF
Asymptomatic mass (new or no old films available) in smoker	Stable mass on CXR, <2 years of observation	Stable mass or scarring, >2 years observation
New solitary pulmonary nodule in smoker or older patient	Solitary pulmonary nodule, <2 years of observation	Solitary pulmonary nodule: >2 years observation, or pattern of benign calcification

preventive care task force recommending routine screening for lung cancer, even in high-risk populations. In part, the controversy arises from the high number of false positives generated by the screening process leading to invasive and expensive testing. It is likely that refinement of testing procedures and better definition of target populations will eventually lead to an accepted screening program.

Treatment: Treatment for bronchogenic carcinoma relies on surgery, radiation therapy, chemotherapy, and palliative care. In patients with nonsmall cell disease, surgery *when feasible* offers the best chance for survival. However, many patients with lung cancer often present with disease that is too advanced to benefit from operation. Many of these patients have comorbid conditions such as heart disease and/or COPD that render them inoperable. The practitioners who are the initial point of contact (usually the primary care clinician in concert with the pulmonary physician) must answer three questions: Will the patient benefit from removing the tumor? If so, is the tumor resectable from a technical standpoint? If the tumor is technically resectable, can the patient withstand the operation and removal of lung tissue?

1. Will the patient benefit from removing the tumor?
   Generally, patients with small cell carcinoma do not benefit from surgery, and treatment is based on chemotherapy and radiation. With the exception of patients with very early stage small cell carcinoma (limited stage), surgery is usually not offered to the patient, and patients with that histologic diagnosis depart the NSCLC treatment planning algorithm at the time of diagnosis. Patients with NSCLC are staged according to a lung-specific TNM system as seen in Table 6.3. Patients with NSCLC do not benefit from surgery if there is extrathoracic tumor spread, or intrathoracic metastases. Most authorities agree that NSCLC patients do not benefit from surgical therapy if there is spread of tumor to the contralateral mediastinal lymph nodes (III-b disease). There is debate over the value of surgery for patients with ipsilateral mediastinal lymph node involvement (III-a disease) with some surgical centers offering surgery in conjunction with radiation and chemotherapy, and other centers offering a conservative approach. All authorities agree that surgery may benefit patients with lymph node involvement at the hilar and intrapulmonary stations, and patients without any evidence of nodal involvement. Current staging depends upon CT scanning and PET scanning to evaluate such factors as direct mediastinal invasion, chest wall invasion, extrathoracic disease, and mediastinal lymph node

Table 6.3 TNM Staging of Lung Cancer

Primary Tumor Characteristics	T1	T2	T3	T4
Size Endobronchial location	≤3 cm No invasion proximal to lobar bronchus	>3 cm Main bronchus, ≥2 cm distal to carina	Any size Main bronchus, <2 cm distal to carina	Any size Does not matter
Local invasion	Surrounded by lung or visceral pleura	Visceral pleura	Chest wall, diaphragm, mediastinal pleura, parietal pericardium	Mediastinum Trachea Heart great vessels Esophagus Vertebral body Carina
Other	None	Atelectasis **OR** Obstructive pneumonitis extending to hilum but not involving entire lung	Whole lung atelectasis **OR** Obstructive pneumonitis	Malignant pleural or pericardial effusion **OR** Satellite tumor nodule(s) within the ipsilateral primary-tumor lobe of lung

Note:
T1: Size **AND** location **AND** invasion criteria must all be met.
T2: Size **OR** location **OR** invasion **OR** atelectasis/pneumonitis criteria must be met.
T3: Location **OR** invasion **OR** atelectasis/pneumonitis criteria must be met; size immaterial.
T4: Invasion **OR** effusion **OR** satellite tumor criteria must be met; size immaterial.

(continues)

Table 6.3 (continued)

Node Class.	Supra clavic	Scalene	Contra med.	Ipsi med.	Sub carinal	Contra hilar	Ipsi hilar	Ipsi peribronch.
N0	(–)	(–)	(–)	(–)	(–)	(–)	(–)	(–)
N1	(–)	(–)	(–)	(–)	(–)	(–)	(+)	(+)
N2	(–)	(–)	(–)	(+)	(+)	(–)	DM	DM
N3	(+)	(+)	(+)	DM	DM	(+)	DM	DM

Note: Supra clavic = supraclavicular; contra med. = contralateral mediastinum; ipsi med = ipsilateral mediastinum; contra hilar = contralateral hilar; ipsi hilar = ipsilateral hilar; ipsi peribronch. = ipsilateral peribronchial; DM = does not matter.

Metastases:

M0 = Distant metastases are absent.

M1 = Distant metastases are present. Metastatic tumor nodules within the same lung but not in the same lobe as the primary are considered M1 disease.

Stage	IA	IB	IIA	IIB	IIB	IIIA	IIIB	IV
T status	T1	T2	T1	T2	T3	up to T3	up to T4	any
N status	N0	N0	N1	N1	N0	N2	N2	any
M status	M0	M0	M0	M0	M0	M0	M0	M1

Note: Staging matrix: Note that IIB disease may be defined by T3/N0 or T2/N1. Capitalized, bolded conjunctions are used as logical operators.

involvement. Mediastinal involvement is an area of particular concern because of both false positives and false negatives with respect to CT and PET scanning.

2. Is the tumor resectable from a technical standpoint? The tumor must be separable from the mediastinum and chest wall (there is more leeway with the latter), and the surgeon must be able to develop a cuff to close the bronchus. Tumor at or within 2 cm of the main carina or within the trachea precludes operation.

3. Can the patient withstand the resection of lung tissue and the insult of the operation? Efforts to be precisely inclusive (operate on all patients who can survive the operation and who will have adequate pulmonary postoperative function, and operate on none of the patients who will not) have been extensively researched. Tests including cardiopulmonary exercise testing, pulmonary artery occlusion testing, 6-minute walks, and pulmonary function testing have been used to assess the likelihood of chronic respiratory failure as a consequence of surgery. In a majority of cases, an adequate decision regarding operability can be made on the basis of pulmonary function studies. Some patients may require quantitative lung perfusion scan to help predict postoperative pulmonary function, and a small group may benefit from CPET as well. In my practice, CPET has been necessary rarely; most patients don't want to chance chronic respiratory failure and a bed-to-chair existence. Quantitative lung perfusion scanning permits the clinician to attribute the fraction of FEV_1 measured in spirometry to the right and left lungs. The clinician can then accurately predict the postoperative FEV_1 by subtracting the component attributable to the lung to be resected.

Figure 6.1, parts 1 and 2, are algorithms followed in one form or another by most pulmonary physicians in advising their

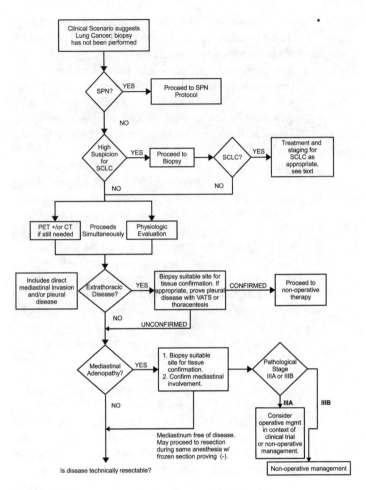

Figure 6.1(a) Lung cancer evaluation algorithm (Part 1).

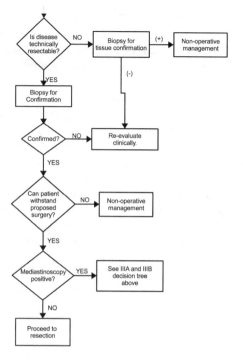

Figure 6.1(b) Lung cancer evaluation algorithm (Part 2).

patients regarding the initial treatment and staging of lung cancer. Although presented as an algorithm, many steps are performed simultaneously. When a patient is suspected of having lung cancer, the tissue diagnosis, clinical staging, and evaluation of the patient's physiologic status occur concurrently. Patients with obviously advanced, extrathoracic disease are subjected to appropriate biopsy and directed toward nonoperative care. Depending upon their physiologic status, they may be further directed toward comfort care, palliative chemotherapy and radiation therapy, or curative therapy. Nonoperative management is generally organized by the primary clinician along with the radiation and/or medical oncologist. Simultaneous with the assessment for extrathoracic disease is estimation as to the likelihood of small cell lung cancer. If the patient has a high likelihood of SCLC (extensive central disease, bulky lymphadenopathy, presentation with superior vena cava syndrome) the patient is biopsied rather than staged. SCLC patients are defined as having limited or extensive disease, and SCLC treatment will be reviewed below. If the patient has neither extrathoracic disease nor SCLC, they will usually undergo PET scanning (and CT scanning if not already done). PET helps further evaluate for extrathoracic disease. If extrathoracic disease is discovered, the patient reverts to the nonoperative arm of the decision tree. PET and CT help define the status of the patient's mediastinum. Mediastinal involvement with direct tumor extension and mediastinal lymphadenopathy are the two most difficult situations for the treating clinicians. This stems from the inexactitude of CT and PET scanning. Direct mediastinal invasion with tumor excludes surgery. In practice, it is sometimes difficult to determine precisely if the mediastinum has been invaded from CT, and the resolution of current PET scanners is insufficient to be of value in this setting. With respect to mediastinal lymphadenopathy, false positives and false negatives occur with both PET and CT at sufficiently high frequency to justify tissue confirmation of nodal status. In this case, PET and CT are used to guide further biopsies. In addition to mediastinoscopy, VATS examination of the mediastinum, endobronchial ultrasound-guided bronchoscopic lymph node needle biopsy, esophageal ultrasound-directed lymph node biopsy, and "blind" (e.g., carinal puncture with knowledge of CT appearance) subcarinal lymph node biopsy are used to determine the patient's stage. If a patient is found to be free of mediastinal disease by imaging (and if necessary, biopsy), it is common for the patient to undergo anesthesia, have mediastinoscopy with frozen section pathology for final confirmation, and then proceed to tumor resection immediately. As indicated in the algorithm and stated previously, Stages IIIA and IIIB disease present clinical difficulties. There is universal agreement that contralateral mediastinal lymph node involvement (IIIB) excludes operation. Current recommendations regarding IIIA disease are mixed, but the most recent recommendations from the American College of Chest Physicians (see general references) recommend surgical treatment of IIIA disease only in the context of a clinical trial. Other clinical trials are evaluating the efficacy of adjuvant or up-front radiation or chemotherapy to try and "convert" IIIA or IIIB disease to operable stages. Depending upon final pathologic findings, adjuvant chemotherapy and/or radiation may be recommended after operation. Typical scenarios include unanticipated pleural involvement or identification of microscopic disease in the mediastinum on final pathology. Most authorities recommend a multidisciplinary evaluation of lung cancer patients at least once in their course. Staging matrix and physiologic evaluation algorithm are presented in Table 6.3 and Figure 6.2, respectively. Some texts refer to nodal stations; current nomenclature subdivides various nodal locations in the lungs and mediastinum into specific named groups, or stations. Although not used for staging currently, they are of value to surgeons and pulmonary physicians in communicating about nodal location, and it is likely that more precise staging will use the station taxonomy in the future.

Current techniques for lobectomy and pneumonectomy include VATS-assisted procedures to reduce the size of the thoracotomy wound. Formal thoracotomy may be necessary if adequate exposure cannot be achieved or unexpected anatomy or operative findings are encountered. At present, lobectomy is the minimum standard "cancer operation." Segmental resection or subsegmental resection in conjunction with adjuvant radiation or chemotherapy is under investigation. Since many tumors occur in the upper lobes, often the site of extensive emphysema, the

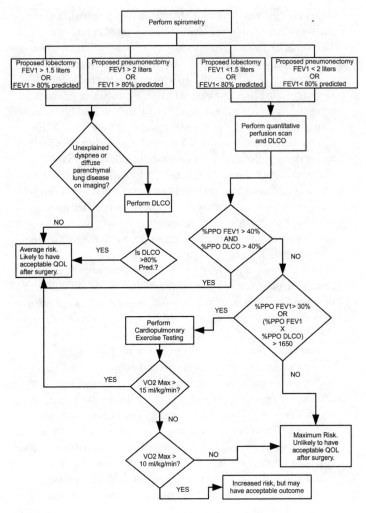

Figure 6.2 Physiologic assessment algorithm for lung cancer resection.

unfavorable physiologic effect of surgery may be tempered by an LVRS-like effect, permitting the patient to withstand the operation better than would be expected.

Nonoperative therapy relies primarily on radiation and chemotherapy. Radiofrequency ablation of small tumors has also been used. Aggressive palliation (attempts to prolong life significantly without effecting cure) and attempts at cure are generally based on accelerated, hyperfractionated radiotherapy and platinum-based chemotherapy regimens. Radiation alone can be used for palliation; it is effective for hemoptysis, cough, and obstructive symptoms. Bronchoscopic ablation of large, unresectable tumors causing symptoms can be achieved with radiofrequency probes, cryotherapy, or laser therapy. Stenting of airways can also provide temporary (but effective) relief of symptoms. At our hospital, patients with Stage IIIB and IV disease (and sometimes IIIA) are introduced to the palliative care team early in the course of their treatment to make the eventual transition to comfort care a natural part of the disease treatment process.

Small cell carcinoma presents a different clinical picture. The patient often has a large disease burden at presentation, and widespread metastasis at presentation is common. Untreated, survival is measured in weeks. Limited-stage disease is defined as disease limited to the ipsilateral hemithorax with a volume of disease burden that can safely withstand radiation therapy; extensive disease encompasses all other patients. Very early disease (e.g., SPN) is very rare. Limited-stage disease is treated with combination radiation therapy to the main tumor burden and platinum-based chemotherapy, often in combination with etoposide. Extensive-stage disease is treated with chemotherapy alone. Extensive-stage disease patients may be offered consolidation radiation if they achieve extrathoracic complete remission combined with intrathoracic complete or partial remission. Patients with limited-stage disease and extensive-stage disease who appear to have complete remissions are often offered prophylactic cranial irradiation, as the risk of brain metastasis disease is very high. SCLC patients must be cared for in a multidisciplinary setting.

For both NSCLC and SCLC patients, end-of-life palliative care may be a major component of management. Efforts have been made to improve and standardize this aspect of treatment (Chest 2007;132:368S).

6.2 Mesothelioma

Ann Oncol 2005;16 Suppl 2:ii240, Nat Clin Pract Oncol 2007;4:344, Chest 2004;126:1318, Cancer Control 2006;13:255, Clin Chest Med 2006;27:335

Epidemiology: Incidence ranges between 15 (United States) and 40 (Australia) cases per million population. Eighty percent of patients are male. In almost all patients with mesothelioma, exposure to asbestos can be documented or reasonably postulated by virtue of geographic location, occupational or environmental exposure, or exposure through other means (wife shakes out and cleans clothes of husband who works with asbestos). It is felt that incidence in the United States has peaked, but incidence will continue to increase in Western Europe (peak 2020) as previously asbestos-exposed patients complete their latency period, which is usually 20 years or more. There is a dose-response relationship between fiber exposure and probability of the disease, and patients with even low-grade exposure have an increased (albeit still small) risk of the tumor.

Pathophysiology: Straight, long, pointed, thin fibers of asbestos (amphibole type) penetrate the lung and lodge in the pleura, where the carcinogenic mechanism is unknown. There are some other inorganic substances, including a zeolite fiber similar in structure to amphibole asbestos found in Turkey that can also cause mesothelioma. These fibers are cleared only slowly, and carcinogenic effect appears due to physical more than chemical characteristics. Some researchers believe that a virus, SV 40 (simian virus 40), may be a cofactor in carcinogenesis, although this is controversial. The disease usually begins on the parietal pleura and is locally invasive. Metastasis is rare. Death and disability occur from superior vena cava syndrome, cardiac tamponade, pulmonary entrapment with pneumonia, and spinal cord compression. Generalized wasting is common, and mesothelioma may track along sites of medical procedures and instrumentation, producing subcutaneous nodules. Spread to the contralateral hemithorax and peritoneum occurs in 20% of cases. Miliary spread to the lung has also been described.

Symptoms: The typical patient with mesothelioma complains of chest pain and dyspnea. Patients with abdominal disease may have distention and bloating from ascites. Chest X-ray often shows an effusion or pleural thickening. As the illness progresses, paraneoplastic wasting becomes apparent. Chest wall pain in these patients is difficult to control, as is recurrent effusion with dyspnea. Pleural effusions are usually bloody.

Course/Prognosis/Complications: This is a uniformly fatal illness. Survival without treatment is ~9 months, and with treatment perhaps 2 years. Pain, wasting, and dyspnea are frequent and difficult to control. Successful palliation requires much skill, compassion, and an organized approach to comfort care and hospice management. Some patients and families may be entitled to awards from various asbestos lawsuit settlements, and seeking legal advice may be appropriate for some patients and their family.

Imaging: On chest X-ray, parenchymal lung disease is usually absent, and an effusion and/or pleural thickening is visible. CT scan often shows an effusion with "lumpy-bumpy" tumor deposits over the pleural cavity. Mesothelioma is metabolically active on PET scanning, and this has also been used to define extent of disease.

Laboratory: There are no serum tests that are in clinical mainstream practice for this illness. Soluble mesothelin-related protein (SMRP) appears to hold the greatest promise for future use. Mesothelioma cells can be recovered in 30–80% of pleural effusions in affected patients. Conclusive cytological identification is difficult, and use of immunohistochemical markers has improved the diagnostic accuracy of pleural fluid cytology. Cytology advances notwithstanding, the majority of patients with mesothelioma have the diagnosis made by biopsy, and most authorities feel that a directed VATS pleural biopsy is superior to a blind, closed Abrams or Cope needle biopsy. Immunohistochemical staining and electron microscopy are used to identify conclusively the tissue as mesothelioma.

Diagnosis: The middle-aged or older patient with chest pain and bloody pleural effusion with pleural CT abnormalities should be suspected of having mesothelioma. These patients should be promptly subjected to thoracentesis and/or biopsy. The clinician often must coax forward appropriate work or exposure history. Asbestos was used widely in the mid-1900s as a thermal insulator, and the substance was found in pipe insulation in ships, boilers, railroad locomotives, many industrial processes, and commercial buildings. Many skilled and unskilled trades worked either directly with the insulation or were present while it was being applied (e.g., the electrician wiring the hull of a WWII Liberty ship next to the pipefitter insulating the steam lines), lived near or worked in asbestos mines, or had secondary exposures (as the wife described above). A small number of patients have either spontaneous mesothelioma or developed the disease from very low-grade asbestos exposure. The common point of differential diagnosis is that of pleural metastases with effusion. In patients without a known primary cancer, it can be difficult to distinguish some histological forms of mesothelioma from metastatic adenocarcinoma of unknown primary. Benign pleural fibrous tumor should also be considered. In my experience, patients with true pleural masses almost never have a benign diagnosis. Bloody pleural effusions have a broad differential diagnosis (see **Pleural Disease**) and it is the combination of pleural mass and effusion that is the diagnostic finding.

Treatment: This is a dreadful disease that responds poorly to treatment. Efforts at treatment are preceded by TNM staging from T1a (ipsilateral parietal pleura without visceral pleural involvement) to T4 (locally advanced, technically unresectable tumor), N0–N3 (contralateral mediastinal, internal mammary, or supraclavicular [ipsilateral or contralateral] nodes) and Mx–M1. All treatment is palliative, even aggressive surgery, and cure should not be presented to the patient as a realistic outcome. Larger centers will undertake aggressive pleural resections (extrapleural pneumonectomy) with chemotherapy. Surgery is unsuitable for most patients because of the early spread of tumor along serosal surfaces, and even "suitable" candidates inevitably recur after resection. Radiation can be used for targeted palliation of problem areas and prophylaxis of needle tracks. Treatment of the entire pleural surface of a lung would be unacceptably toxic. Chemotherapy is modestly successful in some patients, with pemetrexed, a new antifolate agent, having an ~40% partial response rate and an average increase in survival from 9 to 12 months. Gemcitabine has also been used. Pleurodesis can prevent effusion recurrence. Standard techniques for cancer palliation and advanced lung disease palliation should be employed. These patients need particular attention paid to pain control, with early use of narcotics and epidural catheters. Percutaneous cervical cordotomy has been advocated to destroy pain fibers; this requires an experienced center.

Chapter 7

Diffuse Parenchymal Lung Disease

7.1 Inorganic Dust Pneumonitis

Introduction

Diseases caused by inorganic dusts are also known as pneumoconioses. Although the pathology varies among the diseases, they share a common feature of being a consequence of inhaling inorganic dust and that diffuse parenchymal damage and fibrosis is seen. Many, if not most, of these illnesses are related to occupations, and as such may present legal problems. All are capable of causing debility and death. The incidence of these illnesses is dropping as improved surveillance and respiratory protection is encouraged, cajoled, and enforced by state and federal governments, unions, and advocacy groups.

A substantial portion of patients will not provide a detailed occupational history spontaneously, and it is the clinician's task to elicit the necessary information. If an occupational exposure is a consideration, the patient's *entire* occupational history must be sought. Try obtaining complete job descriptions, as exposures can sometimes be hidden in otherwise benign-sounding situations.

This book reviews asbestos-related lung disease, coal workers' pneumoconiosis, silicosis, and berylliosis as prototypical diseases. There are many other inorganic dust offenders, including mica, kaolin, and hard metal (tungsten carbide), and the reader is encouraged to review one of the major pulmonary medicine or occupational medicine texts for a more complete treatment.

Finally, a brief review of aerosols (see **Inhaled Medications**) may be worthwhile because small airway and alveolar deposition of dust is necessary for tissue injury.

Radiographics 2006;26:59 has beautiful photomicrographs of pathology and high-quality reproductions of CT scans of the diseases covered in this section.

Asbestos-Related Lung Disease

http://www.thoracic.org/sections/publications/statements/pages/eoh/ asbestos.html 2003;2007, N Engl J Med 1989;320:1721, Chest 1989;95:1304, Am Fam Physician 2007;75:683

Epidemiology: Asbestos-related lung disease occurs in patients who have inhaled asbestos particles. The mineralogy of asbestos fibers is described in the references. Some forms of asbestos are more toxic than others. In the United States legislative control of asbestos exposure in the workplace was implemented in 1971. Prior to this date, asbestos was used extensively as an insulation material in buildings, boilers, ships, brakes, and industrial processes involving heat. Exposure occurred from mining or living near mines as well. The degree of exposure is significant. Although there is a dose–response relationship between mesothelioma and asbestos exposure, fibrotic asbestos lung disease (asbestosis) requires a considerable lung burden of fibers before disease will occur. Therefore, characterizing the degree of exposure is important. Exposure can occur by working directly with the materials, by being present when the materials were applied (electrician working next to a pipe fitter), or handling asbestos-contaminated implements or clothes where the asbestos is aerosolized again. Intact, in-place insulation that is properly covered poses little or no health hazard. The occupational and exposure history should include a detailed job description. Degree of exposure is difficult to quantify, but time on the job, visible dust, and proximity to the source of contamination are all helpful. There is a latent period between exposure and manifestation of the asbestos-related condition, often in excess of 15–20 years. In general, asbestos-related lung disease is on the decline in the United States as affected patients die and occupational interventions have markedly reduced new cases.

Pathophysiology: Asbestos causes five significant separate syndromes. Mesothelioma (see **Mesothelioma**) is a malignancy of serosal surface mesodermal tissue, the pleura, and/or the peritoneum. Asbestos is the only known risk factor. Pleural disease is more common than peritoneal disease. Asbestos raises the risk of lung cancer (see **Bronchogenic Carcinoma**) multiplicatively in concomitant smokers, and smoking cessation is one of the components of treating and counseling patients with asbestos exposure. Although asbestos exposure is best known for causing parenchymal and pleural disease, small airway injury and obstructive has been identified. The most common manifestation of asbestos exposure is benign pleural disease with calcified pleural plaques and diffuse pleural thickening and fibrosis. The mechanism of this pleural disease is unknown. Another pleural manifestation is benign pleural effusion of asbestos exposure, which is different from most other asbestos-related diseases in that it has a shorter (often <10–15 years) latency than the other benign and malignant diseases. Asbestosis is a fibrotic diffuse parenchymal lung disease. Pathologically, it is indistinguishable from pulmonary fibrosis secondary to usual interstitial pneumonitis (see **Usual Interstitial Pneumonitis**). Asbestos bodies (asbestos fibers coated with iron and protein, also called ferruginous bodies) are seen inconsistently; the ability to see uncoated asbestos fibers by light microscopy is limited. When inhaled, asbestos fibers lodge in bifurcations in terminal bronchioles and injure lung cells producing an inflammatory cascade and release of oxygen and nitrogen free radicals. Unlike UIP, asbestosis progresses slowly, and manifestation of illness from the time of exposure usually is over 20 years.

Symptoms and Signs: See **Bronchogenic Carcinoma** and **Mesothelioma** for the presentation of these diseases. The patient with benign pleural effusion of asbestos exposure will have dyspnea and pleuritic chest pain. Patients with asbestosis have insidious but progressive dyspnea on exertion. Dry, Velcro-type rales can be heard at the lung bases. Cough is common. Clubbing can be seen, as well as right heart failure in advanced illness. Dyspnea out of proportion to physical findings and pulmonary function abnormalities is a distinctive finding.

Course/Prognosis/Complications: Patients with symptomatic asbestosis develop progressive dyspnea and debility. Weight loss, loss of appetite, immobility, right heart failure, and dependence on oxygen all complicate the illness. Lung cancer, particularly with concurrent tobacco use, can be a lethal complication. Prognosis is similar to that of other interstitial fibrotic lung diseases at the same stage of illness, but asbestosis will progress more slowly.

Laboratory: There are no specific serum tests for the diagnosis of asbestos-related lung disease. Recovery of asbestos fibers from lung tissue at biopsy and/or BAL can help diagnosis. Hypoxia can be seen on blood gases, and pulmonary function testing demonstrates restriction. Small airways disease can be seen as a manifestation of the small airways inflammation. Although "monitoring" of pulmonary function testing and X-rays is recommended by many authorities, there are no effective therapies even if disease is identified. If a biopsy is performed, the histopathology is indistinguishable from that of UIP.

Imaging: CT and X-ray appearance of asbestosis are indistinguishable from UIP/pulmonary fibrosis: increased and thickened interstitial markings, scattered areas of confluent fibrosis, loss of volume, basilar predominance, and honeycombing. X-rays are also interpreted using a standardized system of abnormality type and severity; professionals who are certified for this activity are termed B readers(http://www.cdc.gov/niosh/topics/chestradiography/default.html 2006;2007). Because of overlap between public health, legal, and patient management, there is controversy surrounding this system (Acad Radiol 2004;11:843, Chest 1998; 114:1740).

Diagnosis: Any patient who presents with DPLD requires full accounting of their occupational and exposure history. Patients with asbestosis may be confused with UIP or other fibrotic lung diseases. Many authorities feel that a biopsy is not necessary if there is a characteristic HRCT and a history of an appropriate occupational or environmental asbestos exposure. Asbestosis will have a latency, generally of 20 years or greater, between exposure and illness, and this latency should be sought (asbestos exposure 2 years ago does not cause fibrotic lung disease). Asbestosis will progress much more slowly than UIP or the other idiopathic fibrosing lung diseases.

Treatment: There is no disease-altering treatment for asbestosis. Oxygen, control of right heart failure, control of dyspnea, pulmonary rehabilitation, and, when appropriate, palliative care are all that can be offered. Most patients are too old at the time of presentation to be eligible for lung transplantation.

Coal Workers' Pneumoconiosis (CWP)

Chest 2004;126:622, http://www.cdc.gov/niosh/pdfs/95-106d.pdf 1995;2007, Am Rev Respir Dis 1976;113:531

Epidemiology: CWP is a pattern of X-ray, pathologic, and clinical findings found in patients who are exposed to coal and mine dust. The majority of these patients are miners. The illness can be seen also in workers who do not work at the rock face, but handle coal in transport or are end users (such as the "black gang" in steamship engine rooms). In the United States, the number of miners continues to drop as mechanization progresses in the mines. Coal continues to be mined in Eastern and Western Europe as well as the U.K., where industrial hygiene is similar to that in the United States. Coal mining in developing countries (China, India, South America) carries higher risk of CWP (and other mine mishaps). In the United States, <5% of miners have radiographic evidence of CWP.

Pathophysiology: Inhalation of mine dust presents respirable coal, mica, silica, and other minerals to the terminal bronchioles and alveoli. The role of silica in development of CWP, after study, has been discounted. It is felt that coal dust itself is responsible for the lesions of CWP, but that silicosis can coexist with CWP. Coal dust, which is relatively inert, collects until a macrophage response is triggered producing the coal macule, a small (<4 mm) lesion consisting of dust and dust-filled macrophages with surrounding focal emphysema. The coal nodule is a larger, palpable lesion that contains both coal and silica. Progressive massive fibrosis can occur with development of masses of fibrotic material and loss of lung volume. Patients with coal exposure and rheumatoid arthritis can develop large (up to 5 cm) necrobiotic nodules. These nodules may cavitate or calcify. Vasculitis can be seen in these lesions as well. Interstitial fibrosis and chronic bronchitis with airflow obstruction can be seen in coal exposure. For many patients, the obstructive component is the more troublesome aspect of the disease (Am J Respir Crit Care Med 1998; 157:1390).

Symptoms: Patients who have only coal macules may be without symptoms and only have radiographic findings. As the illness progresses, the patient may have dyspnea and cough.

Course/Prognosis/Complications: If patients progress to progressive massive fibrosis, there is progressive loss of exercise tolerance. Patients with obstructive symptoms will have a course similar to that of COPD. Unlike silicosis, there is no predilection to super-infection. Respiratory failure can occur as the disease progresses. Simultaneous rheumatoid disease and CWP can produce very large nodules (Caplan's syndrome).

Laboratory: There are no specific serum markers for CWP. Pulmonary function testing may show reduced FEV_1 and FVC, hyperinflation, and reduced DLCO. If a rheumatoid pneumoconiosis is suspected (Caplan's syndrome), standard markers of this disease (rheumatoid factor, complement levels, etc.) may be elevated.

Imaging: X-ray findings are divided into simple CWP with small irregular or rounded nodules. Coal nodules are larger, and PMF is considered to be present when parenchymal lesions are 1 cm or greater in diameter. PMF can progress from large nodules to large masses of fibrous tissue reducing the amount of normal lung present. PMF fibrosis and nodules can cavitate. Rheumatoid pneumoconiosis can have large, round nodules. Because of the standardization of X-ray interpretation for occupational lung disease ("B" reading), CT is not used extensively for diagnosis (Am J Respir Crit Care Med 1996;154:741).

Diagnosis: Heavy, occupational coal exposure is an absolute prerequisite for diagnosis. Many patients with abnormal X-rays showing coal macules will not have symptoms. Differential diagnosis will include sarcoidosis, malignancy, silicosis, pulmonary vasculitis, and hypersensitivity pneumonitis.

Berylliosis

J Thorac Imaging 2002;17:273, Am J Respir Crit Care Med 2005; 171:54, Lancet 2004;363:415

Epidemiology: Unusual illness confined to individuals exposed to inhaled beryllium. Beryllium is a strong, light metal that has the benefit of not sparking; it is used in the defense industry, aerospace, electronics, nuclear weapons manufacture, ceramics, machine shops, and other high-tech industries that require light, strong metals. Original description of disease was in fluorescent lightbulb manufacturing workers after WWII.

Pathophysiology: Interesting illness in that the metal elicits a hypersensitivity pneumonitis response with populations of sensitized lymphocytes. Noncaseating granulomas identical to those seen in sarcoid are seen on biopsy. Patients with certain HLA-DPβ1 variants have enhanced susceptibility to sensitization of lymphocytes and development of disease.

Symptoms: Pulmonary manifestations are nonspecific with cough, dyspnea, and constitutional symptoms. Airway involvement can cause symptoms similar to asthma. If beryllium has penetrated the skin in the course of exposure, cutaneous nodules can be seen.

Course and Prognosis: Some patients with exposure and abnormal proliferation test may remain disease free. Other patients may have a fulminant course; the best correlation appears to be with the percent of lymphocytes in BAL fluid (Am J Respir Crit Care Med 1994;150:135). Some patients will relapse when steroids are stopped.

Laboratory: There is a specific test that is used for surveillance and diagnosis, the beryllium lymphocyte proliferation test. BAL-derived or peripheral blood mononuclear cells are exposed to graded concentrations of beryllium salts, and proliferation is measured by radionuclide-tagged thymidine uptake by these cell populations. A positive result is laboratory dependent; there is no universal definition. Pulmonary function tests will show obstruction, DLCO abnormalities, and restriction late in the illness.

Imaging: Pattern is very similar to that of sarcoidosis with hilar adenopathy and a variety of manifestations of DPLD with interstitial thickening, subpleural nodules, and ground glass opacities.

Diagnosis: The main alternative diagnosis is sarcoidosis. If beryllium disease is a consideration, occupational history and beryllium lymphocyte proliferation test will make the diagnosis. Exposure history, abnormal beryllium lymphocyte proliferation test, and noncaseating granulomas on lung biopsy are required for diagnosis.

Treatment: There are no controlled trials to support this recommendation, but steroids are recognized to be effective (Clin Immunol Immunopathol 1994;71:123). Doses of prednisone in the 40 mg every other day range have been noted to be effective, and should be continued for 3–6 months and then tapered to the lowest effective suppressive dose. Complete withdrawal may cause recurrence. Patients with positive proliferation test but without symptoms or pulmonary function findings should be started on medication when there is ~10% reduction in pulmonary function compared to baseline. Alternatives to steroids include methotrexate.

Silicosis

Hazard Review 2002;145, Occup Environ Med 2002;59:723, Chest 2002;122:721, Chest 1997;111:779, Chest 1997;111:837, Am J Respir Crit Care Med 1997;155:761

Epidemiology: Silicosis is a fibrotic pulmonary disease that is caused by significant exposure to respirable crystalline silica. Many different minerals contain potentially injurious silica. The most common mineral is quartz. Silica dust is found in many industrial, service, and repair industries, and is found in a number of home environment and hobby situations as well. High-exposure industries include quarrying and stone cutting, foundry work, and industrial processes where sandblasting is used for finishing. Silica is used in building cleaning, bridge repair (sandblasting), and concrete work (cutting and finishing). Road repair often includes cutting of pavement and concrete, and is a source of exposure. A NIOSH document provides a helpful list of exposure sources (Hazard Review 2002;145). There does not appear to be any racial or gender predilection to disease. Incidence is declining, but a significant number of cases are still identified and reported each year in the United States. Workers in developing countries have a higher risk and incidence of the disease in the absence of mandated effective respiratory protection.

Pathogenesis: Respirable crystalline silica particles (amorphous silica, such as glass, does not cause tissue injury/disease) deposit in terminal bronchioles and alveoli. They are engulfed by macrophages and cause physical injury to the cells, releasing inflammatory cytokines and producing oxygen radicals. The chemicals cause further tissue injury and fibrosis. The process perpetuates because the same particles are repeatedly phagocytized (they are never destroyed) and cause more injury until the inflammation subsides or they are expectorated or otherwise cleared. Depending upon the intensity of exposure, the disease is classified as chronic, accelerated, or acute silicosis, with chronic disease manifesting after 10 years of exposure, accelerated <10 years of exposure, and acute presenting within months to years after massive exposure. The initial lesion is that of multiple small (<10 mm) nodules that in time coalesce to larger nodules. As these nodules coalesce, large clumps of fibrous tissue, retraction of the hila, and emphysema can be seen. For reasons that are not understood, silicosis creates an environment that makes the host susceptible to tuberculosis and other granulomatous infections. There is a relationship between silica exposure and development of autoimmune disease, both intra- and extrapulmonary. This is felt to be possibly due to the adhesion of various host proteins to the silica particle, and presentation of these proteins as an antigen to the patient's immune system is facilitated. Some authorities feel that there may be a relationship between lung cancer and silica exposure, although this relationship may be confounded by concomitant smoking history. Chronic bronchitis has been described in silica-exposed populations. Patients with a short, massive exposure may develop pulmonary silicoproteinosis, a condition with extensive filling of alveoli with proteinaceous material.

Symptoms: The precise nature of presentation varies. Some patients have few if any symptoms. These tend to be patients with simple silicosis (see below). Patients with progressive massive fibrosis have dyspnea and cough. Individuals with a short massive exposure who develop acute silicosis may have severe constitutional symptoms as well as cough and dyspnea. Patients with silicosis may also present with mycobacterial infection or autoimmune disease. Specific symptoms may be lacking.

Course/Prognosis/Complications: Course of the disease is variable and depends on the intensity, and to a lesser extent length, of exposure. Some patients may have only X-ray abnormalities; others can progress to respiratory failure or other complications. Patients with silicosis are susceptible to granulomatous infection, particularly tuberculosis, and the patient should be monitored and treated if that disease is detected. Many authorities feel that there is an increased risk of lung cancer in these patients. Scleroderma, rheumatoid arthritis, Wegener granulomatosis, and lupus have been recognized to occur with increased frequency. Risk of TB in patients with silica exposure, particularly in developing countries with a high HIV prevalence (e.g., South African miners) creates a public health hazard as well as presenting a grave danger to the patient.

Laboratory: There is no specific serum test for silicosis. Patients with silicosis, with even relatively mild X-ray findings, can have significant PFT abnormalities.

Imaging: Silica exposure on X-ray is classified into simple silicosis (profusion of nodules <10 mm) and progressive massive fibrosis (coalescing nodules ultimately forming "bat wings" of dense fibrosis emanating from the hilum) with upward retraction of the hilum. Emphysema can be seen. Cavitation of massive fibrosis should raise concern for mycobacterial infection. Patients with silicoproteinosis have a pattern of diffuse alveolar infiltrates. Mediastinal and hilar adenopathy is common, and so-called eggshell calcification of hilar and mediastinal lymph nodes, along with pulmonary nodules or PMF, should raise the possibility of silicosis. Eggshell calcification and a PMF-type X-ray may also be seen in sarcoidosis. Interestingly, there is controversy over whether HRCT imaging provides an advantage in diagnosis and management.

Diagnosis: As with other occupational illnesses, an adequate exposure history must be present. There will be geographic variability in prevalence depending upon local industry. Exposure history, symptoms, and compatible X-ray are the basis of the diagnosis; biopsy is not usually necessary, but may be required if a conclusive diagnosis cannot be achieved otherwise. Silicosis must be distinguished from miliary tuberculosis, sarcoidosis, and other immune diseases. PMF can be asymmetric and can mimic lung cancer.

Treatment: There is no recognized, nonexperimental therapy for this condition. As respiratory failure ensues, treatment with oxygen and measures for control of cor pulmonale and pulmonary hypertension are appropriate. Lung transplantation has been considered for some patients.

7.2 Radiation-Induced Lung Injury

Chest 1997;111:1061 (excellent review); Radiographics 2004;24:985 (beautiful CT scans)

Epidemiology: Radiation-induced lung injury (RILI) occurs in patients who have been exposed to therapeutic ionizing radiation directed at the chest. The lung is a radiosensitive organ and can be injured in the course of treating lung cancer, lymphoma, breast cancer, or thyroid cancer, the most common reasons for irradiating the chest. Incidence of symptomatic RILI is approximately 7–10%. This should be differentiated from radiographic changes, the incidence of which is much higher, probably 70–100%. Predisposition to symptomatic lung injury relates to total dose (in localized areas of treatment, injury almost inevitable with dose >40 Gy, uncommon <25–30 Gy, and intermediate in the interval), total volume of lung irradiated (30 Gy is fatal in whole lung irradiation), preexisting pulmonary conditions, dose fractionation, prior irradiation, concomitant chemotherapy (bleomycin, cyclophosphamide, and Adriamycin, among others), and steroid withdrawal. Two kinds of injury are seen in RILI, radiation pneumonitis and radiation fibrosis.

Pathophysiology: Ionizing radiation causes high-density energy to be delivered to the cellular structures, causing disruption of proteins, DNA, and release of free radicals. There is vascular damage, especially to alveolar capillaries, and type II pneumocytes are susceptible to injury, immediately reducing surfactant. Tissue injury invokes an inflammatory response with multiple cytokines mediating the response. This inflammatory response can progress to fibrosis. Inflammation occurs early, and fibrosis is usually seen in a 6–24-month interval. Symptoms will depend in part on the patient's underlying lung function as well as the volume of lung involved, as patients with poor preexisting lung function have less reserve. A small number of cases of a typical pattern (clinical and radiographic) of BOOP have been reported, and these patients respond to steroids (Radiographics 2004;24:985).

Symptoms: Usually occur anywhere between 1 month and 2 years after treatment. Symptoms are dyspnea, low-grade fevers, and cough. In cases of fibrosis, chronic respiratory failure, pulmonary hypertension, and cor pulmonale may occur. Rales and findings of consolidation such as dullness to percussion and bronchial breath sounds may be heard over affected areas. Skin changes consistent with radiation exposure may be present.

Course/Prognosis/Complications: Radiation pneumonitis can resolve spontaneously. Fibrotic changes that are present at 18–24 months will generally not regress further. Impaired gas exchange, chronic respiratory failure, and dyspnea may be chronic.

Laboratory: Nonspecific. Pulmonary function testing will show restriction. Mild leukocytosis may be present.

Imaging: The typical chest X-ray of RILI is that of an infiltrate that (1) is consistent with fields of prior radiation and (2) does not obey anatomic boundaries. I have found the latter to be a useful finding. "Sympathetic" inflammation in nonradiated portions of the lung has been seen, and with multiple oblique ports, such as that used in breast cancer treatment, a straight line cutoff between affected and unaffected lung may be absent. Early changes may be an indistinct infiltrate or vascular congestion, while fibrosis may cause a dense infiltrate with volume loss and mediastinal shift. Radiation to the mediastinum causes other problems such as fibrosing mediastinitis, pericarditis, pericardial fibrosis, and premature atherosclerosis. CT scanning can be striking.

Diagnosis: Patients receiving radiation therapy by definition have comorbidities, and the differential diagnosis can be broad. RILI will be suggested by prior history of radiation, time course, and imaging. RILI should be differentiated from infection, malignancy, and heart failure as the three most common alternatives.

Treatment: Careful planning by the radiation therapist can minimize risk; this includes dosing, ports, and fractionation. Many practitioners use steroids (prednisone, 60 mg or ~1mg/kg IBW) for 2 weeks and taper to zero over 2–3 months. Pentoxifylline has been used experimentally for prevention, as well as amifostine.

7.3 Drug-Induced Pulmonary Disease

Eur Respir J 2000;15:373, Mayo Clin Proc 2005;80:1298, Clin Infect Dis 2004;39:1724, Am J Hematol 2007, Cancer 2002;94:847, Am Rev Respir Dis 1970;101:408, Chest 2001;120:617, Ann Pharmacother 2001;35:894, Clin Chest Med 2004;25:65, Br J Dis Chest 1978;72:327, Dis Chest 1969;55:170, Chest 2003;124:406

Epidemiology: Drug-induced pulmonary disease is an important cause of diffuse parenchymal lung disease, and should be one of the considerations when confronted with a patient with DPLD/ILD. Effective treatment, when possible, depends upon identification of the offending agent, cessation of toxic treatment, and reversal of inflammation when appropriate. Multiple agents have been identified as etiologies of drug-induced lung disease, but generally fall into the categories of chemotherapeutic agents, antibiotics, biologicals, and cardiovascular agents. See Table 7.1.

Table 7.1   Drugs Associated with Pulmonary Toxicity

Antineoplastic	
Methotrexate	(Eur Respir J 2000;15:373)
Taxanes	(Cancer 2002;94:847)
Busulfan	(Am Rev Resp Dis 1970;101:408)
Bleomycin	(Chest 2001;120:617)
Cyclophosphamide	(Ann Pharmacother 2001;35:894)
Antibiotic	
Nitrofurantoin	(Mayo Clinic Proceedings 2005;80:1298)
Cardiac	
Amiodarone	(Clin Chest Med 2004;25:65)
Procainamide	(Dis Chest 1969;55:170)
Propranolol	(Br J Dis Chest 1978;72:327)
Biological Agents	
Rituximab	(Am J Hematol 2007, epub)
Interferon*	(Chest 2003;124:406)

Note: We recommend searching www.pneumotox.com.
*Pegylated interferon alpha is often administered with ribavirin when used for the treatment of hepatitis C. This list is not complete.

Pathophysiology: The mechanism of injury varies from agent to agent. *Methotrexate* is a form of hypersensitivity pneumonitis, but is also associated with a rapidly progressive pulmonary fibrosis that is partially dose dependent. *Busulfan's* mechanism is unknown and is hypothesized to be direct cell injury. *Nitrofurantoin* is a hypersensitivity-type reaction with a potential for progression to fibrosis and/or chronic inflammation. *Beta blockers* cause bronchospasm. *Procainamide* is associated with drug-induced lupus, and the patient may go on to develop symptoms of pulmonary lupus. *Amiodarone* toxicity is common, perhaps more so than my cardiology colleagues would like to concede, and pathogenesis is incompletely understood. Hypotheses include direct cell injury and hypersensitivity. *Taxanes* are associated with hypersensitivity and direct cell toxicity. *Bleomycin* is a prototypical pulmonary toxin, and one relevant observation is the absence of bleomycin-hydrolyzing enzyme in the lung. There appears to be a dose–response relationship between the drug and injury. Most chemotherapeutic protocols include pulmonary function monitoring. *Interferon/ribavirin* has been associated with severe pulmonary toxicity, but the mechanism has not been described. *Rituximab* has been associated with severe and fatal pulmonary injury, albeit uncommonly. As use increases in both malignant and nonmalignant conditions, incidence may increase. Many of these agents are associated with alterations of the immune system predisposing the patient to pulmonary infection.

Signs and symptoms: Nonspecific. Fevers, cough, chills, chest pain, dyspnea, rales predominate. Wheezes are possible. Some drugs may have associated laboratory findings.

Prognosis and Course: Variable. Prognosis and course will be dictated by the degree of reversible inflammation present and the underlying illness(es).

Laboratory: Nonspecific. A few of the drugs will induce a specific pattern of laboratory abnormality. Drug-induced lupus will have a positive ANA and the presence of anti-histone antibodies is strongly correlated with drug-induced lupus. Chemotherapeutic agents may be associated with anemia, thrombocytopenia, and neutropenia. Drugs with a prominent allergic component (e.g., nitrofurantoin) may produce eosinophilia.

Imaging: Nonspecific. Plain chest X-ray and HRCT may show different patterns including ground glass, reticular, nodular, reticulonodular, and areas of dense consolidation. I do not think there is sufficient specificity in the pattern of presentation to permit use of imaging to differentiate among agents. Patients who have had substantial exposure to amiodarone may have a hyperdense liver on CT scanning. This is not related to pulmonary effects.

Diagnosis: A patient in whom a pulmonary drug reaction is suspected has at minimum the comorbid condition for which he or she is being treated. Many patients are being treated for serious conditions that may cause pulmonary disease itself, there may be other drugs involved, and opportunistic or conventional infections may be possible. As part of the evaluation of a patient with DPLD/ILD, a drug history should be elicited. *These drugs should then be researched. We recommend the use of a high-quality, continuously updated source such as UpToDate for common agents or www.pneumotox.com.* Pneumotox.com in particular permits searches by radiographic pattern, brand name, or generic name. The possible drug reaction should be differentiated from infection or exacerbation and/or progression of the underlying illness. In my experience, drug toxicity should be considered when: (1) there is a plausible agent, (2) subacute time course, (3) absence of fever and leukocytosis, (4) no response to antibiotics, and (5) reasonable assurance that the underlying disease is controlled or in remission. These rules are not hard and fast. In many cases, surgical lung biopsy may be necessary. This is especially important if other treatable causes of lung injury are in the differential diagnosis.

Treatment: Treatment consists of withdrawal of the offending agent. Steroids may be used as an adjunct in the conditions that have an inflammatory component. Regimens are disease specific and are available in previously mentioned resources. Surprisingly, I have been unable to secure the help of some pharmaceutical manufacturers in accessing diagnostic and treatment strategies for drug reactions.

7.4   The Lung and Recreational and Illicit Drug Use

West J Med 1990;152:525, Curr Opin Pulm Med 2001;7:43, Am J Physiol Lung Cell Mol Physiol 2007;292:L813, J Intensive Care Med 2004;19:183, Clin Chest Med 2004;25:203

Epidemiology: Understanding the mechanisms of addictive and self-destructive behavior and developing truly effective interventions is one of the greatest health challenges of our time. The lung often suffers along with the rest of the body. Epidemiology is difficult to define because of wide geographic variation in drugs of choice and routes of administration. This article will focus on crack/cocaine, opiates, marijuana, and alcohol.

Pathophysiology:

Alcohol: The effects of alcohol ingestion have been studied extensively. The primary pulmonary effect of alcohol is to degrade pulmonary defense mechanisms, increasing the risk of infection and severity of infection. Alcohol consumption impairs consciousness and may contribute to aspiration pneumonia, foreign body aspiration, and lung abscess. Alcohol's effect on other organs, such as causing pancreatitis, may lead to ARDS. The socioeconomic downslide caused by alcoholism may lead to exposure to tuberculosis. Alcohol impairs judgment and may lead to unsafe sexual practices, leading to HIV and its attendant lung complications. Alcohol withdrawal may complicate the treatment of an otherwise uncomplicated CAP. Inexperienced drinkers (often seen on college campuses) may drink to respiratory depression and loss of airway control, necessitating intubation and mechanical ventilation.

Cocaine: Usually inhaled as crack or snorted as a powder. A syndrome of pulmonary infiltrates, eosinophilia, and dyspnea occurring after acute cocaine inhalation is termed "crack lung." Chronic use may lead to pulmonary fibrosis, BOOP/COP, diffuse alveolar damage, and pulmonary hemorrhage syndrome. Pulmonary vascular spasm has been reported. Pulmonary hypertension can occur. Contaminated cocaine may cause talc granulomas when inhaled.

Opiates: Injected or inhaled. Heroin and oxycodone are current favorites. Inhalation may lead to foreign body granulomas. Reduced consciousness may lead to aspiration. Addiction may lead to needle sharing and sex in exchange for money or drugs, both of which are significant risk factors for HIV infection. Suppression of respiratory drive and loss of airway control may lead to need for intubation and mechanical ventilation. Abrupt injection of heroin may lead to histamine release with bronchospasm and an anaphylaxis-like picture. Heroin-induced pulmonary edema has been described. With any injected agent, endovascular infection may result in septic emboli.

Marijuana: Smoked. A link between marijuana use and COPD is suspected, and measurable changes in pulmonary function have been noted. Smoking 3–4 marijuana cigarettes per day is thought to be equivalent to a pack of tobacco cigarettes per day, probably because of the difference in how the smoke is inhaled. Marijuana may impair judgment and lead to unsafe sexual practices leading to HIV.

Signs and Symptoms: Highly variable. Patients may have cough, wheeze, dyspnea, hemoptysis, rales, and respiratory failure.

Course/Prognosis/Complications: Many patients will have chronic dyspnea if they have had an episode of acute lung injury.

Pulmonary hypertension from chronic hypoxia or vascular occlusive disease is also a concern. The most serious medical complications have more to do with chronic hepatic injury (alcohol) and development of chronic infection such as HIV. Ultimately, prognosis may rest more upon engaging the patient in rehabilitation and reestablishment of healthy interpersonal relationships than efficacy of inhaled steroids.

Laboratory: The presence of drugs of abuse is confirmed with urine toxicology screens and blood levels (alcohol). The clinician should have a working knowledge of the screening system used by his or her laboratory. Some commercial opiate screens will not identify oxycodone in the urine, which in some areas of the country is the opiate of choice. Eosinophilia may be present in some syndromes. Many patients with chronic drug and alcohol problems will have evidence of liver disease, anemia, comorbid infections, and some may be HIV positive. Hypoxia may be evident on blood gases or saturation oximetry, and hypercapnea may be present when respiratory drive is suppressed. Pulmonary function testing abnormality may be either restrictive or obstructive.

Imaging: Variable, depends upon agent, route of administration, and chronicity of use. Foreign body granulomatosis (Am Rev Respir Dis 1983;127:575) has a defined spectrum of radiology (Am J Roentgenol 2000;174:789). Patterns of diffuse alveolar and interstitial infiltrates may be present, and areas of consolidation may be seen when infection or BOOP/COP are present. Bullous changes have been identified with chronic inhalation of drugs. Cavitating lesions or multiple areas of patchy infiltrates should raise the possibility of septic emboli.

Diagnosis: Patients with known or suspected pulmonary injury from drugs need systematic and thorough evaluation. With the exception perhaps of ARDS, pulmonary hemorrhage, or overwhelming infection, the patient's other organ system problems may be more pressing than chest X-ray abnormalities. Support of respiratory failure, treatment of possible infection, and support of other failing organ systems takes precedence over the differential diagnosis of the X-ray findings. Once the patient is stable, the patient can be assessed for how much of the respiratory problem is due to the drug(s) themselves or comorbid conditions. If ARDS is present, evaluation for sepsis or trauma should be considered as well as direct drug effect.

Treatment: Prevention of further exposure to the drug and general supportive measures are the mainstay of treatment. Some authorities advocate the use of steroids in "crack lung." If a patient is bronchospastic from histamine release or has chronic airways obstruction, bronchodilators are appropriate.

7.5   Eosinophilic Lung Disease

Am J Respir Crit Care Med 1994;150:1423, Annu Rev Med 1992;43:417; Radiographics 2007;27:617 (has gorgeous imaging and histopathology).

Eosinophilic Pneumonias

Introduction: The combination of pulmonary infiltrates and blood, BAL fluid, and/or pulmonary tissue eosinophilia encompasses multiple illnesses. Classification of diseases is by necessity arbitrary. In this section, we will cover acute and chronic eosinophilic pneumonia, Loeffler's syndrome, and tropical eosinophilia. Churg-Strauss syndrome is reviewed with entries on pulmonary vasculitis. Drug-induced eosinophilic lung disease is covered with drug-induced pulmonary disease, and allergic bronchopulmonary aspergillosis (ABPA) is reviewed with asthma.

Epidemiology: Tropical eosinophilia is an immune response to *Wuchereria bancrofti* and, less commonly, *Brugia malayi*, which are microfilariae. The disease is confined to individuals who have traveled or lived in endemic regions. Loeffler's syndrome is due to pulmonary passage of several different kinds of helminths, including ascaris (most common), hookworms, and strongyloides. Exposure to these agents is a precondition to the illness. Acute eosinophilic pneumonia is a disease of uncertain etiology, but is felt by many experts to be the consequence of an environmental exposure. Chronic eosinophilic pneumonia is a different entity, also of unknown etiology. Both of these illnesses are uncommon.

Pathophysiology: Tropical filarial pulmonary eosinophilia occurs in a small percentage (<1%) of patients with lymphatic filariasis. The patient develops an immune response to the filaria, and the helminths are trapped in the lungs, where they elicit a response of infiltrates and inflammation. Time from infection to illness is months. Long-standing untreated disease can lead to fibrosis. Loeffler's syndrome is a transient response to the pulmonary passage of helminths such as ascaris, which pass through the lungs as part of their life cycle. The illness causes little morbidity. Acute eosinophilic pneumonia is a disease of unknown etiology, but reports suggest an inhalational exposure that results in a severe and diffuse eosinophilic infiltrate in a short period of time (usually less than 1 week, always less than 3 weeks). Chronic eosinophilic pneumonia is of unknown etiology. There are alveolar collections of eosinophils and histiocytes. Fibrosis is not generally seen.

Symptoms: Tropical pulmonary eosinophilia presents with cough and some wheezing. Outright dyspnea is uncommon. Patients can have constitutional symptoms. Loeffler's syndrome presents with cough and low-grade fevers. A small percentage of patients may have hemoptysis, or may expectorate helminths. Acute eosinophilic pneumonia has a more aggressive picture, with progression to respiratory failure the norm. These patients are severely ill, with high fevers, severe dyspnea, and cough. Nonspecific constitutional symptoms, such as myalgias and night sweats, are also seen. Chronic eosinophilic pneumonia often has cough, fevers, night sweats, and weight loss. Onset can be abrupt, with a progressive illness. Many patients with chronic eosinophilic pneumonia have antecedent asthma.

Course/Prognosis/Complications: Tropical pulmonary eosinophilia is a slowly progressive disease, with an eosinophilic infiltrate developing after about 1 month of exposure. Early treatment (first few years of disease) permits regression of disease changes toward normal. Late treatment or no treatment can result in fibrosis. Loeffler's syndrome is a benign condition where morbidity and mortality result from extrapulmonary manifestations of the worms. Treatment is directed primarily at preventing intestinal obstruction, etc. AEP is often a fatal illness unless treated, with a picture of ARDS and diffuse alveolar damage. CEP has a slower course and is rarely fatal. It can, however, be debilitating with dyspnea and constitutional symptoms. Long term, there may be irreversible pulmonary fibrosis. In terms of complications, AEP is probably the worst of the lot, with the capability to cause significant pulmonary damage and death. Tropical pulmonary eosinophilia is but one manifestation of lymphangitic filariasis, which has multiple manifestations and consequences (http://whqlibdoc.who.int/trs/WHO_TRS_821.pdf 1992;18 June). Ascaris infestation can cause intestinal obstruction, and coughing up worms is really bad for your social life. CEP, although less destructive than AEP, can be debilitating with a reduction in sense of well-being and functional status.

Imaging: Tropical pulmonary eosinophilia shows diffuse increase in interstitial markings and small, almost miliary markings. Poorly defined, mottled lower lobe opacities can be seen. Loeffler's syndrome has round or oval infiltrates that may coalesce, and they are often migratory. Acute eosinophilic pneumonia has a variety of presentations, with ground glass opacities, reticular changes, and Kerley B lines. Some patients will have isolated alveolar infiltrates. Chronic eosinophilic pneumonia has a classic appearance of a photographic negative of pulmonary edema, with infiltrates confined to the periphery of the lung, and central sparing.

Laboratory: All of these syndromes are associated with pulmonary eosinophilia. Peripheral blood eosinophilia is not an absolute prerequisite for diagnosis, and the absence of blood eosinophilia does not exclude any of these diagnoses. Tropical pulmonary eosinophilia usually has elevated IgE levels, and blood eosinophilia can be seen. Loeffler's syndrome usually has blood eosinophilia, and antibodies against the offending helminth may be identified. In AEP, IgE and sedimentation rate may be elevated; blood eosinophilia is usually found. In CEP, blood eosinophilia, an elevated ESR, and anemia may be seen.

Diagnosis: History is important: underlying medical conditions (asthma and CEP, ABPA, or Churg-Strauss syndrome), drugs (nitrofurantoin, minocycline), and travel (helminthic infections). If a drug or another specific etiology is suspected, an invasive workup is not indicated, particularly if the patient responds well to intervention. Patients with helminth infection will often have other manifestations of infection and can usually provide a travel or exposure history. Ascaris infection should be documented by larvae in respiratory secretions or gastric aspirates. BAL may be necessary. Tropical pulmonary eosinophilia does not require an invasive evaluation; the presence of eosinophilia, pulmonary infiltrates, travel/residence in an endemic area, and elevated antifilarial titers are sufficient for diagnosis. Both CEP and AEP usually require a BAL to demonstrate the presence of pulmonary eosinophilia. AEP is confirmed by the presence of BAL eosinophils >25%, respiratory failure, fever, rapid course, and exclusion of alternative etiologies. CEP has such a distinct X-ray picture that BAL eosinophilia with a reverse batwing pattern is considered conclusive.

Treatment: Tropical pulmonary eosinophilia: diethylcarbamazine. In the United States, consultation with infectious disease is recommended since the drug can only be obtained from the CDC. Loeffler's syndrome: the most common offender is ascaris, which is treated with mebendazole (100 mg bid × 3 d or 500 mg once); US alternative is pyrantel (11 mg/kg, do not exceed total dose of 1 gram). AEP responds rapidly to high-dose steroids (Am J Respir Crit Care Med 1999;160:1079). Prednisone (40–60 mg/day) may be used if respiratory failure is not present, otherwise methylprednisolone (60 mg q 6 h × 2–3 days) with conversion to prednisone. High doses should be continued for 4–6 weeks with subsequent weaning to zero over ~8 weeks. CEP responds rapidly to prednisone in the 40–60 mg/day range. Relapse is common if steroids are stopped altogether. My experience and that of others is that a slow taper of prednisone from this initial level to a minimum dose that suppresses symptoms and normalizes the sedimentation rate is most appropriate. Often, this will be <10 mg/day. I periodically stop steroids altogether (perhaps once a year) to see if they are still required.

Eosinophilic Bronchitis

These patients will present with a chronic cough and have many of the manifestations of cough variant asthma. However, they do not manifest the functional and physiologic abnormalities of airways obstruction and bronchial hyperreactivity. Methacholine challenge testing is negative. Sputum contains high concentrations of eosinophils. Bronchial biopsy (if performed) demonstrates eosinophilic infiltration of the bronchial mucosa. These patients respond well to inhaled corticosteroids. Some authorities believe that this condition, in some fraction of patients, may represent a precursor to clinical asthma. In one study, 1 year follow-up showed that ~50% of patients remained stable, ~35% had resolution of the illness, and ~15% progressed to asthma (Thorax 2002; 57:178).

7.6 Hypersensitivity Pneumonitis (Extrinsic Allergic Alveolitis)

Fraser and Pare 1999;3:3076, Mayo Clin Proc 2007;82:812, Orphanet J Rare Dis 2006;1:25, Respirology 2006;11:262, pp. 2362-3

Epidemiology: The overall incidence of HP is unknown. There are subpopulations of individuals who will have a higher incidence of illness, such as farmers and bird fanciers. Incidence is related to exposure, making it difficult to predict attack rates. Even though this is a relatively uncommon illness, recognizing the condition and intervening can make a great difference for the patient.

Pathophysiology: HP is an immune-mediated response to the inhalation of an antigenic molecule. Unlike the pneumoconioses, the mechanism is a response to an antigen, rather than physical injury to respiratory tissue with resulting nonspecific inflammation. The immunopathogenesis is incompletely understood. Most authorities believe that the illness arises from a combination of type III and type IV immune responses implied by elevated IgG levels and granulomas respectively. For this reason, the majority of HP scenarios involve organic or biological molecules. Small molecules such as some anhydrides and isocyanates have also been implicated, and it is not clear why they are antigenic. Many different occupational, environmental, and leisure/hobby scenarios have been associated with HP. From a populational standpoint, the two most common situations are farmer's lung stemming from exposure to molds and complex bacteria in moldy hay, and bird fancier's lung, resulting from exposure to bird dander and droppings. Occupational situations where the patient is exposed to aerosolized organic material present a risk. Environmental situations may include homes with chronic water damage with mold and fungi in the walls. Leisure scenarios have included "hot tub lung," secondary to antigenic response to mycobacterium avium. See Table 7.2 for a longer, nonexhaustive list. The disease has

Table 7.2   Antigens Known to Cause Hypersensitivity Pneumonitis with Common Disease Name

Antigen	E	O	H	Disease Condition
Thermophilic bacteria	•	•	•	Farmer's lung, humidifier lung, building assoc. HP (1)
Avian proteins (serum, excreta, feathers)		•	•	Bird fancier's lung
Rodent sera, proteins		•		Laboratory worker's lung
Mycobacterium avium	•		•	Hot tub lung
Bacillus subtilis		•		Detergent-worker's lung
Penicillium sp.		•		Cheese-worker's lung
Trichoderma konigii		•		Sawmill-worker's lung
Thermoactinomyces sacchari		•		Bagassosis (2)
Pseudomonas sp.		•		Machine-operator's lung (3)
Aspergillus clavatus		•		Malt-worker's lung
Isocyanates		•	•	Isocyanate-induced lung disease (4)
Trimellitic, phthalic anhydrides		•		Anhydride-induced lung disease
Shellfish protein		•		Prawn-worker's lung
Alternaria		•		Wood pulp-worker's lung

Notes: E = environmental, O = occupational, H = hobby.
(1) Humidifier lung and building associated HP (*not* sick building syndrome) are associated with other agents such as fungi.
(2) Sugar cane-miller's disease.
(3) Contaminated cooling fluids for drilling/milling metal.
(4) Also produces isocyanate-related asthma.

three clinical presentations, with acute, subacute, and chronic forms. In the acute variety, often precipitated by a single heavy exposure to antigen, there is an intense inflammatory response with a clinical picture similar to atypical pneumonia. Resolution occurs when the patient is separated from the offending antigen. Subacute disease results from repeated, episodic exposures to antigen and development of a picture suggestive of a wasting illness with cough, fever, night sweats, and weight loss. These patients will recover well if the offending antigen is identified and avoided. Chronic HP implies permanent, anatomic structural injury as well as a chronic inflammatory infiltrate. Removing the antigen will prevent further damage but permit only incomplete resolution of symptoms.

Symptoms: Acute HP occurs 4–6 hours after exposure and is associated with dyspnea, cough, and fevers. Rales, but not wheezing, are heard on exam, and tachypnea is present. The illness resolves in anywhere from 12 hours to several days. Subacute HP has the appearance of a wasting illness with weight loss, cough, fever, night sweats, fatigue, and anorexia. Rales and tachypnea are noted on exam. Resolution occurs over weeks to months, but results in complete resolution of symptoms. Chronic HP presents with cough, dyspnea, and weight loss. Separation from the antigen results in slow and incomplete recovery.

Course/Prognosis/Complications: The prognosis is good for patients with acute and subacute disease if the condition is identified early and the patient has no further antigen exposure. Patients with chronic HP may go on to have respiratory problems up to and including chronic respiratory failure. Patients with extensive parenchymal injury can have superinfection (e.g., mycetoma, see **Aspergillosis**), and chronic steroid use may lead to iatrogenic Cushing syndrome. I have been struck by the effect of the illness on the personal lives of the patients affected. Patients have been forced to give up hobbies, beloved animals, and even their occupation. Several farmer patients have been forced to use elaborate respiratory protection devices (military-grade dust respirators) to keep their farms; they were too heavily in debt to sell out. However, for the majority of patients, diagnosis brings relief and a swift response to the offending agent.

Laboratory: Much has been made of serologic testing for HP, with many laboratories having hypersensitivity pneumonitis profiles testing for thermophilic actinomycetes, pigeon dander, micropolyspora faeni, etc. Presence of a positive precipitin finding is helpful, but absence of a precipitin finding does not exclude disease. Routine testing may show elevated CRP/ESR. Pulmonary function testing will show restriction, not obstruction, and DLCO abnormalities may be present. BAL, if performed, may show lymphocytosis and eosinophilia. Many patients may come to biopsy. Acute HP will show noncaseating granulomas (more likely poorly formed than the well-formed granulomas of sarcoidosis) and peribronchial lymphocytic infiltration. As the disease progresses to a subacute stage, the granulomas may be better formed. Chronic HP is a complex histologic picture with granulomas, BOOP/COP, and fibrosis.

Imaging: Plain film X-rays may be normal in early disease. HRCT may show ground glass appearance and micronodules, both in acute and subacute disease. Advanced disease shows upper lobe fibrosis, emphysema, areas of ground glass appearance, and sometimes honeycombing.

Diagnosis: Most texts and articles about HP go through a litany about how the diagnosis should be anticipated by taking a careful history at presentation, etc. This may be true for acute HP, where the exposure is easily identified and recalled by the patient. In this setting, the differential diagnosis includes viral or atypical pneumonia, metal fume fever (Emerg Med J 2002;19:268), asthma, or inhalational injury such as silo filler's disease (Mayo Clin Proc 1989;64:291). This is less true in subacute and chronic illness, where often the patient presents as an undifferentiated case of dyspnea and cough with abnormal HRCT scan. An initial interview (Do you have birds? Do you work on a farm?) provides no guidance, and the patient proceeds to surgical lung biopsy (usually VATS) that shows hypersensitivity pneumonitis. At this point, I will usually order my hospital's hypersensitivity pneumonitis panel (although I have yet to have a positive finding) and take an exhaustive history, recalling the patient (hopefully along with a voluble family) to the office for a long appointment where we go over the workplace in detail, all leisure activities, and the home environment (see **The Pulmonary History**). Etiologies discovered in this manner have included moldy hay ("We don't have a farm, we have horses."), bird dander (previous tenants of an apartment had used it as an illegal parrot breeding rookery; site was so contaminated with droppings and dander it was almost impossible to clean), and mycobacterium avium ("hot tub lung" from a poorly drained and sanitized hot tub).

Treatment: Treatment relies on identification of the offending antigen and preventing further exposure to the patient. Steroids are used by many clinicians (myself included) to hasten recovery, but there is no evidence that steroids influence prognosis. Courses often consist of prednisone, 30–40 mg/day for 2–3 weeks followed by a gradual taper to zero over a further 6–8 weeks. In patients with chronic HP, steroids may be needed for longer periods of time, and the lowest effective dose to stabilize clinical, pulmonary function, and X-ray findings is used.

7.7 Bronchiolitis Obliterans with Organizing Pneumonia (BOOP) and Cryptogenic Organizing Pneumonia (COP)

Clin Chest Med 2004;25:12, Am J Respir Crit Care Med 1994;149:1670

Introduction: Currently recognized terminology uses *bronchiolitis obliterans with organizing pneumonia* (BOOP), *organizing pneumonia*, and *cryptogenic organizing pneumonia* (COP). BOOP is used when a combination of clinical findings, radiographic findings, and pathology is typical and there is a known etiology. Organizing pneumonia is used when only the pathologic pattern is seen as an incidental finding. COP, the majority of cases, is appropriate when an etiology cannot be identified.

Epidemiology: 6–7/100,000 hospital admissions is reported. This probably represents underdiagnosis. Male and female incidence is the same. Patients are usually in their 5th or 6th decade. There is usually a delay in diagnosis, often of weeks.

Pathophysiology: COP represents a poorly defined immunologic response to sometimes known (BOOP) and sometimes unknown agent(s) (COP). It is distinct from other parenchymal lung diseases in that it is often reversible. Pathology shows temporally uniform proliferative bronchiolitis with bronchiolar plugging and associated surrounding alveolar inflammation. Distribution of lesions is patchy and peribronchial. Severe fibrosis and granulomas are rare at presentation. Symptoms arise from interference with gas exchange and airways obstruction and irritation. Clin Chest Med 2004;25:12 provides an excellent review and includes a list of known etiologies.

Symptoms: Chronic nonproductive cough, dyspnea. Fever, weight loss, general malaise, and fatigue are common. Rales are common on exam, but wheezing is rare.

Course/Prognosis/Complications: Respiratory failure is rare. Two thirds of patients have eventual full radiologic and symptomatic remission.

Imaging: "Classic" is bilateral alveolar opacities that look like masses or pneumonia. Lesions generally are more peripheral and can be migratory. Diffuse, bilateral interstitial opacities, nodules, and single large consolidation also can be seen. HRCT confirms both alveolar and interstitial nodular disease. Unlike some other forms of ILD, COP does not have a signature HRCT appearance. Severity of symptoms correlates with degree of involvement on imaging (Fraser and Pare 1999;3:3076, pp. 2344–2348).

Diagnosis: Often presents as nonresolving pneumonia (see **Nonresolving Pneumonia**). Lung mass or diffuse infiltrates may be identified from chest X-ray that has been obtained to evaluate respiratory symptoms. Differentiation from malignancy often is the greatest concern. Nonbacterial pneumonias (fungal, myco-bacterial) are other diagnostic alternatives. In interstitial/ nodular form, the gamut of interstitial lung disease, and eosinophilic pneumonia should be considered. Conclusive diagnosis requires biopsy. TBLB not recommended: lesion is patchy and can suffer from sampling error because of the small sample size of TBB. Surgical lung biopsy (usually VATS) is preferable.

Laboratory: Findings are nonspecific: increased ESR, CRP, and WBC, with few other findings. PFTs may show restriction and reduced DLCO. Hypoxia is common.

Treatment: Steroids are the mainstay of treatment. High-dose IV treatment is appropriate for rapidly progressive disease (125 mg q 6 h methylprednisolone/day for 3–5 days); prednisone 0.5–1.0 mg/kg day may be used for less aggressive disease. Clinical response is difficult to predict. Most clinicians taper the steroids after 4–6 weeks of therapy. If there is a flare, steroids are restarted, and the patient is treated for another 4–6 months; a taper is then tried again. This cycle should be tried every 4–6 months for 4–5 cycles. Successful cessation of steroids is unlikely if steroids are still necessary after 18–24 months of disease (Am J Respir Crit Care Med 2000;162:571). Approximately one third of patients get better within 6 months, one third within 18 months, and one third need extended prednisone. Cyclophosphamide can be used as a steroid-sparing agent. Relapse is common, and relapse early on does not imply a poor prognosis. It is generally felt that COP has better prognosis than BOOP.

7.8 Sarcoidosis

Lancet 2003;361:1111, Clin Chest Med 2004;25:521, Am Fam Physician 2004;70:312

Epidemiology: Sarcoidosis is a relatively common multisystem illness, with prevalence in the United States of 10–20/100,000. Prevalence and incidence in the United States in African-Americans are 3–4 times higher than that of European ancestry population. Disease tends to be more acute and more severe in African-Americans. There does appear to be some HLA correlation and family clustering (Lancet 2003;361:1111).

Pathophysiology: The precise mechanism of damage and etiology of this disease remains one of the frustrating and most researched areas in pulmonary medicine. In the lung, the primary lesion is a CD4+ T-lymphocyte alveolar inflammation. The alveolitis progresses to a noncaseating granulomatous inflammation, which in turn can either resolve without sequelae or can progress to scarring and fibrosis (Semin Respir Crit Care Med 2007;28:3). Treatment with interferon may precipitate the illness, suggesting a mechanism relating to that molecule (Int J Clin Pract 2006; 60:201). Although classified as a parenchymal pulmonary disease, sarcoid lesions are peribronchial and can be intrabronchial. As a result, both damage to the airway and the pulmonary parenchyma is possible with obstructive and restrictive (or combined) pulmonary physiology. Although many (if not most) researchers believe that sarcoid has an infectious etiology, there has been no confirmation of a specific agent, even using DNA-based probes. Sarcoid attacks multiple other organs, with skin (erythema nodosum, "apple jelly" lesions), ocular (uveitis, vasculitis), cardiac (conduction abnormalities, heart failure, ventricular and atrial arrhythmias), CNS (basilar meningitis), splenic (sequestration syndromes with thrombocytopenia, neutropenia, and anemia in varying proportions), hepatic (granulomatous hepatitis), and arthritic (sarcoid arthritis) manifestations seen regularly. Sarcoid causes abnormal calcium metabolism, with hypercalcemia a relatively common manifestation of the disease. Patients may have poorly defined constitutional symptoms including fatigue, anorexia, and low-grade fevers. Lymph node involvement is very common. As pulmonary disease progresses, progressive respiratory failure can occur, and there can be chronic superinfection of cysts and bronchiectatic areas. Pulmonary artery hypertension can occur when there is progressive hypoxia and damage to the pulmonary parenchyma.

Symptoms: Sarcoid has multiple well-defined presentations. One of the most common is that of asymptomatic X-ray findings. Lofgren's syndrome consists of fever, erythema nodosum, arthralgias, and bilateral hilar adenopathy. This constellation of findings is a special case that will be discussed under the diagnosis and treatment sections. Patients with symptomatic pulmonary disease will present with cough and dyspnea. Chest pain when present is poorly defined and located in the center of the chest. Hemoptysis is uncommon. Unless there is a great delay in diagnosis or presentation, clubbing and manifestations of pulmonary artery hypertension are uncommon. Extrapulmonary findings include malaise, anorexia, and fever. Cardiac symptoms, particularly arrhythmias and heart failure, may occur. Uveitis will present with eye pain and reduced visual acuity. Conjunctivitis can be present, and granulomas may be seen in the conjunctiva. Basilar meningitis may present with altered mental status and headache; cranial nerve palsies may be present. Diabetes insipidus (central) and hypopituitarism may be seen, as well as typical meningitis findings of stiff neck, etc. Spinal fluid demonstrates lymphocytes. Joint and muscle aches are common. Palpable adenopathy may be present. Splenomegaly and/or hepatomegaly are present in a minority of patients, but should be sought. Skin lesions are common with erythema nodosum a "classic" (Am Fam Physician 2007;75:695). Waxy, pink nodular lesions may be seen, and a maculopapular rash seen on the face and eyelids is typical. Plaque lesions may be seen, and a specific purple discoloration of the skin, lupus pernio, is typical but uncommon. Although these manifestations vary among ethnic groups, ages, and sex, all are possible in all patients (Semin Respir Crit Care Med 2007;28:83, Semin Respir Crit Care Med 2007;28:53).

Course/Prognosis/Complications: Patients who have no or limited pulmonary parenchymal involvement at presentation have a spontaneous remission rate in excess of 70% over the course of 5 years. Patients with extensive parenchymal lung disease at presentation have a 30% probability of 5-year remission. The overall death rate from sarcoid is <5%. Poor prognostic factors include dyspnea at presentation, African descent, progressive pulmonary infiltrates, multisystem involvement, skin lesions, and arthritis. Asymptomatic presentation and European descent are good prognostic factors, as is the presence of erythema nodosum. The difference between patients of African and European descent in disease course and outcome is considerable, and I counsel my patients to make sure that what they look up on the Internet applies to their ethnic background (Clin Chest Med 2006; 27:453). Patients with prolonged courses may have relatively good preservation of lung function and functional status if they are compliant and capably treated. Complications include chronic respiratory failure, cor pulmonale, and fungal (aspergillus) mycetomas in sarcoid cavities. These latter lesions can be associated with massive hemoptysis (see **Aspergillosis**).

Laboratory: There is no specific diagnostic test for sarcoidosis. Lung biopsy or other tissue biopsy will demonstrate noncaseating granulomas. ACE (angiotensin-converting enzyme) levels may be elevated but are nonspecific and do not play a role in diagnosis. Analysis of BAL fluid demonstrating elevated lymphocyte content and elevated CD4/CD8 ratio is felt by some to be a useful adjunct to biopsy. Anemia and leukopenia are present but uncommon. Eosinophilia is described in ~25% patients acutely. Elevated ESR, nonspecific hypergammaglobulinemia, and skin testing anergy are commonly noted. ECG may be normal or show conduction abnormalities. Pulmonary function testing is often normal, but when abnormal will show restriction and often obstruction. There is often a "disconnect" between the patient's symptoms and severity of pulmonary function abnormalities. Hypercalcemia may be seen. Echocardiography may show evidence of valve injury or stiff or dilated ventricles from granulomatous infiltration. The Kveim test is of historical interest only and will not be discussed.

Imaging: Chest X-ray "classic" is bilateral hilar lymphadenopathy, with or without parenchymal infiltrates. Occasionally, patients may have parenchymal infiltrates without adenopathy. Infiltrates are usually reticular opacities and are upper lung zone predominant. In advanced disease, there can be upper lung zone conglomerations of fibrosis similar to progressive massive fibrosis of silicosis (see **Silicosis**), and like silicosis, there may be eggshell calcification of hilar and mediastinal adenopathy. Although there is a staging system for chest X-rays in sarcoidosis, I confess that I have survived the last 30+ years in medicine without using it or referring to it. HRCT will demonstrate hilar and mediastinal adenopathy, irregular thickening of the bronchovascular bundles, nodules along the bronchovascular bundles, and nodules in the subpleural regions. Areas of ground glass opacity suggest active inflammation, and cyst formation is a consequence of scarring. Fibrosis and traction bronchiectasis are seen in advanced cases.

Diagnosis: How does one come to the diagnosis of sarcoid in the setting of this hodgepodge of clinical scenarios? Sarcoid, although technically a diagnosis of exclusion (correct clinical setting and histology in the absence of a good alternative diagnosis), in practice is often easily identified as the most likely diagnosis. However, there is a significant list of alternatives. For patients with primarily lymph node manifestations, lymphoma is the most serious alternative. Patients with parenchymal lung disease as well may have both infectious and noninfectious diffuse parenchymal lung disease. With the presence of adenopathy, mycobacterial infections and HIV illness (both primary and immunocompromised infections) should be considered. HP and EG can be confused with sarcoid initially, and investigation for beryllium exposure is warranted given the indistinguishable histological appearance (see **Berylliosis**). Many patients present with asymptomatic bilateral hilar lymphadenopathy (BHL). In these individuals, a careful search for other illnesses and an appropriate biopsy will be all that is necessary. In patients who are symptomatic, or who have an atypical chest X-ray or HRCT, biopsy will play an important role, and other illnesses will need to be excluded with a greater level of confidence. Patients with Lofgren's syndrome arguably can be excluded from biopsy; the pattern is so specific and the prognosis so good that a presumptive diagnosis is justified. In patients who are judged likely to have sarcoid, we do a complete physical examination including fundoscopy and full skin exam. A full, detailed review of systems is important. Basic chemistry profile, CBC with diff, EKG, urinalysis, and HRCT of the chest are usually all the testing that is necessary. Examination and this initial data will define the biopsy site. Accessible skin lesions, salivary glands, or lymph nodes are easily biopsied. Patients who have primarily thoracic disease may require mediastinoscopy or bronchoscopy with transbronchial lung biopsy; the sarcoid lesion is at such high density and uniformity that TBLB is feasible (Apmis 2001;109:289). It is less certain how to approach the patient if only mediastinal and hilar adenopathy is visible (no parenchymal disease even on HRCT); the yield of TBLB vs. mediastinoscopy in this setting has not been reported in the literature.

Treatment: The natural history of sarcoid is that most cases resolve spontaneously leaving few or no sequelae. Treatment usually involves the use of moderately high to high doses of steroids. We would like to avoid exposing patients to 40 mg of prednisone a day for several months if they were going to get better anyway. Despite decades of research, there is still no universally accepted approach to treatment across the spectrum of disease. My approach, which is mainstream, is to categorize patients into must treat, might treat, and no treatment needed categories. There is universal agreement that patients with cardiac sarcoidosis (echocardiographic findings or conduction delays), severe constitutional symptoms, meningeal symptoms, hypercalcemia, severe hematologic abnormalities, severe pulmonary disease, and ophthalmic disease *must* be treated with steroids. Some authorities recommend placement of an AICD in patients with significant cardiac sarcoid. There is equally good agreement that patients with normal pulmonary function, no extrapulmonary manifestations, and simple bilateral hilar adenopathy do not need treatment. Patients with an incidental finding of granulomas on liver biopsy do not need treatment. Patients with Lofgren's syndrome and arthropathy need little more than NSAIDs. "Might treat" is the difficult category. How bad must disfiguring skin lesions become before resorting to prednisone? How rapidly must the patient lose lung function to warrant steroids?

Once a diagnosis of sarcoid is made, we obtain full pulmonary functions, a full eye exam by an optometrist or ophthalmologist, and other testing (MR brain, echocardiogram) as indicated by the patient's presentation. If any findings drive the patient into the must-treat category, we initiate steroids (usually ~0.5 mg/kg/day), sustain this level of treatment for 6–8 weeks, and then taper to the lowest dose that maintains clinical gains. My threshold for consultation for serious extrapulmonary disease is low. If a patient falls into the "no treatment needed" category, we reassure the patient and develop a surveillance program of exams, lab work, X-rays, and pulmonary functions beginning at an interval of every 2–3 months and gradually lengthening to once per year over the course of 5 years.

Patients who fall into might-treat category are referred for consultation as appropriate for extrapulmonary disease if decision making is uncertain. For pulmonary disease, we discuss the pros and cons of steroid treatment, and my assessment includes consideration of comorbid conditions as well as the views of the patient and family. We will develop a similar plan of surveillance to evaluate response to therapy or evidence of clinical deterioration whether treatment is started or not. Decision making is dynamic, and the patient is comprehensively reassessed at each encounter.

Treatment decisions for pulmonary disease are difficult. Most pulmonary physicians integrate chest X-rays, symptom reports, and pulmonary function testing results to formulate a treatment decision. Although there has been investigation of ACE levels, gallium scans, and BAL analysis to guide treatment decisions, none of these tests have been shown to be any more useful than simpler clinical decision making. In my own patients, I will initiate therapy at presentation if a patient is severely dyspneic or has a vital capacity of 60% predicted or less. I am less swayed initially by chest X-rays. If a decision is made initially not to treat, the patient will return in 3 months for retesting. If there is more than a 10–15% drop in FVC or TLC, or more than a 20% drop in DLCO, I will initiate therapy. I will also initiate therapy on the basis of pulmonary function testing data if there are successive drops in lung function over the course of observation even if the difference between one test date and the next is <10%. I will also start therapy for worsening symptoms and worsening X-rays.

Treatment with systemic steroids starts at ~0.5 mg/kg/day for 4–6 weeks and is then tapered slowly over the course of several months. We find the lowest dose that stabilizes disease and stay there. Every 6–12 months I will attempt a further reduction in dose to see if there has been spontaneous resolution of the illness.

Alternatives to systemic steroid therapy include inhaled steroids (I use this particularly in patients with evidence of airway disease and relatively mild illness) and cytotoxics such as methotrexate and azathioprine. Cyclosporine, judging by mechanism of action, should theoretically work well, but it doesn't. TNF antagonists do not appear to be effective either. Cytotoxics should be considered as steroid-sparing agents in patients who have limited tolerance for the side effects, have experienced bad side effects, or are going to be on steroids for prolonged periods of time. Patients with severe, advanced sarcoid pulmonary disease are appropriate candidates for consideration of lung transplantation (Chest 2005;127:1006, Cochrane Database Syst Rev 2006;3: CD003536, Cochrane Database Syst Rev 2005;CD001114, Expert Opin Pharmacother 2007;8:1293).

7.9   Langerhans Histiocytosis

Thorax 2000;55:405, Clin Chest Med 2004;25:561, Chest 2003; 123:1673

Introduction: Langerhans histiocytosis is preferred over the older term of *eosinophilic granuloma*. Many clinicians use these names interchangeably.

Epidemiology: Precise incidence is unknown. The disease tends to be seen in younger individuals (peak incidence 20–40 years old) and seen almost exclusively in smokers.

Pathophysiology: The Langerhans cell is derived from the macrophage-monocyte line. The inciting event is unknown, but proliferation of Langerhans cells occurs in the lung in the peribronchial region. These proliferative centers can extend into the parenchyma. There can be perivascular inflammation and desquamation of cells into the alveoli. The mechanism is unknown, but as the disease progresses characteristic upper lung zone cysts may form and fibrosis may occur. This structural lung damage translates into multiple pulmonary symptoms, the most prominent of which are cough and dyspnea. Because the integrity of some alveoli have been compromised, spontaneous pneumothorax may occur. As the disease progresses, there may be extensive parenchymal damage with very few inflammatory cells. This "burned out" picture is difficult to differentiate from other forms of end-stage lung disease.

Symptoms: Often the patient will present with an asymptomatic abnormal X-ray. When symptoms are present, dyspnea and cough (nonproductive) are the most common complaints. Fatigue, weight loss, and fever may be present. Spontaneous pneumothorax may occur because of the cysts.

Course/Prognosis/Complications: Prognosis is variable, with some patients having asymptomatic X-ray changes and others progressing to respiratory failure. Patients may have repetitive pneumothoraces. Some patients may have pulmonary vascular disease. In some patients Langerhans histiocytosis is a systemic illness with skin, brain (hypothalamus with diabetes insipidus), and bone involvement. Extrapulmonary disease, particularly hypothalamic disease, is a poor prognostic finding.

Laboratory: There are no specific serologic markers, and routine blood testing abnormalities may be nonspecific. BAL may show a high fraction of Langerhans cells. Often, the patient will undergo biopsy for diagnosis, and surgical lung biopsy is preferred over TBB. Histologic changes can be difficult to interpret, particularly in the face of progressive disease as the number of identifiable Langerhans cells decreases. Immunohistochemical (S-100, CD1a antigen) staining has supplanted electron microscopy for identification of Langerhans cells. Pulmonary function testing results are variable, with both restrictive and obstructive patterns seen. Diffusing capacity is reduced.

Imaging: Plain chest X-ray may show a "classic" pattern of stellate ~1 cm nodules, extensive upper lobe cyst formation and honeycombing, and an underlying reticulonodular pattern. HRCT will confirm these findings, showing a profusion of small nodules, cysts, and interstitial thickening. There will be upper and mid-lung zone predominance.

Diagnosis: These patients are initially evaluated using the algorithm for interstitial lung disease/diffuse parenchymal lung disease. A young smoker with a typical HRCT picture arguably does not need a biopsy. In most other circumstances, surgical lung biopsy will likely be employed for a diagnosis.

Treatment: Smoking cessation. Steroids are of limited benefit, as are cytotoxics. Patients with advanced disease may be candidates for lung transplantation.

7.10 Idiopathic Interstitial Pneumonias

Introduction to Idiopathic Interstitial Pneumonias

Since the mid 1930s, physicians have recognized a group of diseases that produce diffuse parenchymal lung disease. These illnesses are largely confined to the interstitium, are progressive and often fatal if untreated, and have limited therapeutic options. Histologically, the lesion is one of replacement of normal lung tissue with fibrosis and various forms of inflammation in varying proportion.

Initially, these diseases were grouped together as idiopathic interstitial pneumonia or idiopathic pulmonary fibrosis. Plain chest X-rays showed obvious lung injury and scarring, but it was difficult to differentiate among patterns. Surgical lung biopsy was difficult and dangerous, and pathologic data came mostly from autopsy specimens. However, autopsy specimens were misleading because of the tendency toward convergence of all the different illnesses toward a final common pathway of nonspecific end-stage lung disease.

In 1969, Liebow and Carrington proposed a pathologic staging system that was the predecessor of current classification. In 2001, ATS and ERS developed a consensus statement (Am J Respir Crit Care Med 2002;165:277) that further subdivided and classified the idiopathic interstitial pneumonias. Currently, there are six generally accepted classes of disease: idiopathic pulmonary fibrosis/usual interstitial pneumonitis, nonspecific interstitial pneumonitis, acute interstitial pneumonitis, respiratory bronchiolitis associated interstitial lung disease, desquamative interstitial pneumonitis, and lymphocytic interstitial pneumonia.

While this exercise of division and subdivision may seem academic, this is not the case. Three components of care have converged to make precise classification and diagnosis clinically relevant. First, treatment and prognosis differ among the illnesses. This is important to remember when reviewing older literature. Many older articles addressing prognosis are potentially misleading because of cross-contamination of diagnostic groups. Second, the development of HRCT scanning has revolutionized imaging of these diseases. Clinical-pathologic-radiologic correlation has bestowed upon HRCT considerable diagnostic (and sometimes prognostic) value and has obviated the need for biopsy in a number of cases. Third, VATS lung biopsy is a safe and effective means of obtaining lung tissue in sufficient quantity to permit detailed pathologic examination. Transbronchial lung biopsy was often unhelpful, and OLB through a formal thoracotomy was a painful and morbid procedure. Currently, even relatively frail patients can be given a tissue diagnosis.

Unfortunately, the missing piece is still effective treatment. Numerous false leads have disappointed physicians and patients alike, and occasionally have caused some embarrassment to various pharmaceutical companies. Effective treatment of fibrosing pulmonary disease remains one of the elusive goals of pulmonary medicine.

Usual interstitial pneumonitis/idiopathic pulmonary fibrosis is the most common of these conditions and will be reviewed in the greatest detail. The other five conditions will also be summarized.

Patients with any of these conditions or with new pulmonary interstitial disease should be seen by a pulmonary physician, at least once and preferably regularly. These are sick, high-maintenance patients often with serious comorbidities. Consultation regarding appropriate evaluation and exploration of alternative treatable conditions is often helpful.

There are many excellent references on this topic. I would recommend most highly the issues of *Clinics in Chest Medicine* from September and December 2004 (vol 25, issues 3 and 4). These two issues provide a comprehensive review of both idiopathic and non-idiopathic interstitial lung disease, superb pathology images, and superb CT scan images. Newer materials should be reviewed for treatment options as well as these two volumes. King provides an overview of the last 100 years, which is of some historical interest (Am J Respir Crit Care Med 2005;172:268).

Usual Interstitial Pneumonitis (UIP)

Am J Respir Crit Care Med 2002;165:277

Epidemiology: Most common of the idiopathic pneumonias. Incidence in one study was 25–30/100,000. Incidence increases with age, sharply increasing over 70. Approximately 75% of patients are smokers or ex-smokers. The older term of *idiopathic pulmonary fibrosis* is used interchangeably with UIP.

Pathophysiology: The primary abnormality seen in UIP is fibrosis. There is a minor, chronic interstitial inflammatory component, but the primary finding is that of fibroblasts, honeycombing, and scarring. The inflammatory component is not the primary problem. Rather, there appears to be a primary fibrosing process present. Multiple cellular mechanisms have been proposed for the pathogenesis and etiology (Clin Chest Med 2004;25:749). From a clinical standpoint, pulmonary fibrosis increases the stiffness (reduces the compliance) of the respiratory system and causes an increase in the work of breathing. Obliteration of alveolar capillary units interferes with gas exchange. Both hypoxia and stiff lungs lead to dyspnea and tachypnea. As the disease progresses, coalescence of destroyed alveoli into larger cystic structures causes the X-ray appearance of honeycombing. Pulmonary fibrosis may lead to bronchiectasis because of increased radial traction on the airways. Chronic hypoxia and obliteration of the cross-sectional area of the alveolar capillary bed and arterioles eventually lead to pulmonary hypertension and cor pulmonale. As with many chronic lung diseases, there may be impressive clubbing. These patients may suffer episodes of exacerbation, sometimes caused by infection, but sometimes of uncertain etiology. Death is often from respiratory failure or overwhelming pulmonary infection.

Symptoms: Typical presentation is that of relentlessly worsening dyspnea and cough (months to years). Wheezing is absent. Dyspnea and exercise intolerance are universally present. Exam may show clubbing and/or cyanosis. UIP/IPF has the "classic" finding of so-called Velcro rales, a dry crackling sound usually more prominent at the bases. It really does sound like pulling apart Velcro. Evidence of right heart failure (edema, right heart S3) may also be present.

Course/Prognosis/Complications: UIP/IPF is a fatal disease with at least a 50% 5-year mortality. In addition to respiratory failure and pulmonary hypertension, there is an increased incidence of bronchogenic carcinoma. Many of my patients with this illness have been overwhelmed psychologically by the prognosis and the severe distress caused by unrelenting dyspnea.

Laboratory: Both anemia of chronic disease and erythrocytosis of hypoxia may be seen. Hyponatremia may be present from SIADH. Hypoxia is universally present, if not at rest then at exercise. ANA, rheumatoid factor may be weakly positive. Pulmonary function tests show reduced vital capacity, reduced total lung capacity, and reduced diffusing capacity consistent with a restrictive pattern. Presence of some obstruction may be due to smoking-related injury as well.

Imaging: Plain chest X-rays show a fine reticular pattern with a predominance at the bases. Adenopathy is absent. HRCT is felt by some experts to be pathognomonic for UIP/IPF when the reticular pattern is seen along with septal thickening, honeycombing, basilar predominance, and little ground glass appearance.

Diagnosis: UIP/IPF is a diagnosis of exclusion. A pattern of interstitial lung disease on X-ray and HRCT is not pathognomonic, and other idiopathic and nonidiopathic diseases of the pulmonary parenchymal may be in the differential diagnosis. Interstitial pulmonary fibrosis may be produced by RA, scleroderma, drugs, and environmental exposures (e.g., asbestos). I favor the approach of taking a pulmonary history and doing an HRCT as my first steps. If the images are not typical of UIP, I usually recommend some form of tissue sampling. This may be transbronchial lung biopsy (suspicion for sarcoid), bronchoalveolar lavage (infection, carcinomatosis, chronic eosinophilic pneumonia) but most often surgical lung biopsy (usually VATS procedure). If the HRCT suggests UIP and the patient does not have a known predisposing condition, I will obtain basic laboratory testing to assess the presence of collagen vascular disease (ANA, RF) although it is unlikely for an UIP/IPF picture to be the presentation of one of those diseases. Pulmonary history is reviewed looking for possible drug etiology. I will obtain a surgical lung biopsy for the patient if they are healthy enough to withstand surgery. In older, infirm patients I am more willing to use a compelling HRCT picture as sufficient evidence of disease.

Treatment: There is currently no uniformly effective treatment for UIP/IPF. A minority of patients will have a favorable response to corticosteroids in moderate to high doses (0.5–1 mg/kg/day prednisone). I use pulmonary function testing to provide objective evidence of response, using a 1 month interval between baseline testing and retesting after initiation of prednisone. If there is clinical and objective improvement, I will continue the medication at the lowest dose possible to sustain improvement. Many authorities recommend the simultaneous use of a cytotoxic agent as well as a steroid, although review of the literature suggests little incremental benefit (Am Rev Respir Dis 1991;144:291, Am J Respir Crit Care Med 2000;161:646). Current studies are under way to address UIP/IPF with antifibrosis agents. One sustained investigation involved interferon gamma-1b, heavily marketed by the manufacturer on the basis of limited clinical data, an episode reviewed in depth by the *New York Times* (New York Times 2003). An RCT failed to show clear benefit (N Engl J Med 2004; 350:125), and a second study was terminated early because of excessive mortality (http://www.fda.gov/cder/drug/advisory/interferon_gamma_1b.htm 2007;2007). Several novel agents are under investigation (Proc Am Thorac Soc 2006;3:330). Oxygen therapy, pulmonary rehabilitation, aggressive treatment of exacerbations with steroids, and antibiotics can improve the quality of life. End-stage patients may benefit from lung transplantation (see **Lung Transplantation**), and UIP/IPF is an indication for this intervention. Patients may benefit from palliative care as their disease worsens.

Other Idiopathic Interstitial Pneumonias

Respiratory Bronchiolitis and Respiratory Bronchiolitis Interstitial Lung Disease (RB) and (RBILD)

Respiratory bronchiolitis is a common pathologic finding in heavy smokers, implying inflammation around respiratory bronchioles. This is a pathologic finding rather than clinical illness. In some patients, RB can progress to RBILD, which is a clinical illness manifested by similar inflammation in the bronchioles along with inflammation in the alveoli. RBILD causes symptoms and pulmonary function abnormalities. HRCT findings show centrilobular nodules and ground glass appearance. There can be some septal wall thickening. RB/RBILD is strongly associated with smoking. Patients present with cough and dyspnea. Differentiation from other interstitial pneumonias will be on the basis of HRCT. However, lung biopsy may be necessary and surgical lung biopsy is preferred. Overall prognosis is good, with some patients having spontaneous remission (particularly, in my experience, with smoking cessation), and the illness does appear to be at least partially steroid responsive (Clin Chest Med 2004; 25:717).

Desquamative Interstitial Pneumonitis (DIP)

DIP is felt by many experts to be closely related to RBILD, and some authors think that these two illnesses are just different points on the same disease's spectrum of presentation. Histopathology is distinct, with intense desquamation of macrophages into the alveoli. Abnormalities are diffuse and not necessarily bronchocentric. There may be septal thickening. As with RBILD, there is a strong association with smoking. HRCT has findings of ground glass and small peripheral cystic spaces. Traction bronchiectasis may be seen. Patients with DIP typically present with cough and dyspnea. Differentiation from other interstitial diseases will be on the basis of HRCT, and it is likely that a surgical lung biopsy will be needed for diagnosis. These patients respond well to steroids and smoking cessation, and there is in excess of a 70% 5-year survival (Clin Chest Med 2004;25:717).

Acute Interstitial Pneumonia (AIP)

AIP is also known as Hamman-Rich syndrome. It is a rapidly progressive illness with a high mortality (~70%). Symptoms are usually present for weeks or less. The patient typically has a flulike prodrome with progressive respiratory failure. Histologically, the picture is that of diffuse alveolar damage, similar to ARDS. Treatment is primarily supportive (mechanical ventilation, etc.) but researchers have tried steroids, cytotoxics, and interferon. AIP looks like many other acute infectious and noninfectious respiratory diseases that cause acute respiratory failure. X-ray/HRCT pictures are similar to viral pneumonia, ARDS from other causes, acute eosinophilic pneumonia, drug-induced lung disease, inhalation injuries, or acute presentations of collagen vascular illnesses. AIP is a diagnosis of exclusion, and other treatable causes of ARDS and respiratory failure *must* be excluded before reaching this diagnosis. In an acute setting, BAL may be helpful in looking for infection, hemorrhage, etc., if the patient is too ill for surgical lung biopsy. Prognosis is similar to that of ARDS, with many patients dying, some patients surviving without sequelae, and some patients surviving with chronic respiratory insufficiency of one degree or another (Clin Chest Med 2004;25:739).

Nonspecific Interstitial Pneumonitis (NSIP)

NSIP is a relatively new subcategorization that is primarily one of histology. In 1994, it was proposed that there should be a category of interstitial pneumonia for biopsy specimens that did not fit neatly into one of the defined patterns. This proposal has been accepted, and NSIP is the result. Because it is a nonspecific category, there is no specific histology. Patients with primarily inflammatory and primarily fibrotic lesions as well as mixed lesions can be seen. Although this may seem like an abstract exercise with little clinical relevance, the purpose of this new category was to sharpen criteria for other diagnoses. In particular, UIP is now well defined and observations regarding prognosis, treatment, and mechanism are made from a uniform group of patients. The number of patients reported in the literature with this diagnosis is still relatively small. Prognosis and treatment are poorly defined. Prognosis is probably most related to the degree of inflammation (and hence susceptibility to treatment) present (Clin Chest Med 2004;25:705).

Lymphoid Interstitial Pneumonitis (LIP)

LIP is a very interesting histologic classification and almost certainly represents a disease mechanism that is different from the other interstitial pneumonias. LIP is characterized histologically by infiltration of the interstitium by lymphocytes and plasma cells as well as histiocytes. Larger architectural elements such as noncaseating granulomas and germinal centers may also be seen. LIP is classified both as an idiopathic interstitial pneumonia and a nonmalignant lymphoproliferative disorder. Typical presentation is nonspecific, with fevers, dyspnea, and cough. Laboratory findings usually include dysproteinemias, with a polyclonal hypergammaglobulinemia the most common.

X-ray imaging shows lower lung zone predominant reticular or reticular-nodular pattern. HRCT shows centrilobular nodules, septal thickening, ground glass regions, and cyst formation. Lymph node enlargement is usually absent. Surgical lung biopsy is often required for diagnosis. LIP is associated with Sjögren's syndrome and HIV infection, and a diagnosis of LIP should prompt evaluation for these conditions (although it is likely that the Sjögren's or HIV will already be evident). LIP must be distinguished from other lymphoproliferative disorders and MALT lymphoma. LIP is thought to have a good prognosis and is usually steroid responsive. Spontaneous remission occurs, so it is difficult to fully attribute resolution of the illness to treatment. Approximately 5% of patients may have transformation to a systemic lymphoma (Chest 2002;122:2150).

7.11 Rheumatologic Lung Disease

Introduction

A number of collagen vascular diseases affect the lung. Rheumatoid arthritis, scleroderma, and systemic lupus are prototypical. Mixed connective tissue disease has manifestations of all three conditions. Ankylosing spondylitis, Sjögren's syndrome, and Behçet's syndrome are among other illnesses that can cause pulmonary symptoms. Rheumatoid arthritis is the most common, and scleroderma and lupus are the most destructive.

The patient with pulmonary symptoms and collagen vascular disease must be assessed with care. The patient may indeed have a pulmonary complication of the underlying illness. Each condition can cause multiple pulmonary abnormalities, and parenchymal, pleural, vascular, and airway involvement are possible. The drugs that treat these illnesses can have pulmonary toxicity. Immune suppression both from the illness and its treatment render the patient at high risk for opportunistic infections. One illness does not confer immunity to other conditions, and the mundane diseases we all know and love can always crop up.

Rheumatoid Lung Disease

Epidemiology: RA is a common illness. Depending upon the ethnic/sex population investigated, incidence of the illness is between 0.1% and 5% of the population. Some studies suggest that ~30–50% of patients may have some degree of DPLD (not necessarily symptomatic) and that rates of pleural involvement may be even higher (although again, not necessarily symptomatic). Women are affected approximately twice as frequently as men.

Pathophysiology: The cellular biology of RA involves T-cells, B-cells, cytokines, and antigen–antibody interactions. A discussion of the mechanisms involved is beyond the scope of this text. It is appealing to speculate that the synovial surface bears some chemical resemblance to the pleural surface, and the frequent involvement of the pleura makes some sense. Pleural disease is common, and effusions and pleural thickening may be seen. Rheumatoid nodules (necrobiotic nodules) are pathologically similar to RA subcutaneous nodules. No other collagen vascular disease produces this abnormality. Two variants include rheumatoid nodulosis, where nodules are widespread, and Caplan's syndrome, where the interaction of coal dust exposure and RA causes formation of bilateral cavitating nodules (see **Coal Workers' Pneumoconiosis**). Interstitial lung disease is common in RA and may take the form of any of the interstitial pneumonias. NSIP and UIP are the most common. ILD is associated with a higher level of disease activity and a less favorable prognosis. BOOP is noted frequently and, like other forms of BOOP/COP, responds to therapy. Airway obstruction from involvement with RA is common. Bronchiectasis can be seen, and true bronchiolitis obliterans with rapidly progressive reduction in airflow is a rare but life-threatening complication. Pulmonary vasculitis and pulmonary hypertension are rarely seen with RA lung disease. One indirect effect on the respiratory system is cricoarytenoid arthritis with hoarseness and dyspnea from airway obstruction when the condition is severe. Kyphoscoliosis and arthritis of rib articulations may impair respiration.

Course/Prognosis/Complications: With the exception of ILD and rapidly progressive bronchiolitis obliterans, RA lung disease generally has a benign course. BOOP, although capable of causing considerable morbidity, usually responds to treatment. Occasionally, very aggressive BOOP can be seen (Am J Respir Crit Care Med 1994;149:1670). Nodules are generally associated with a good prognosis. Pleural effusions can be controlled. RA ILD generally has a better prognosis than idiopathic ILD, but is still capable of serious injury and death (J Rheumatol 2006; 33:1250). Rapidly progressive bronchiolitis obliterans has a poor prognosis, with one series having no survivors. Complications include drug toxicity, infection as a consequence of immune suppression, hemoptysis from necrosis of a nodule, and spontaneous pneumothorax. Progressive ILD can result in respiratory failure.

Symptoms: The patient's complaints and physical findings can vary widely. Pleural effusions and pleural involvement may be clinically silent, or cause dyspnea and pleurisy. Interstitial lung disease may cause cough and dyspnea, and rales are often present. Nodules are often without symptoms. BOOP related to RA manifests as other forms of BOOP/COP with cough, fever, dyspnea, and constitutional symptoms. Bronchiolitis obliterans is associated with rapidly progressive airflow obstruction resulting in severe, progressive dyspnea. (J Rheumatol 2006;33:1250, Clin Chest Med 1998;19:667, Arthritis Rheum 2006;54:628).

Laboratory: It is uncommon that pulmonary involvement will be the first manifestation of RA, and primary diagnosis of RA will not be discussed. Rheumatoid factor titers have limited linkage to disease activity. CRP and ESR determinations may be helpful in assessing disease activity. Pleural fluid analysis typically shows a yellow-green fluid, either serous or opaque. Rheumatoid effusions are not bloody. Low blood glucose levels are "classic," and one study cites statistics that over 70% of rheumatoid effusions have glucose content <30–40 mg/dl. Anaerobically collected pleural fluid pH is low, often <7.2. Complement levels in the pleural fluid are decreased, and rheumatoid factor may be detected. Cell count should be less than 10,000 and PMNs predominate (Clin Chest Med 2006;27:309). Pulmonary function testing may show restriction from DPLD, kyphoscoliosis, or pleural effusions; obstruction from bronchiolitis obliterans or larger airways obstruction; and diffusing capacity abnormalities from DPLD.

Imaging: Radiologic manifestations vary with disease presentation. Pleural effusion and pleural thickening are common. Radiographic presentation of BOOP/COP (see **BOOP/COP**) most frequently has the appearance of a patchy or consolidated pneumonia. Rheumatoid nodules are round, well-defined nodules. DPLD associated with RA will demonstrate diffuse basilar interstitial abnormalities. The appearance of the abnormalities is indistinguishable from the same illnesses not associated with RA. Honeycombing may be present in long-standing disease, and ground glass appearance may be seen in areas of active inflammation. HRCT can, in some circumstances, provide a diagnosis without biopsy. Bronchiolitis obliterans can be associated with hyperinflation, and CT scanning may enhance identification of areas with air trapping (Radiographics 2002;22 Spec No:S151).

Diagnosis: The patient with rheumatoid lung disease will present either with pulmonary symptoms or an abnormal chest X-ray. It is likely that the diagnosis of RA will already have been established. Many of these patients have been on cytotoxic agents and are middle aged or older. Rheumatoid arthritis, drug toxicity, immunocompromised pneumonia, malignancy (primary and metastatic), heart failure, and other forms of obstructive lung disease can be causes of both symptoms and X-ray findings. With perhaps the exception of unequivocal HRCT findings of interstitial lung disease without inflammation (no ground glass areas), the assumption that symptoms and X-ray changes may be attributed to RA is potentially dangerous. Drug toxicity and infection are important to identify, as one of those diagnoses will change treatment. Intercurrent illnesses such as cancer or heart failure may cause changes in treatment or prognosis. Serologic studies are poor markers of disease activity and cannot be used reliably. If infection is a consideration, bronchoscopy with BAL may be helpful, but masslike lesions may require either TTNB (e.g., nodule) or surgical lung biopsy (e.g., ground glass lung). A significant new pleural effusion should be sampled to assure that infection is not present.

Treatment: Although rheumatoid arthritis affecting the joints increasingly is treated with anticytokine therapy, steroids and steroid-sparing agents such as methotrexate and azathioprine are used for pulmonary RA. At present, there are no RCT data to confirm efficacy of anticytokine therapy for RA lung disease. Interestingly, there are also no RCT data for steroid or cytotoxic therapy. For interstitial lung disease, high-dose (0.5 mg/kg prednisone or higher) steroids are used for several months, supplemented or replaced by methotrexate or azathioprine. Symptomatic pleural effusions can be treated with steroids in similar doses, but for shorter intervals. Recurrent effusions may require pleurodesis. BOOP/COP of RA should be treated the same as BOOP/COP of other etiologies. Nodules generally do not need treatment. Rapidly progressive bronchiolitis obliterans is treated with high-dose steroids.

Systemic Lupus Erythematosus and the Lung

Radiographics 2002;22 Spec No:S151 (gorgeous pictures), Thorax 2000;55:159

Epidemiology: SLE is a relatively common illness with incidence rates in the range of 40–50/100,000. This can be lower or higher depending upon the subpopulation studied. The disease is more common in women than men. Most patients are diagnosed when they are young or middle aged. The rate of pulmonary involvement (detectable, not necessarily clinically significant) is high, well over 50% in most series.

Pathophysiology: There appears to be a genetic predisposition to the illness as expressed by haplotype. From an immunologic standpoint, there are numerous defects in immune regulation including T-cell–mediated down-regulation of immune response, increases in T-cell helper activity, nonspecific increases in B-cell stimulation, and dysfunctional cell surface receptor signaling. Which of these findings are primary abnormalities and which are secondary is unknown. These defects lead to premature cell death and exposure of cell contents to the immune system, resulting in the development of antinuclear antibodies. In turn, these antibodies cause further injury, resulting in clinical manifestations of disease. Pulmonary manifestations are diverse, with all pulmonary tissues affected. Pleural involvement is the most common, with effusion being the primary manifestation. Parenchymal involvement includes acute lupus pneumonitis and alveolar hemorrhage syndrome. Chronic interstitial lung disease is less common than in other collagen vascular diseases, but occurs with sufficient frequency to warrant consideration. BOOP/COP has been seen with lupus. A syndrome of acute reversible hypoxemia without demonstrable parenchymal infiltrates has been described, thought to be secondary to transient vascular plugging. Pulmonary hypertension is well described and occurs at relatively low frequency, perhaps 10% of patients. Pulmonary thromboembolism is associated with the antiphospholipid antibodies often seen in lupus (so-called circulating lupus anticoagulant, obviously misnamed). Respiratory muscle involvement by lupus is common, and the shrinking lung syndrome is probably related to respiratory muscle weakness. Airway involvement is uncommon. Upper airway involvement, such as that seen with Wegener granulomatosis (see **Wegener Granulomatosis**) is rare (Clin Chest Med 1998;19:641).

Symptoms: Unlike other collagen vascular diseases, fulminant pulmonary disease may be the first manifestation of lupus. Symptoms vary widely, with chest pain, dyspnea, cough, hemoptysis, fever, and constitutional symptoms all possible. Examination may demonstrate rales, bloody sputum, tachypnea, tachycardia, fever, and profound dyspnea. At the other end of the spectrum, the patient may have some mild chest pain or discomfort from pleural irritation.

Course/Prognosis/Complications: Depends largely on form of involvement. Pleural disease has little effect on survival and prognosis and survival will be driven by severity of other organ system involvement. Parenchymal lung disease can be devastating, with pneumonitis and hemorrhage associated with short-term mortality of 30–60%. Pulmonary hypertension is associated with a poor prognosis with one study indicating <50% 5-year survival. A wide spectrum of manifestations of the antiphospholipid syndrome makes it difficult to provide prognostic information. Patients with chronic interstitial lung disease are refractory to treatment and have persistent symptoms. The major complications of SLE are infections and consequences of treatment, including iatrogenic Cushing syndrome. The prognosis for patients with lupus has improved over the last 50 years, but some of this may be because of a greater number of patients with mild disease (due to more aggressive and sensitive testing).

Laboratory: Because lung involvement may be the first sign of SLE, a brief review of serologic testing is warranted. Antinuclear antibodies are the hallmark of SLE. However, low positive titers (<1:160) can often be seen in other autoimmune illnesses, and a small proportion of normal patients may have a low positive titer. The higher the titer, the more likely that the finding is a true positive and related to lupus. Anti-double-stranded DNA and anti-Smith antibody (anti-dsDNA, anti-Sm) are specific to lupus, but are not as sensitive. Most institutions offer a panel of autoantibody testing, and assistance from a rheumatologist is appropriate. Nonspecific markers of inflammation are also elevated (CRP, ESR) (Semin Arthritis Rheum 1995;24:323). Anemia, neutropenia, and thrombocytopenia can be seen, and hypoxia will be present if there is significant pulmonary involvement. Unlike rheumatoid arthritis, pleural fluid may be blood tinged, pH is usually normal, and glucose levels are not reduced. Antinuclear antibodies can be detected in some pleural fluid, and LE cells can be seen on microscopy (although this test is now performed rarely, if at all). If parenchymal lung biopsies are performed, H&E staining may be nonspecific, and some tissue should be reserved for immunohistochemical staining. From a practical standpoint, direct communication with the pathologist and submission of unfixed tissue has the highest likelihood of satisfactory tissue handling. Pulmonary function testing may show restriction and reduction of diffusing capacity. If airway disease is present, nonreversible obstruction may be seen.

Diagnosis: Patients may present with symptoms and signs consistent with lupus pulmonary involvement both with and without an established diagnosis. Presentations consistent with lupus lung involvement are also plausible presentations of neoplastic disease, infectious disease, and other autoimmune illnesses that require different treatment. Acute lupus pneumonitis and lupus-related pulmonary hemorrhage are life-threatening critical illnesses with double-digit mortality even with treatment. Patients with lupus are immunosuppressed by their illness and its treatment, and incidence of infection, opportunistic and otherwise, is high. New pleural effusions should be sampled and drained if feasible; neoplasm or infection are plausible alternatives. Pulmonary hypertension should raise the possibility of primary pulmonary hypertension or secondary pulmonary hypertension (see **Pulmonary**

Hypertension). Patients with a positive ANA and pulmonary hypertension may also have scleroderma. Pulmonary thromboembolism may be due to antiphospholipid antibodies or a more mundane reason. Chronic interstitial infiltrates can be associated with SLE but are less common than in other autoimmune illnesses. A low positive ANA can be associated with UIP, RA, and scleroderma. Dyspnea may have multiple causes, including cardiac/pericardial involvement with lupus, anemia, etc. Dense consolidations and cavitating lesions are infectious until proven otherwise. Both conventional and opportunistic infections are seen, and patients with SLE have a propensity to develop nocardia infections. Acute, diffuse infiltrates, with or without hemoptysis are an emergency and require rapid diagnosis and treatment. These patients should be hospitalized and in the ICU. Infectious etiologies should be considered and treated prophylactically even while the patient is receiving therapy directed against the immune illness. Pulmonary hemorrhage should raise the consideration of ANCA positive or anti-GBM illness (see **Pulmonary Vasculitis, Pulmonary anti-GBM Disease**). The presence of concomitant renal disease should heighten concern for these two diseases. Drug-induced lupus may be a consideration if the patient has had an appropriate exposure (hydralazine is the classic, along with procainamide).

Treatment: Agents used to treat SLE include steroids, antimalarial drugs, NSAIDs, and cytotoxics such as methotrexate, azathioprine, and cyclophosphamide. Mycophenolate has been used successfully (Expert Opin Investig Drugs 2008;17:31). Steroids and cytoxics are reserved for "significant" disease, and most authorities feel that pulmonary involvement meets that test. Lupus pneumonitis and pulmonary hemorrhage require the use of 1–2 mg/kg/day of prednisone equivalent, and some practitioners will use higher doses. Plasmapheresis is used by some practitioners for pulmonary hemorrhage. Patients with antiphospholipid antibody require anticoagulation, and patients with symptomatic pleural disease may respond either to NSAIDs or modest doses of gluco-corticoids (Chest 2006;130:182, Chest 2000;118:1083).

Pulmonary Scleroderma

Radiographics 2002;22 Spec No:S151 (gorgeous pictures), Curr Opin Rheumatol 2003;15:761, Curr Opin Rheumatol 2003;15:748, Medicine (Baltimore) 2002;81:139, Clin Chest Med 1998;19:713

Epidemiology: Scleroderma is less common than RA or SLE. Current estimates suggest an incidence of 3–4/1,000,000. The incidence of pulmonary involvement is high, on the order of 70% or greater. Women are more frequently affected than men. The disease is also termed *progressive systemic sclerosis* (PSS).

Pathophysiology: Scleroderma is a progressive, multisystem disease with fibrosis of multiple tissues and organs as well as vascular damage and vasoconstriction. Cellular mechanisms of disease are incompletely understood. Skin, renal, pulmonary, cardiac, and gastrointestinal involvement define the illness. Pulmonary involvement can involve pulmonary fibrosis, pulmonary artery hypertension, and/or occasionally aspiration pneumonia when severe esophageal dysfunction is present. Scleroderma pulmonary fibrosis can occur with both limited and systemic disease, as can pulmonary artery hypertension. Extensive pulmonary fibrosis can lead to traction bronchiectasis and all of the complications of chronic airway infection. Severe fibrosis can lead to spontaneous pneumothorax. It is unusual for there to be pleural involvement. The majority of patients with scleroderma lung disease already have been diagnosed; it is very uncommon for respiratory problems to be the presenting complaint.

Symptoms: The primary manifestations of scleroderma lung disease are dyspnea and cough. Patients with bronchiectasis may have chronic sputum production. Examination may show rales, right-sided P2 on cardiac auscultation, and a right ventricular heave. Oxygenation may be compromised. Patients will have the usual skin manifestations of Raynaud's phenomenon; digital ulceration; telangiectasia; tough, shiny skin with impairment of joint mobility; and sometimes scleroderma.

Course/Prognosis/Complications: This is a bad disease when it affects the lungs. One study showed a 30% survival at 9 years with pulmonary involvement, and a 70% survival in the absence of pulmonary involvement. Pulmonary disease is often a cause of death in patients with scleroderma. Two major complications include opportunistic infection as a result of the disease and its treatment, and malignancy. Lung cancer occurs in this group of patients at five times the rate seen in the general population.

Laboratory: Multiple autoantibodies are seen in scleroderma. ANA is frequently positive. Anti-centromere antibody is strongly associated with limited disease, but is specific to scleroderma. Anti-topoisomerase I antibodies (previously termed scl-70) are seen almost exclusively in scleroderma and are associated with pulmonary involvement. Oxygenation will be abnormal, and the patient may have evidence of renal insufficiency and anemia of chronic illness. Echocardiography may show PAH and right ventricular dysfunction. Primary manifestations of scleroderma cardiac involvement may also be present. Pulmonary function testing will reflect the presence of parenchymal lung disease with restriction and impaired diffusing capacity.

Imaging: Interstitial lung disease of scleroderma will have the same appearance as that of other inflammatory and fibrotic interstitial disease. On HRCT, a reticulonodular pattern will be present in areas of fibrosis, and ground glass will be seen in areas of more active inflammation. Areas of dense consolidation suggest infection or malignancy. There is no specific parenchymal pattern associated with PAH, although so-called pruning of vessels (truncated, plump pulmonary artery shadows) may be seen on plain X-ray.

Diagnosis: Most patients who present with scleroderma lung disease have already been diagnosed. Diagnosis concerns have to do with a change in X-ray or change in symptoms. Change may represent progression of the disease, aspiration pneumonia from esophageal dysfunction, opportunistic infection, drug toxicity, or malignancy. Fluid overload from renal insufficiency or cardiac disease may account for X-ray changes. Biopsy is rarely necessary for the de novo diagnosis of scleroderma interstitial lung disease, but may be required if opportunistic infection or malignancy is possible. New areas of dense consolidation should prompt a search for infectious or malignant complications.

Treatment: Treatment of interstitial lung disease of scleroderma is frustrating both to the clinician and patient. Patients with evidence of ground glass changes on HRCT or a BAL analysis indicating active inflammation may derive benefit from immunosuppressive therapy with prednisone and a cytotoxic agent such as cyclophosphamide. Patients on this regimen should receive PCJ prophylaxis. At present, there are no agents that can reverse fibrosis. Most authorities recommend treatment of scleroderma-associated pulmonary hypertension in a manner similar to that of primary PAH with pulmonary vasodilators such as iloprost, bosentan, and sildenafil. These patients should be treated at a center with special expertise in the treatment of PAH. In both forms of lung disease symptomatic and general supportive care are appropriate, with pulmonary rehabilitation, appropriate vaccinations, oxygen therapy, and adequate nutrition helping to improve outcomes.

Other Connective Tissue Diseases

Radiographics 2002;22 Spec No:S151, beautiful CT scans and histology. This text has covered RA, SLE, and PSS in greater detail because they are relatively common and define the spectrum of collagen vascular disease from a pathophysiologic standpoint. There are several other conditions that should be mentioned.

Mixed Connective Tissue Disease (MCTD): This disease has been recognized since the early 1970s and has several names, the most enlightening of which is *overlap syndrome*. The patient typically has manifestations of several connective tissue diseases, including dermatomyositis, RA, SLE, and PSS. The patient may have pleural effusion, interstitial fibrosis, pulmonary hypertension, and pulmonary hemorrhage. Thromboembolic disease may be seen, and these patients are at risk for opportunistic infections. Autoantibody patterns are different in this condition, with high titers of speckled ANA (>1:1000), and presence of anti U1 snRNP antibody (previously termed *extractable nuclear antigen [ENA] antibody*). Anti-sm is usually absent. Treatment consists of steroids and cytotoxics, with varying degrees of success reported (Clin Chest Med 1998;19:733, Am J Med 1972;52:148).

Polymyositis/Dermatomyositis: This is a multisystem disease that affects primarily the muscle and skin. Patients usually present with proximal muscle weakness and any of a number of dermatologic findings. There is a high incidence of pulmonary involvement (~40%) with interstitial pneumonitis. In the early course of the pulmonary disease, the patient may have inflammatory histology. Later in the course, the histology may be that of fibrosis. HRCT in some instances has taken the place of biopsy. Patients may also have respiratory muscle weakness with chronic respiratory failure. Complications may include infection and drug-induced lung disease. Autoantibody patterns may include anti-Ro, anti-Jo, anti-Sm, and anti-La antibodies detected. Treatment consists of steroids and cytotoxics (Semin Arthritis Rheum 1995; 24:323, Clin Chest Med 1998;19:701).

Sjögren's Syndrome: This is a common illness (~0.1% of population) that presents with the triad of dry mouth, dry eyes, and arthritis.

Pulmonary involvement has been reported at varying frequencies. The histologic hallmark of the illness is lymphocytic infiltration, and this can occur in the lungs. Lymphocytic interstitial pneumonia has a strong association with Sjögren's syndrome; other authors have reported patterns consistent with UIP. Lymphocytic infiltration (pseudolymphoma) and MALT lymphoma (mucosa-associated lymphoid tumors) of the lung have been seen in this condition. Sjögren's syndrome is considered both primary (no evidence of any other autoimmune illness) or secondary (evidence present for another autoimmune illness). A variety of different autoantibodies may be seen, including ANA, anti-Ro, and rheumatoid factor (among many others). Treatment of pulmonary complications is aggressive, using steroids and cytotoxics. Newer therapies include rituximab and other anti-B lymphocyte antibodies (Clin Chest Med 1998;19:687, Mayo Clin Proc 1989;64:920, Arthritis Rheum 2007;56:1371).

Ankylosing Spondylitis: This autoimmune illness affects the joints of the axial skeleton. Of historical interest, it was one of the first illnesses to be associated with a specific HLA antigen, HLA B27. Diagnosis is made on the basis of clinical and X-ray findings, as this is a seronegative disease. Pulmonary involvement occurs on the basis of chest wall restriction and apical fibrobullous disease. Physiologic impairment caused by these two disease manifestations is usually quite limited. Superinfection of upper lobe fibrobullous disease with fungi and mycobacteria (*Aspergillus*, atypical mycobacteria) can occur and is usually managed as conservatively (noninvasively) as possible. Underlying joint disease can be managed with NSAIDs and anti-TNF alpha drugs such as infliximab and etanercept (Clin Chest Med 1998;19:747, Ann Rheum Dis 2006;65:316, Ann Rheum Dis 2003;62:817).

7.12 Pulmonary Vasculitis

Ann Intern Med 1992;116:488, Lancet 2003;361:587, Rheum Dis
Clin North Am 1995;21:949, Clin Chest Med 1998;19:18, Am J
Med 2004;117:39

Introduction: Several disease processes may produce a picture of vasculitis and affect the lung. Three diseases merit particular attention because they share some components of pathogenesis and are relatively common in comparison to other entities. Wegener granulomatosis, microscopic polyangiitis, and Churg-Strauss syndrome affect the lung frequently and will be covered here. Diseases such as polyarteritis nodosa and giant cell arteritis rarely affect the lung and are best left to other texts.

Epidemiology: Wegener granulomatosis, microscopic polyangiitis, and Churg-Strauss syndrome have been reported to occur in white populations in the frequency of 8/1,000,000 (Wegener) to 2/1,000,000 (Churg-Strauss) with polyangiitis somewhere in between. The disease is less common in nonwhite populations. Patients tend to be middle aged with 50s predominating but the disease can be seen in both younger and older patients. Fifty percent or more of patients with Churg-Strauss syndrome have preexisting asthma. There is some concern that use of leukotriene-receptor blockers such as zafirlukast and montelukast may be associated with the development of Churg-Strauss, but most experts think that the addition of a non-steroid treatment reduces steroid use and then unmasks preexisting disease. There do not appear to be predisposing factors for the other illnesses.

Pathophysiology: These three conditions share detectable anti-neutrophilic cytoplasmic antibodies (ANCA). Antibodies are directed against proteinase-3 (PR3) and myeloperoxidase (MPO). There are a number of technical issues associated with testing that are beyond the scope of this text. Immunofluorescence assays mix patient serum with ethanol-fixed human neutrophils, and antigen antibody complexes are identified. Cytoplasmic pattern ANCA (C-ANCA) is usually associated with anti-PR3 antibodies, and perinuclear pattern ANCA (P-ANCA) is usually associated with myeloperoxidase antibodies. The distinction is important, in that a P-ANCA has a broader association with immune disease, and a C-ANCA positive titer is more tightly associated with Wegener or Churg-Strauss (Wegener has a much higher positive rate than Churg-Strauss). For reasons that are unclear, shielded antigens (epitopes) in the polymorphonuclear cell become exposed immunologically and antibodies form against granule proteins, primarily MPO and PR3. It is thought (although not proven) that an infectious or environmental agent, superimposed on a genetic predisposition to the illness, initiates the chain of events that leads to disease. It is also not clear that ANCA is the offending antibody, and it may be an epiphenomenon. The actual mechanism of injury to tissue involves both T- and B-cell immunity. Endothelial cells appear to participate in the injury process, explaining the presence of vasculitis. Respiratory tract (upper and lower), renal, eye, joints, skin, and neural tissue are the most common sites of disease. The histologic lesion is granulomatous inflammation with vasculitis.

Symptoms: Patients with Wegener and polyangiitis often present with bloody or purulent nasal discharge, nasal ulcers, ocular ulcers, or sinus pain. The trachea and larynx may be involved, causing upper airway obstruction. The patient may have hemoptysis and dyspnea as well. Frank respiratory failure with need for mechanical ventilation may be seen. Skin involvement (nodules, typical vasculitis lesion of palpable purpura) and renal involvement are common, and rapidly progressive renal failure may be associated with the illness. Joint tenderness may also be present. Churg-Strauss syndrome has a somewhat longer course with often years of antecedent asthma, succeeded by blood and organ (pulmonary,

GI tract) eosinophilia, and a final phase of vasculitis with manifestations similar to that of WG and MPA. Neurologic involvement is more common with CSS, and pericardial disease may occur as well. Wegener may be be associated with an alveolar hemorrhage syndrome.

Course/Prognosis/Complications: Morbidity and mortality in these conditions arise from the diseases themselves and the treatment. Aggressive immunosuppression makes the host susceptible to PCJ, fungal illnesses, conventional pneumonia, and mycobacterial disease. Some studies have identified 40–50% of patients having complications from treatment (Ann Intern Med 1992;116:488). Pulmonary hemorrhage, respiratory failure from diffuse pulmonary disease, renal failure, and damage to other affected structures such as the eye, nose, sinuses, airways, heart, and central nervous system arise from the illness. Gastrointestinal involvement may occur. Renal, CNS, and cardiac disease are the most feared and worsen prognosis. Survival from appropriately diagnosed and treated WG is approximately 80%, but may include serious sequelae such as end-stage renal disease and respiratory insufficiency.

Imaging: X-ray and CT findings may show nodules (classic is cavitating), alveolar infiltrates, pleural effusions, and diffuse hazy infiltrates. On CT scan peripheral vascular structures may be enlarged and thickened in comparison to companion bronchi. These findings are similar for all three diseases.

Laboratory: CSS may be associated with eosinophilia and elevated IgE as well as anemia. All three diseases may have thrombocytopenia and elevated ESR. All three illnesses have a high incidence of positive ANCA titers. WG most frequently has a positive C-ANCA correlating with anti-PR3 antibodies (90% positive ANCA), while MPA is more often associated with P-ANCA titers (anti-MPO, 70–80% positive ANCA). The overall frequency of a positive ANCA in CSS is somewhat lower (70%), but a preponderance of patients have a C-ANCA finding.

Diagnosis: The triad of nasal ulcers, pulmonary infiltrates, and renal failure should bring to mind the possibility of WG. Any patient with simultaneous pulmonary disease and renal disease should have WG and MPA in the differential diagnosis. Patients who have cavitating nodules in the absence of malignancy and infection also have a significant likelihood of having one of these three illnesses. A patient with a long history of asthma who then develops pulmonary infiltrates with peripheral eosinophilia should raise the possibility of CSS. With all three of these illnesses, diagnosis is hastened by keeping an open mind and being alert to the idea that a nonresolving pneumonia may not be infectious or malignant. Once the consideration of vasculitis is raised, the patient should have ANCA titers measured. A positive ANCA greatly raises the possibility of one of these three diseases, but all authorities I reviewed (1) do not feel that a positive ANCA is conclusive and (2) strongly believe that a tissue diagnosis is mandatory. Any accessible lesion may be sampled. However, kidney biopsies are frequently performed because the nature of the glomerulonephritis seen carries prognostic information. As implied earlier, the primary differential diagnosis for lung-related illness includes infection and malignancy. Antibasement membrane disease (Goodpasture syndrome) has considerable overlap with WG, and many pulmonary clinicians will order anti-GBM and ANCA testing simultaneously as a routine. WG may need to be differentiated from other pulmonary hemorrhage syndromes. Finally, injudicious use of ANCA testing may be confusing because positive ANCA titers are noted in a variety of clinical settings including other autoimmune illnesses and some drug reactions.

Treatment: All three of these conditions are life threatening and require consultation with a pulmonary physician, nephrologist, and/or rheumatologist. Of the three illnesses, WG presents the most serious threat. Multiple studies indicate that initial treatment with cyclophosphamide and steroids induces the quickest and most durable remission. Data suggest that ~90% of patients achieve remission, and ~75% do so within 3 months of starting therapy. WG has a tendency to relapse, and maintenance therapy is often required. Because of the toxicity of long-term cyclophosphamide, maintenance with methotrexate or azathioprine is sought. Steroids do not appear to play a major role in maintenance management. Maintenance therapy is usually continued for 12–18 months. If a relapse occurs when therapy is stopped, therapy is restarted. Multiple relapses often indicate a need for indefinite therapy. Microscopic polyangiitis is treated similarly. MPA has considerably less propensity to relapse. Alternative therapies are available for induction and maintenance, but are beyond the scope of this article. CSS responds well to steroids alone (0.5–1.5 mg/kg/day for 6–8 weeks) and relapses infrequently.

7.13 Pulmonary Anti-GBM Disease

Ann Intern Med 2001;134:1033, Kidney Int 1996;50:1753, Kidney Int 2003;64:1535, Am J Kidney Dis 1986;8:31

Introduction: Although pulmonary anti-glomerular basement membrane disease is rare, it is of interest because of the mechanism of injury and the seriousness of the illness. Survival requires rapid identification of the problem and prompt treatment. Goodpasture syndrome is the eponym given to the triad of pulmonary hemorrhage, rapidly progressive glomerulonephritis, and detectable anti-GBM titers.

Epidemiology: Rare, <1/1,000,000. Primarily seen in whites. Male predominance.

Pathophysiology: An unknown stimulus produces antibodies against the basement membrane present in the alveoli and glomeruli.

Antibody production is short lived, and for that reason if the patient can survive the initial illness the likelihood of recurrence is low. Research has demonstrated that the antibody is directed against a segment of the type IV collagen molecule in the basement membrane. It is unclear why some patients may have only pulmonary disease, renal disease, or both. Specific HLA types (DR2, DRw15, and DRw16) are associated with the disease. Immunochemical staining of the glomerulus (and less commonly the alveoli) shows linear deposition of antibody in the basement membrane. This causes loss of integrity of the alveoli and glomeruli with hemoptysis, respiratory failure, and glomerulonephritis with renal failure.

Symptoms: Pulmonary manifestations of disease include hemoptysis (probably over 90% of patients will have hemoptysis at one point or another in the illness), dyspnea, chills, fevers, and weight loss. Chest pain can also be seen. Many patients will have associated rapidly progressive renal failure.

Course and Prognosis: Untreated, mortality is at least 50% and may be as high as 90%. Death occurs by respiratory failure and/or renal failure. Current therapy has improved mortality and hemodialysis-free survival, but a substantial number of patients still are left with renal insufficiency. Patients who go on to have renal transplantation may have evidence of linear deposition of anti-GBM in the allograft glomeruli, but clinical illness is not seen.

Laboratory: The sine qua non of diagnosis is evidence of circulating anti-GBM. The literature raises concerns regarding specificity and sensitivity of various test kits, and communication with your laboratory may be important if a patient is thought to have the disease. Anemia and evidence of renal failure ($\uparrow$ BUN, $\uparrow$ creatinine) are often present. Elevation of ESR may be mild. Urinalysis will demonstrate evidence of glomerulonephritis with microscopic hematuria, red cell casts, and proteinuria.

Imaging: Chest X-ray is nonspecific, with evidence of diffuse infiltrates, patchy areas of infiltrates, and confluent infiltrates commonly referred to as "whiteout."

Diagnosis: A patient with acute hemoptysis and renal failure should immediately raise the possibility of Goodpasture syndrome. Rapid initiation of therapy is critical, and differentiation from other conditions may be lifesaving. Wegener granulomatosis can have a similar presentation, and most pulmonary physicians order anti-GBM and ANCA titers simultaneously. Any process that causes acute renal failure may produce volume overload, and hemoptysis can occur in that setting. Anti-GBM antibodies may be seen concurrently with ANCA. If questions persist about the diagnosis despite serologic testing, renal biopsy, rather than lung biopsy, is preferred as the disease affects the kidneys more than the lungs, and the histology is more specific.

Treatment: These patients are sick and require subspecialist management immediately, typically from a nephrologist/pulmonary physician team. Treatment with immunosuppressive agents alone was unsuccessful. Current practice employs plasmapheresis, cyclophosphamide, and steroids simultaneously. Because of the urgency for treatment, many practitioners will initiate therapy for Goodpasture while awaiting test results. Plasmapheresis can be terminated if the patient is determined to have WG or another condition. Therapy appears to be most effective when serum creatinine is less than 6–8 mg/dl and oliguria is not present. Therapy is usually continued for 6 months.

7.14 Diffuse Panbronchiolitis

Sarcoidosis Vasc Diffuse Lung Dis 2004;21:94, Clin Chest Med 1993;14:765

Introduction: Although uncommon, this illness is of sufficient scientific interest to warrant discussion. Response to macrolide antibiotics in the absence of a defined infectious agent has led to the use of macrolides in other chronic airway diseases such as cystic fibrosis. The relatively narrow ethnic spectrum makes this illness ripe for disease mechanism analysis.

Epidemiology: The majority of cases occur in Japanese men, although the illness has been reported in other ethnic groups. Familial case patterns have been recorded, and there are HLA types associated with the illness (HLA-Bw54 and HLA-A11). Cofactors are probably involved in pathogenesis, as the illness is rarely seen in Japanese living abroad. The disease is most common in nonsmokers.

Pathogenesis: The primary lesion is an intense inflammatory infiltration of the bronchial walls and sinuses with lymphocytes, neutrophils, plasma cells, and "foamy macrophages" that are lipid laden. Chronic airway and sinus inflammation leads to physical damage to the airways and sinuses, which in turn leads to bronchiectasis and chronic sinusitis. Superinfection with *Pseudomonas* and *Haemophilus* species is common, and the patient eventually develops a picture of bronchiectasis.

Symptoms: Sinusitis may precede lung disease by years or decades. Cough, sputum, dyspnea, and constitutional signs of chronic infection such as weight loss may be present. Patients are typically nonsmokers.

Course/Prognosis/Complications: Without treatment, 5-year survival is stated to be 50%. Macrolide antibiotics improve this prognosis, but the precise effect is unknown. Progression to the usual complications of bronchiectasis with respiratory failure and chronic infection is common.

Laboratory: Evidence of chronic infection with positive sputum cultures for *Pseudomonas* and *Haemophilus* is common. ANA and RF titers may be positive. IgA levels may be elevated, as well as positive cold agglutinins. Pulmonary function test results are varied, with obstructive and obstructive-restrictive patterns both found. Hypoxemia is present. DLCO will be reduced.

Imaging: X-rays are nonspecific with small nodular shadows in all lung fields and sometimes hyperinflation. HRCT has a "tree-in-bud" pattern of centrilobular nodules and branching opacities. Air trapping is common. Although the CT scan may be suggestive of diffuse panbronchiolitis, it is not specific (High-Resolution CT of the Lung 2001;629, pp. 538–540).

Diagnosis: The disease should be differentiated from other airway and bronchiectatic diseases. Cystic fibrosis and Kartagener syndrome would be viable alternatives. The illness should be considered in Asian ancestry men who are nonsmokers with bronchiectasis and sinusitis. Surgical lung biopsy is necessary for a conclusive diagnosis.

Treatment: Macrolide antibiotics are clinically effective in this illness. Long-term low-dose erythromycin has effects that are unrelated to the drug's antibacterial properties. Changes in CD4/CD8 ratios, reduction of neutrophil superoxide production, and other alterations in cellular function appear to be the relevant mechanisms. Length of treatment (and if the drug can be stopped at all) is unknown. Aggressive treatment of infection, pulmonary toilet, and other strategies used in bronchiectasis are appropriate (Am J Respir Crit Care Med 1998;157:1829).

7.15 Pulmonary Alveolar Proteinosis

Clin Chest Med 2004;25:593, Am J Respir Crit Care Med 2002; 166:215

Epidemiology: Rare, <0.5 cases/1,000,000. There is an association between disease and smoking. 2:1 male preponderance. There is possibly a slightly increased risk for African-Americans. Although some cases are associated with malignancy, the majority is idiopathic. The unique mechanism of disease (excessive surfactant production) and its treatment (whole lung lavage) warrant discussion of this illness.

Pathophysiology: Abnormal regulation of surfactant production in the lung produces alveolar filling with proteinaceous material and lipids. Macrophages containing lamellar bodies (surfactant material as found in type I pneumocytes) are present. Etiology of this abnormal regulation is unknown, although mouse strains that do not produce granulocyte-macrophage colony-stimulating factor have a high incidence of a pulmonary alveolar proteinosis-like condition. Diffuse alveolar filling with this material leads to abnormal respiratory mechanics, impaired gas exchange, and fertile ground for infection.

Symptoms: Dyspnea is most prominent. Cough is present ~75% of the time. Constitutional symptoms such as fever, weight loss, and generalized fatigue are seen. Hemoptysis and chest pain are occasionally present but uncommon. Exam is often normal or minimally abnormal with basilar rales.

Course/Prognosis/Complications: Modern survival rates for this illness are high, approaching 100% with early diagnosis and lavage. The primary complication seen is infection. *Nocardia* species appear to have a particular affinity for PAP afflicted patients, and these agents should be among the primary considerations in a PAP patient with pneumonia.

Laboratory: LDH elevations; hypoxia on blood gases; abnormal diffusing capacity and mild to moderate restriction on pulmonary function testing. Bronchoalveolar lavage fluid has a characteristic milky appearance, and microscopic examination shows acellular protein material and macrophages that stain for high concentrations of lipid.

Imaging: Chest X-ray shows bilateral diffuse alveolar densities. HRCT has a "crazy paving" appearance—there is scattered/diffuse ground glass appearance with superimposed linear opacities from interlobular septal thickening and intralobular lines. Although the pattern is suggestive, it is not diagnostic.

Diagnosis: This is a rare illness and should not be the prime diagnosis. Numerous infectious and noninfectious illnesses are more common and more acute: viral pneumonia, PCJ pneumonia, ARDS, pulmonary edema, interstitial pneumonitides, BOOP/COP, etc. If "crazy-paving" is present on HRCT, PAP should be considered more strongly. The diagnosis is secure if BAL shows a milky, turbid fluid with lipid-laden macrophages and acellular protein material in the washings.

Treatment: Since the early 1960s, treatment has consisted of sequential whole lung lavage. A double lumen endotracheal tube is placed, isolating one lung from the other, and while relying on single-lung ventilation, the other lung is flooded with saline and then drained. Typical total volumes are 20–40 liters before the returned fluid is clear to visual inspection. Some patients can have both lungs lavaged in a single anesthetic session, while others may require a longer period of recovery and separate procedures. Relief from symptoms with this intervention may last for months to years, with repeat lavage performed based on symptomatic and radiographic worsening. Some centers will use other techniques such as bronchoscopic instillation of the lavage fluid. Smoking cessation is necessary.

7.16 Lymphangioleiomyomatosis (LAM)

Eur Respir J 2006;27:1056, Chest 1998;114:1689

Epidemiology: LAM is a rare disease that affects women of childbearing age. Incidence is not known precisely, but estimated to be 1 per million. Occurrence in postmenopausal women is uncommon, and only one case has been identified in a man. Postmenopausal LAM may be associated with HRT (hormone replacement therapy).

Pathophysiology: LAM is a multisystem disease characterized by benign atypical smooth muscle proliferation. In the lung, smooth muscle proliferation leads to airway obstruction, pulmonary venous hypertension, and dilation/rupture of intrapulmonary lymphatics and enlargement of thoracic lymph nodes. Progressive distention of the alveoli and distal bronchioles leads to cyst formation. Injury from smooth muscle proliferation may lead to fibrosis. The disease appears to be dependent upon estrogen stimulation. Other organs may be involved, including renal angiomyolipomas. Retroperitoneal lymphadenopathy may be seen. As the lung is progressively injured by cyst formation and fibrosis, there is loss of gas exchange and progressive respiratory failure. The pathologic appearance of LAM is identical to that of tuberous sclerosis when it affects the lung, suggesting that LAM may be a *form fruste* of tuberous sclerosis.

Symptoms: Include pneumothorax, progressive dyspnea, pleural effusions, hemoptysis, and occasionally chyle in the sputum.

Course/Prognosis/Complications: LAM is a progressive illness with a variable course. Different series describe varying survival rates (78% at 10 years, 26% at 8.5 years), but the most recent paper quotes 70% 10-year survival. Because of the frequent delay in diagnosis, it is difficult to describe a typical course. The young age of the patients, often with a young family, makes for a socially and emotionally taxing illness. There are no accepted benchmarks for marking disease progression, and pulmonary function testing, radiographic evaluation, and clinical evaluation are used collectively. In addition to progressive respiratory failure, pneumothorax, chylous effusions, chylous ascites, hemoptysis, and retroperitoneal bleeding (from angiomyolipomas) can complicate the illness.

Imaging: Chest X-ray may show pneumothorax and multiple patterns associated with DPLD. Effusions may also be present. HRCT is more useful, and the presence of numerous thin-walled cysts surrounded by normal parenchyma is the "signature" of this disease. In advanced disease, there may be evidence of fibrosis. When ground glass appearance is seen, this may be associated with intrapulmonary hemorrhage as a consequence of pulmonary venous hypertension. Adenopathy may be seen (High-Resolution CT of the Lung 2001;629, pp. 429–435).

Laboratory: Pulmonary function tests will show low diffusing capacity, obstruction, and loss of lung volume. Blood gases will show hypoxemia. There are no specific serum tests.

Diagnosis: There is often a delay in diagnosis (sometimes years) for these patients, as the disease is confused with asthma, other obstructive lung diseases, or another DPLD. The clinician should develop a high index of suspicion for LAM when a woman of childbearing age presents with a spontaneous pneumothorax or effusion with abnormal pulmonary parenchyma and progressive dyspnea. Although some authorities feel that a definitive diagnosis can be made from HRCT alone, conclusive diagnosis usually rests on a lung biopsy (surgical lung biopsy rather than TBB).

Treatment: There are no controlled trials of treatment. Steroids and cytotoxic agents don't work. Therapies judged to be successful rely on hormone manipulation, with oophorectomy, progesterone administration, and estrogen blockade (tamoxifen) used most frequently. Pregnancy exacerbates the disease, and conception is not recommended. The large number of fragile cysts and physical obstruction of the bronchioles make sudden barometric pressure changes dangerous, and some authorities caution against air travel. Lung transplantation has been used for patients with LAM with varying results. One series appeared to have outcomes similar to patients with other advanced lung disease. Several other studies, however, suggest that these patients may have a more difficult course because of injury to the thoracic cavity from LAM and continued effusions and pneumothoraces in the remaining native lung (in single lung transplantation).

Chapter 8

Adult Respiratory Distress Syndrome and Acute Lung Injury

Clinics in Chest Medicine: Acute Respiratory Distress Syndrome. December, 2006, volume 27, number 4, provides a current overview of accepted practice and areas of investigation in ARDS/ALI.

Epidemiology and Definitions: Acute lung injury is a syndrome of acute and persistent lung inflammation that results in breakdown of the alveolar-capillary membrane and resultant increased vascular permeability. The chest X-ray must show bilateral pulmonary infiltrates. In addition, the PaO_2/FIO_2 ratio is between 201 and 300. This ratio is an attempt at quantification of impaired oxygen transfer present. ARDS is the extreme of this condition, requiring the PaO_2/FIO_2 ratio to be 200 or less. These are arbitrary divisions but permit comparison of data sets and trials. One study cited an incidence of 86 cases per 100,000 person-years (age adjusted) (N Engl J Med 2005;353:1685). ARDS/ALI is seen in all age groups, although the etiology will differ among age groups (more trauma related in the young, more sepsis related in the elderly). As many as 20% of patients who are placed on mechanical ventilation have ALI/ARDS.

Pathogenesis: The pathogenesis of ARDS is not fully understood, although many cellular and biochemical mechanisms have been

401

implicated, investigated, and ultimately found to provide an incomplete or no explanation. There is general agreement that ARDS is a consequence of inflammation. Multiple mediators of inflammation are trapped by the pulmonary circulation and an inflammatory process is induced. There are numerous conditions that can lead to ARDS. The most common causes are listed in Table 8.1. Breach of the alveolar-capillary barrier has specific physiologic consequences. There is contamination of the interstitium and alveoli with fluid. This impairs gas exchange and may also lead to dead space ventilation. Second, production of surfactant is impaired or absent. This leads to collapse of alveoli, which then do not participate in gas exchange, causing shunt physiology. Loss of surfactant and an engorged interstitium lead to stiff, noncompliant lungs increasing work of breathing, causing further collapse of alveoli, and further impairment of gas exchange. Onset of the illness is usually rapid, occurring over a few hours to 2–3 days. The initial damage pattern is that of fluid in the alveoli, stiff lungs, and refractory hypoxia. As the course progresses, there may be resolution of abnormalities or progression to a fibrosing, proliferative phase. Diffuse pulmonary infiltrates, difficult ventilation with high oxygen requirements, and

Table 8.1   Common Causes of ARDS/ALI

Sepsis
Trauma
Aspiration of gastric contents
Pneumonia
Massive transfusion
TRALI
Drugs and alcohol
Organ transplantation
Relief of upper airway obstruction

Note: TRALI = transfusion-related lung injury. This is different from massive transfusion.

need for a mechanical ventilator generally resolve as the condition improves.

Symptoms: Patients at risk for ARDS are easy to identify. In a community hospital setting, a diagnosis of vehicular or penetrating trauma, sepsis, pneumonia, or aspiration are the most common risk factors. Sepsis is the most common etiology. ARDS patients will go on to have tachypnea, tachycardia, air hunger, and sometimes cardiovascular collapse. Both saturations and blood gases will show hypoxia. There are no specific laboratory tests for ARDS, and many of the signs and symptoms will be that of the underlying condition. When intubated, these patients will show normal airway resistance, but marked reduction in compliance.

Course/Prognosis/Complications: At present, the overall death rate from ARDS is in the 30% range. The majority of patients who die *with* ARDS do not die *from* ARDS, but their underlying illness or complications of treatment (pneumonia, IV catheter-related sepsis, multisystem organ failure, etc.). Only ~15–20% of deaths are attributable to respiratory failure. Poor prognostic signs include failure to improve within 72–96 hours and marked elevations of the ventilatory dead space (measure of ventilation of alveoli that are not perfused, wasted ventilation) (N Engl J Med 2002;346:1281). Patients who survive ARDS are often deconditioned and require rehabilitation. Long-term use of paralytics and sedation may cause prolonged muscle weakness and delirium, respectively. Patients often have various degrees of post-traumatic stress disorder. Long-term impairment of lung function is a recognized complication, with obstructive, restrictive, and diffusing capacity deficits identified. Measurements of health-related quality of life are also abnormal (Am J Respir Crit Care Med 2003;167:690).

Imaging: Chest X-ray will show bilateral fluffy, interstitial infiltrates. Patients may occasionally have minimally abnormal X-rays with severe gas exchange abnormalities. CT scans performed on these patients, however, will demonstrate extensive alveolar and interstitial infiltrates.

Laboratory: There are no specific laboratory tests that can conclusively diagnose or exclude ARDS. Laboratory abnormalities will often reflect the precipitating condition. Hypoxia is universal, as it is required for diagnosis. Hypercarbia may be present. In pure ARDS, echocardiography should show normal left ventricular function. Approximately 25% of patients may have pulmonary hypertension.

Diagnosis: The main alternative diagnosis is cardiogenic pulmonary edema: CHF or fluid overload. Treatment strategies for ARDS and CHF diverge, and if there is any question at all as to etiology of dyspnea and pulmonary infiltrates, transthoracic or transesophageal echocardiography, central venous pressure measurement, and/or pulmonary artery catheterization should be performed. Pulmonary hemorrhage, some forms of viral pneumonia, diffuse alveolar damage from inhalation injury, Hamman-Rich syndrome, acute eosinophilic pneumonia, and occasionally malignancy may have the same aggressive appearance.

Treatment: Treatment of ARDS has four goals:
1. Identify and treat the underlying, precipitating process.
2. Defend tissue oxygenation.
3. Minimize injury related to therapy.
4. Prevent complications.

The course and prognosis of ARDS (independent of etiology) have not been influenced by any therapy directed at interruption of the inflammatory cascade. The most studied treatment has been corticosteroid therapy: different flavors, different amounts, different timings. Steroids appear to have no role in the proliferative phase of ARDS. One study suggests that steroids may have some value in early ARDS (Chest 2007;131:954), and a second study suggests that aggressive steroid replacement therapy in patients who appear to have relative adrenal insufficiency may benefit (Crit Care Med 2006;34:22). This second study is a post hoc analysis and needs further evaluation. Patients who have ARDS as a consequence of a specific steroid responsive illness (e.g., acute eosinophilic pneumonia or massive gastric aspiration) should receive steroids.

While receiving physiologic support, the patient should be evaluated for the precipitating cause. Sepsis is the most common etiology, and a search for the source of infection should be undertaken if sepsis is suspected. In a community hospital, the most common sources will be abdomen (biliary tract and soilage of peritoneum with intestinal contents), lung, and urinary tract. Treatment of sepsis seeks to eradicate infection and maintain tissue perfusion while not causing further injury secondary to treatment. The "Surviving Sepsis" campaign has sought to provide guidelines based on evidence and consensus statements addressing the multiple physiologic derangements encountered in septic shock (Intensive Care Med 2007;epub). First published in 2004, some recommendations of the campaign have encountered criticism because of industry funding that may have influenced treatment advice, specifically the use of drotrecogin alfa (recombinant activated protein C for infusion) (N Engl J Med 2006;355:1640). Nonetheless, there are noncontroversial recommendations such as goal-directed fluid resuscitation that offer an effective, structured framework for aggressive treatment. The treatment of ARDS-related respiratory failure is directed at maintenance of tissue oxygenation by providing adequate pulmonary gas exchange and adequate tissue perfusion with oxygenated blood. Oxygenation is achieved with supplemental oxygen and recruitment of alveoli not participating in gas exchange. Positive end expiratory pressure (PEEP) is the best tool available for recruitment. It prevents end-expiratory collapse of alveoli that cannot subsequently reopen (hysteresis induced by lack of surfactant) and because of an unfavorable position on the pulmonary compliance curve. In effect, it "converts" shunt physiology to V/Q mismatch. High FIO_2 and high PEEP respiration for sustained periods is achieved only with tracheal intubation (endotracheal or tracheostomy) and mechanical ventilation. Mechanical ventilation, PEEP, hyperoxia, and the adjunct treatments used carry a high rate of complication and secondary injury. Treatment of respiratory failure, prevention of lung injury, and prevention of complications are addressed in an integrated manner by the ARDS network protocol. This protocol is the result of efforts to reduce macro-barotrauma, micro-barotrauma, and oxygen toxicity. Macro-barotrauma refers to rupture of alveoli leading to pneumothorax and cardiovascular collapse. Oxygen toxicity describes injury to airway and parenchymal lung tissue as a direct result of high oxygen concentrations. Pathologic changes of tissue injury both in animals and humans are recognized as a result of high oxygen tensions. Efforts to minimize this risk must be balanced against the need to defend the patient's tissue oxygenation. Micro-barotrauma refers to a more recently recognized process of tissue injury resulting from ventilation, including alveolar overdistention, end-expiratory alveolar collapse, and initiation of the inflammatory cascade. Collectively, these processes are referred to as ventilator-induced lung injury (VILI) (Clin Chest Med 2006;27:601). Lung-protective ventilation describes low tidal volume (~6 ml/kg) breaths and prevention of plateau pressures greater than 30 cm H_2O. This strategy was found so effective that an NIH-sponsored trial was stopped because of excessive death in the control arm (N Engl J Med 2000;342:1301). Injury and complication prevention are also addressed through other interventions. These include nutrition, meticulous attention to fluid balance, VAP prophylaxis, DVT prophylaxis, gastrointestinal bleeding prophylaxis, glucose control, and avoidance of paralytic agents/minimization of sedation when possible. Hypercarbia is tolerated in the context of lung-protective ventilation and is referred to as permissive hypercapnia; excessive hypercarbia with severe acidosis is treated with bicarbonate buffer; mild acidosis is simply tolerated. Patients with an established diagnosis of ARDS should be treated by a pulmonary or critical care physician or transferred to a center where this expertise is available.

Chapter 9

The Lung and Pregnancy

Introduction: Although not a disease state per se, pregnancy is associated with disease states unique to pregnancy and complicates the treatment of conditions that also occur in the nonpregnant population. Cardiac and pulmonary physiology is altered during pregnancy and must be taken into account in caring for the pregnant patient.

Physiology: Normal pregnancy causes several changes in the mechanics of respiration. The diaphragm is elevated and the shape of the chest wall is altered. This results in a reduction in residual volume and FRC and can lead to V/Q mismatching at the lung base. Higher circulating progesterone levels stimulate ventilation, and $PaCO_2$ is near 30 rather than 40. Oxygenation is preserved and the PaO_2 is usually slightly over 100. There is often a mild compensated respiratory alkalosis. Many patients complain of dyspnea during pregnancy, which is multifactorial in etiology. Vasocongestion of the mucosa of the upper respiratory tract can make instrumentation of the upper airway difficult and more traumatic, and contribute to discomfort and dyspnea (Clin Chest Med 2004;25:299). Cardiovascular changes include elevated heart rate, elevated circulating blood volume, elevated cardiac output, and reduced pulmonary and systemic vascular resistances (Crit Care Med 2005;33:1616).

Pathophysiology: Acute lung injury syndromes are associated with several catastrophic complications of pregnancy. Amniotic fluid em-bolism, preeclampsia (HELLP), air embolism, and

407

chorioamnionitis are among the most serious associated with pregnancy and delivery. ARDS can occur from obstetric hemorrhage, acute fatty liver of pregnancy, and transfusion reactions. Pneumonia and other catastrophic infectious illnesses can precipitate ARDS in the pregnant patient. Pulmonary edema (PE) can occur from tocolytics and pericardium cardiomyopathy. These conditions each have a characteristic presentation, and the lung will not be the only organ involved, with the possible exception of tocolytic pulmonary edema. The effects of both the disease and treatment on the fetus as well as possible need for early delivery of the fetus in the context of critical illness are beyond the scope of this article.

Pneumonia in the pregnant patient is associated with a higher rate of complication than in the nonpregnant patient. Immunologic changes make the patient more susceptible to viral pneumonia, and influenza and varicella pneumonia carry a high mortality. TB is successfully treated during pregnancy. Typical bacterial pneumonia should be treated taking into account the toxicities to the fetus of such drugs as quinolones, sulfas, and tetracyclines.

Peripartum aspiration of gastric contents (Mendelsson's syndrome) can cause a lung injury syndrome or aspiration pneumonia if there is superinfection. Pregnancy creates a high risk environment for venous thromboembolism, and the clinician should be suspicious for this condition. Pregnancy should not create an obstacle to appropriate radiologic evaluation for PE. Coumadin is a Category X drug and is contraindicated in pregnancy. Unfractionated heparin and low-molecular weight heparin are Category B. The cardiovascular changes associated with pregnancy and the stress of delivery can occasionally precipitate cardiovascular decompensation in a patient with occult underlying cardiac disease. Dyspnea or pulmonary edema may be the presenting problem.

In the outpatient setting, asthma will be the most common respiratory illness encountered in the pregnant patient. Some texts state that in terms of asthma activity/severity, 1/3 of OB patients stay the same, 1/3 get worse, and 1/3 improve. The experience of many clinicians (mine included) is that asthma is stable or better in pregnancy, and exacerbation is rare. Aggressive protection of the fetus from hypoxia is warranted and should not be influenced by concerns about medications. Although many asthma medications are technically Category C, in practicality they are safe, including oral corticosteroids. Montelukast and budesonide are both Category B.

Other References: Critical Illness in Pregnancy, Critical Care Clinics Oct 2004; (Murray and Nadel 2005, 2269-77) .

Chapter 10
Pleural Disease

10.1 Introduction

There are relatively few primary diseases of the pleural space. Pleural abnormalities arise from diseases of the cardiovascular system or the pulmonary parenchyma. The pleural space can fill with fluid, air, or tissue. All can cause discomfort and dyspnea. Large amounts of fluid or air, particularly when they accumulate rapidly, can reduce venous return to the heart and cause cardiovascular collapse (i.e., tension pneumothorax). Pleural abnormalities are common in everyday practice.

10.2 Pneumothorax

Air in the space between the visceral and parietal pleura is termed *pneumothorax*. Air entering the pleural space from outside the chest is invariably traumatic (penetrating trauma, thoracentesis, or biopsy needle). Air entering the pleural space from the lung occurs because of disruption of lung tissue and the formation of a bronchopleural fistula. Pneumothorax usually does not occur as a result of the spontaneous rupture of a normal alveolus; the rupture of a normal alveolus usually arises from barotrauma of mechanical ventilation or laceration of the lung from a rib fracture. Rarely, spontaneous rupture of a normal alveolus may be seen as a component of a diving accident. More frequently, the underlying lung tissue that gives way is abnormal. Rupture of bullae associated with COPD is a common source of pneumothorax. Patients who have marked differences in distensibility of various areas of the lung, such as during an asthmatic attack, can have local overdistention of alveoli and sustain a pneumothorax. A number of pulmonary parenchymal conditions and infections give rise to pneumothorax as well. These include AIDS (especially with PCJ pneumonia), TB, cystic fibrosis, sarcoidosis, Langerhans histiocytosis, and lymphangioleiomyomatosis. Malignancy may cause pneumothorax, as may endometrial implants on the pleural surface (catamenial pneumothorax). There is also a syndrome of spontaneous pneumothorax in the absence of known preexisting lung disease. This condition is often seen in tall, thin patients, presenting during the teen years. Examination of the pleural surface in these patients often demonstrates the presence of small blebs and bullae, one of which has ruptured and caused the pneumothorax. In some patients, these abnormalities are not present, and the etiology of pneumothoraces in these patients remains under investigation (Clin Chest Med 2006; 27:369). Initial treatment of a pneumothorax uses insertion of a chest tube (tube thoracostomy) if needed; a small PTX without significant distress may be treated with observation alone. If only air is present and the air leak is small, a small bore tube may be inserted. Larger air leaks, trauma, and/or presence of liquid in the pleural space require the use of a large bore tube. Practice after insertion of the tube can vary widely. The patient may be sent home with a Heimlich (one-way) valve; patients with nonresolving PTX could get surgery in 2 or 3 days, or in 2 or 3 weeks. The ACCP (also the British Thoracic Society) has published guidelines for management of pneumothorax (Chest 2001;119:590). These guidelines include provision for simple aspiration of a small pneumothorax if this is the first event, and surgical intervention after 4 to 5 days of persistent air leak. A proportion of patients will go on to have a second PTX. These patients do not have the option of simple aspiration, and it is recommended that they undergo surgical intervention after ~5 days of conservative therapy. Surgical intervention usually consists of bullectomy (or repair of a visible pleural rupture) and either parietal pleural abrasion or parietal pleurectomy. These two procedures are designed to create a raw, inflammatory surface that will lead to adhesions between the lung and the chest wall.

10.3 Pleural Effusion

Pleural effusion is a common clinical condition. Effusions are classified as transudates or exudates. Transudates are the consequence of hydrodynamic migration of fluid into the pleural space in the face of an intact capillary membrane; exudates are the consequence of fluid entering the pleural space because of a breakdown of the integrity of the capillary membrane. Investigation of a pleural effusion should begin with sampling of the pleural fluid and evaluation of the patient for predisposing conditions and possible diagnoses. Multiple pleural fluid biochemical tests have been proposed to differentiate an exudate from a transudate. The most widely accepted algorithm remains Light's criteria, seen in Table 10.1. Other tests include serum albumin-pleural fluid albumin gradient, pleural fluid cholesterol, and pleural fluid bilirubin. Once the fluid has been determined to be exudative or transudative, the clinician can pursue a diagnosis with a more limited spectrum of possibilities. Common diagnoses for exudates and transudates are listed in Table 10.2. A more comprehensive list of common and not so common etiologies may be found in these two references (Clin Chest Med 2006;27:309, Clin Chest Med 2006;27:285). It is not possible to review the management and diagnosis of all forms of pleural effusion. The three most common effusions will be covered here.

Table 10.1 Light's Criteria for Distinguishing Between Exudates and Transudates

Pleural fluid/serum protein ratio >0.5
  OR
Pleural fluid/serum LDH ratio >0.6
  OR
Pleural fluid LDH >2/3 upper limit of normal serum LDH

Table 10.2   Common Causes of Transudative and Exudative Effusions

Transudate	Exudative
Congestive heart failure	Parapneumonic
Cirrhosis	Malignancy
Peritoneal dialysis	Tuberculosis
	Pulmonary embolism
	Pancreatic disease
	Associated with cardiac injury and/or CABG
	Intra-abdominal pathology
	Rheumatoid illness

Source: Data from Light, 2006, Clin Chest Med 2006 27(2);309.

Congestive Heart Failure

Congestive heart failure is the most common cause of effusion. The effusion is a transudate. Most patients will have evidence of heart failure with depressed left ventricular ejection fraction or diastolic dysfunction on echocardiography, elevated BNP, and enlarged cardiac silhouette and pulmonary vascular engorgement on chest X-ray. There is a tendency for the effusion to be right sided, although this cannot be used as a point of conclusive diagnosis. Often, the effusions are bilateral. Some patients, particularly those who have had aggressive diuresis or in whom the effusions have been long-standing, may have an effusion that has exudative characteristics. A patient with obvious heart failure with effusions does not require thoracentesis for diagnosis or treatment *if* the effusion(s) responds to treatment directed at the heart failure *and* there are no complicating factors such as fever, accompanying pulmonary infiltrate, etc. Treatment is directed at the underlying heart failure with diuresis, afterload reduction agents, beta blockade, and inotropic agents. Occasionally, a patient may have a large effusion from heart failure causing respiratory compromise, and thoracentesis drainage may provide immediate relief and improvement in oxygenation. Prevention of recurrence of the effusion is directed at optimizing treatment of the underlying heart failure. In a small number of patients, pleurodesis may be required (Chest 1992;102:1855). Some authorities recommend repeated thoracenteses over time if tolerated by the patient, but I have seen several patients who have developed an empyema from this practice, and I would recommend it only when other options were not working or were not available.

Empyema and Parapneumonic Effusion

Infections of the pleural space may occur as a consequence of contamination by penetrating trauma (gunshot or knife wound, thoracentesis needle), extension from the mediastinum or abdomen, or more frequently by extension from a pulmonary parenchymal infection. Penetrating trauma or infection by extension from the mediastinum or abdomen will be easily identified and treatment with appropriate antibiotics and surgical drainage will be instituted. Many patients with pneumonia will have an effusion, but not all will need surgical drainage. Some patients will have a sterile parapneumonic effusion that requires drainage. Prompt identification of a parapneumonic effusion requiring drainage is important because early intervention may only require tube thoracostomy, while delay may lead to decortication. Nontreatment of a parapneumonic effusion may cause fibrothorax with trapped lung and chronic effusion and atelectasis if it heals and severe chronic infection if it does not. Refer to Chest 2000;118:1158 for a consensus statement from the ACCP regarding the treatment of parapneumonic effusion. The paper recommends sampling a parapneumonic effusion if loculated pleural fluid and/or free-flowing fluid producing a layer >10 mm in thickness on lateral decubitus is present on chest X-ray. Although differentiation between transudate and exudate employs a variety of tests, differentiation of a sample between a complex and simple parapneumonic effusion requires only pH determination, gram stain, and culture. Table 10.3 outlines the criteria for surgical vs. medical treatment. Pleural fluid for pH determination should be collected anaerobically and tested using a blood gas analyzer. Tuberculous empyema generally should not be

Table 10.3 Categorization of Risk of Unfavorable Outcome for Parapneumonic Effusion

Risk of Poor Outcome	Effusion Status		Culture and Gram Stain		Pleural pH	Drain ?	Notes
Very low	Minimal, free flowing (<10 mm on lateral decubitus)	AND	Results unknown	AND	Results unknown	No	1, 2
Low	Small to moderate free flowing (>10 mm and <½ hemithorax)	AND	Negative culture, negative-gram stain	AND	pH ≥7.20	No	3, 4
Moderate	Large free flowing effusion (>½ hemi-thorax) loculated effusion, or w/ thickened parietal pleura on contrast enhanced CT	OR	Positive culture OR positive-gram stain	OR	pH <7.20	Yes	5
High	Doesn't matter		Pus		Doesn't matter	Yes	

Notes: AND and OR are used as logical operators.
(1) Minimal effusions do not require sampling, and results may be misleading.
(2) Increase in size of effusion or unfavorable clinical course should prompt reassessment including thoracentesis.
(3) Increase in size of effusion or unfavorable clinical course should prompt reassessment including repeat thoracentesis.
(4) Previous use of antibiotics does not influence gram stain and culture result interpretation.
(5) Loculations are associated with a poorer prognosis.
Modified from Colice, Chest 2000 118(4):1158

surgically drained. Treatment of bacterial empyema consists of antibiotics appropriate to the underlying pneumonia (e.g., antibiotics active against anaerobes for aspiration associated pneumonia) and drainage as appropriate. Most authorities recommend 4–6 weeks of antibiotic therapy for an infected pleural space. Additionally, the pleural space should be drained of fluid (no pockets on chest X-ray or CT scan and minimal fluid drainage from chest tube), and the lung should be fully expanded. Drainage options include tube thoracostomy, VATS for destruction of loculations and removal of debris, and formal thoracotomy. The ACCP statement recommends early intervention for loculations, and an obvious empyema with pus on gram stain should prompt an early invasive approach. Often, this can be achieved with VATS-directed destruction of intrapleural septae, mobilization of the lung, and removal of debris. Decortication is a more invasive procedure where the infected pleural peel is removed from the pleural space. Decortication is a major, difficult operation, and from the standpoint of a pulmonary/critical care doctor, these patients get really sick postoperatively when all the endotoxins and inflammatory mediators are unceremoniously dumped into the bloodstream. Early aggressive intervention often obviates the need for decortication. The ACCP statement references the use of fibrinolytics to break up loculations and endorses their use. Subsequent analyses suggest that while fibrinolytic agents are safe, they do not shorten length of stay, reduce mortality, or reduce the need for surgery, and their use is not recommended (N Engl J Med 2005;352:865).

Malignancy

Malignant pleural effusions may be a manifestation of metastasis (or further metastasis) of a known malignancy or the first manifestation of cancer. Primary pleural malignancy is uncommon and is reviewed in the section on mesothelioma (see **Mesothelioma**). Pleural effusion is a common complication of advanced malignancy. Lung and breast cancer, followed by hematologic malignancy such as lymphoma, are the most common cell types. Unfortunately, with the occasional exception of lymphoma, pleural malignancy is a fatal diagnosis. Treatment is directed at palliation of pain and dyspnea and prevention of reoccurrence rather than sterilization of the pleural space. Malignant pleural effusions are exudates. The analysis profile may suggest infection with low glucose and low pH. Bloody or blood-tinged effusions are common, and a bloody pleural effusion in the absence of trauma, pneumonia, or pulmonary embolism should be considered malignant until proven otherwise. Most authorities (and I) believe that a new pleural effusion that is either suspicious for malignancy or appears in the context of a known malignancy should be proven to contain malignant cells by histology or cytology. Reported yields for pleural fluid cytology vary widely, based on type of malignancy and how high a concentration of malignant cells are shed into the pleural fluid; one recent review quoted between 60% and 90%. My experience has been a false negative considerably greater than 10–30%. Closed pleural biopsy with a Cope or Abrams needle is performed infrequently at present, if at all. This is a blind (undirected) sampling with a high false-negative rate and a technique that can only be described as barbaric. Attempts to obtain tissue confirmation of malignancy often employ medical thoracoscopy or VATS sampling. This approach is particularly appealing because sampling error is very low (procedure is performed under direct vision), and pleurodesis using talc poudrage may be accomplished under the same anesthesia if the effusion is obviously malignant. Medical thoracoscopy is not available in all centers, and a VATS-based procedure is usually easier to arrange. Treatment of malignant pleural effusion is palliative. The main symptoms are dyspnea and less often pain or chest discomfort. Direct treatment of the underlying malignancy may or may not be possible. Radiation is not possible because the entire lung would be subjected to radiation, causing extensive damage and even more dyspnea. A variety of sclerosing agents have been introduced into the pleural space including tetracycline and bleomycin. At present, studies favor talc poudrage (talc powder blown into the pleural space through a thoracoscope) as the most effective and least painful procedure. Patients with a poor performance status and whose effusions reaccumulate slowly may benefit from repetitive thoracentesis. Simple tube thoracostomy with introduction of a sclerosing agent or talc slurry may be appropriate in selected individuals. (Am J Respir Crit Care Med 2000; 162:1987 is an excellent general reference.) There is a much greater comfort level with VATS since 2000; therapy recommendations from this older document should be interpreted accordingly.

10.4 Fibrothorax

Nonmalignant obliteration of the pleural space occurs as the consequence of pleural inflammation and subsequent proliferation of fibrous tissue. Fibrosis of the pleural space may produce a uniform rind of fibrous tissue over the lung producing restriction and reduced vital capacity. Alternatively, there may be inhomogeneous fibrosis with severe atelectasis of a single lobe. The latter may lead to chronic infection and localized bronchiectasis. Fibrothorax usually occurs as the consequence of no treatment or incomplete treatment of a pleural process such as hemothorax or empyema. Treatment of this condition (when treatable at all) requires extensive bloody surgery for pleurectomy and lysis of adhesions. In most cases, fibrothorax can be avoided with prompt treatment and diagnosis of inflammatory pleural effusions (Clin Chest Med 2006;27:181).

Reference: Pleural Disease. Clinics in Chest Medicine June 2006 Volume 27, number 2. This is an excellent volume devoted entirely to pleural disease, addressing current issues in diagnosis and treatment.

Chapter 11

Neuromuscular and Ventilatory Control Conditions

11.1 Pulmonary Complications of Neurological and Musculoskeletal Disease

Introduction

The lungs depend on the musculoskeletal system (controlled by the central nervous system and connected to the CNS by peripheral nerves) for the bellows pump function that produces alveolar air exchange. When this fails, alveolar hypoventilation occurs. This produces hypercarbia and hypoxia. Greater degrees of hypoxia than expected by the alveolar air equation (see **Hypoxia**) may be produced by V/Q mismatching produced by atelectasis. Many diseases associated with bellows pump failure may also produce an unprotected upper airway leading to aspiration and pneumonia. Some of these illnesses are progressive and fatal, some may be controlled with medication, and others may spontaneously resolve if the patient is kept alive during the illness.

Central Nervous System

Major stroke or *brain injury* with coma may cause apnea and loss of control of the upper airway. These patients require intubation and mechanical ventilation until there is resolution of the problem or a decision is made to terminate life support. *High cervical spinal cord injury* (C3 or above) interrupts normal neural control signals from reaching the diaphragm and intercostal muscles and hypoventilation results. These patients are apneic and require full ventilatory support despite the presence of intact cervical accessory muscles of respiration (cranial nerve innervation). Lower cervical spine injury (C4 and below) may leave patients able to breathe spontaneously or require only partial ventilatory support. Cervical spine injury patients are at high risk of pneumonia and atelectasis as well as pulmonary embolism (Respir Care 2006;51:853). Acutely, these patients may also suffer neurogenic pulmonary edema. For reasons that are not fully understood, even high cervical cord injury patients regain some bellows function as they recover from their injury. Cough and clearance of secretions is a major problem, and pneumonia is a frequent cause of death in these patients. *Amyotrophic lateral sclerosis (ALS)* is a devastating degenerative central nervous system disease where there is progressive loss of strength of respiratory muscles and loss of control over the upper airway. Shortness of breath, orthopnea, difficulty clearing secretions, aspiration, and difficulty with speech are seen in advanced forms of this illness. Both upper motor neuron and lower motor neuron manifestations of disease are encountered (Respiration 1994;61:61).

Peripheral Neurons

Guillain-Barré syndrome is the prototypical disease in this category. GB syndrome is characterized by an ascending peripheral neuropathy with muscle weakness and ultimately paralysis. Sensory function is often preserved. This illness is unique in that the great majority of cases have recovery of strength and independent respiration over the course of weeks to months. These patients may require tracheostomy, and DVT prophylaxis is appropriate (Arch Neurol 2005;62:1194). *Bilateral phrenic nerve paralysis* is occasionally encountered as a complication of diabetes or collagen vascular disease; it may also be seen as a consequence of chest trauma and rarely as a consequence of cardiac surgery (J Cardiovasc Surg (Torino) 2001;42:785). This condition is a mononeuritis multiplex with preservation of all other neurologic functions. Because the intercostal muscles and cervical accessory muscles are intact, the patient may remain ventilator independent while upright but need assistance when lying down. These patients may derive adequate assistance from NIPPV or a portable negative pressure ventilator (Semin Respir Crit Care Med 2002;23:275).

Muscle

Several different muscle diseases can affect the respiratory system. These include acquired illnesses such as *myasthenia gravis, Eaton-Lambert syndrome*, and *dermatomyositis/polymyositis*. Inherited diseases such as the *muscular dystrophies* and congenital diseases such as the *glycogen storage diseases* may also affect respiration. Many of the diseases in this category affect children and adolescents. These illnesses cause respiratory muscle weakness, instability of the upper airway, and heart failure with cardiomegaly. Patients with myasthenia may have myasthenic crisis, which can lead to acute respiratory failure (Semin Neurol 2004;24:75).

Skeletal

Scoliosis and *kyphosis* refer to abnormalities of the thoracic and lumbar spine. Kyphosis refers to anteroposterior angulation of the spine leading to loss of height of the thoracic cage. Scoliosis describes lateral angulation of the spine that leads to loss of height of the thoracic cage. Both of these conditions impede rib mobility and interfere with intercostal muscle function. Scoliosis is often seen in combination with kyphosis. Kyphosis may be seen exclusively as a consequence of vertebral compression fractures. The majority of cases of kyphoscoliosis (KS) are idiopathic and arise in adolescence. A measurement known as the Cobb angle describes the severity of the abnormality. However, the Cobb angle may not necessarily correlate with the degree of respiratory impairment noted. As patients age, the compliance of the chest wall lessens (becomes more stiff), and the effects of the bony abnormality will be amplified. Patients with symptomatic KS will have reduced lung volumes on PFT testing, and hypoxia, hypercarbia, and reduced exercise tolerance may be seen. At least one report describes bronchial torsion as contributing to respiratory difficulty as well (Chest 1997;111:1134). My personal experience and the literature suggest that NIPPV may have a positive impact on blood gases, exercise tolerance, and quality of life of patients with KS (Chest 1988;94:811, Chest 2003;124:857). General reference: (Am Rev Respir Dis 1979;119:643).

Diagnosis: It is uncommon that dyspnea will be the sole presenting complaint of one of these conditions, with the exception of diaphragm paralysis. Patients with insidious spinal cord lesions may ultimately present as dyspnea, and I have had at least one case of undiagnosed ALS referred to me for dyspnea where in retrospect the patient had been having muscle weakness for months. In patients with unexplained dyspnea and reduced vital capacity/total lung capacity, neuromuscular-skeletal disease should be more than a passing consideration.

Treatment: The cornerstones of treatment of neuromuscular-skeletal respiratory disease are:
1. Defend oxygenation.
2. Treat the underlying condition.
3. Provide mechanical assistance to alveolar ventilation.
4. Know when to quit.

Oxygenation is necessary in these conditions as it is in other diseases. Supplemental oxygen in the face of atelectasis and hypoventilation will improve neurological and cardiac function, reduce pulmonary artery pressures, and if administered properly will not cause carbon dioxide retention. The treatment of these conditions varies widely. At present, there is no effective treatment for ALS or muscular dystrophy. Both Guillain-Barré and myasthenia have specific treatment protocols that are beyond the scope of this book. Myasthenia gravis is of particular interest in that patients may enter a crisis with acute respiratory failure. These patients may require temporary ventilatory support. Guillain-Barré patients may need several weeks or months of mechanical ventilation and still regain independent respiration. Initiation of mechanical support, especially in the early stages of an acute illness such as a myasthenic crisis or GB, has been studied extensively. Initial response to progressive illness will be tachypnea, tachycardia, and loss of exercise tolerance. These patients should have their vital capacity measured regularly (if hospitalized, once per day at least), and ventilatory assistance should be considered when the VC drops below 15 ml/kg. If it is possible to measure inspiratory pressures, support should be considered when the patient cannot generate -20 cm H_2O pressure. Hypoxia and hypercarbia are late findings that imply that the patient has lost all ability to compensate; these laboratory values should not be relied upon to signal the need for a measured, unhurried intervention. In addition to ventilation, protection of the upper airway enters into the decision, and aspiration risk rather than ventilatory failure may prompt intubation (Semin Neurol 2003;23:97). In chronic conditions such as ALS and kyphoscoliosis, NIPPV has been studied extensively. NIPPV improves health-related quality of life and probably prolongs life as well. NIPPV should be considered when the patient's $PaCO_2$ is 45 or greater, the patient has sustained (>5 min 88% sat or lower) hypoxia at night, VC is $<50\%$ predicted, or the patient cannot generate -60 cm H_2O inspiratory pressure. Patients with ALS or muscle disease may lose airway control and not be candidates for NIPPV. This is not an issue with KS (Respiration 1994; 61:61, Arch Neurol 2005;62:1194, Chest 2003;124:857).

Patients who recover ventilatory function should be weaned from mechanical ventilation like any other patient. There should be demonstration of adequate strength, oxygenation, CO_2 elimination, and reserve. Airway control (gag, ability to swallow safely) needs to be demonstrated as well. Patients on NIPPV for ALS or muscle disease must make the difficult decision as to whether to proceed to tracheostomy and invasive ventilation. I don't think there's really a right answer here, and the decision depends greatly upon local resources (e.g., there is no nursing home in the state of Maine that can care for a chronic ventilator patient, but we have superlative hospice services), family resources (care providers and financial), other contributing factors to overall quality of life, and personal philosophy. The clinician's duty here, I believe, is to help the patient and his or her family make an informed decision by providing expert technical knowledge interpreted in the context of the clinician's understanding of the patient. The clinician may be called upon for help in timing the withdrawal of care or redirection of care toward comfort only (see **Palliative Care**). How the clinician makes his or her contribution may vary depending upon the beliefs and values of the practitioner; one clinician may be more willing to offer an opinion than another who wishes to remain value neutral.

11.2 Central Sleep Apnea (CSA)

(Chest 2007;131:595)

Epidemiology: Considerably less common than obstructive sleep apnea (OSA); probably ~5% of the incidence of OSA. High prevalence exists in the congestive heart failure population.

Pathophysiology: Unlike OSA, where there is a respiratory effort against a closed airway, in central sleep apnea there is no stimulus to respiration. The phenomenon is due to a faulty feedback loop between respiratory effort and chemoreceptors. Excessive sensitivity of chemoreceptors for oxygen and/or carbon dioxide, reduced cardiac output slowing arterial blood flow reflecting O_2/CO_2 changes, abnormal processing of appropriate signals (impaired central drive), and abnormal environments such as high altitude can precipitate central apnea. State change, the transition from wake to sleep, can change the feedback loop. CSA has multiple subcategories: periodic breathing of altitude, Cheyne-Stokes respiration, obesity hypoventilation syndrome, and narcotic-induced central apnea. Physiologically, CSA can be classified as hypercapneic or nonhypercapneic. Hypercapneic forms include narcotic-induced blunting of respiratory drive and obesity hypoventilation syndrome, defined as obesity (BMI >30) and P_{CO_2} >45 during wakefulness without alternative explanation. Patients with impaired neuromuscular function may also have reduced response to respiratory drive. Nonhypercapneic forms include Cheyne-Stokes respiration with typical crescendo-decrescendo amplitude of respiration and varying frequency of respiration during the cycle. This form is seen particularly frequently in heart failure. There is a small group of individuals who have idiopathic central apnea as well. There is overlap between OSA and CSA; both are disorders of respiratory control, and there is no "steel door" division between the two pathologies. Previously unrecognized concomitant CSA is often apparent on polysomnography once OSA is treated.

Symptoms: Clinical manifestations of CSA are similar to those of OSA with poor sleep and daytime hypersomnolence. I have informally noted a higher incidence of insomnia in this population than in the OSA population. Headaches are common. Evidence of congestive heart failure, obesity, and impaired memory/cognition are seen. See **Obstructive Sleep Apnea** for a discussion of symptoms.

Course and Complications: A query of NLM PubMed did not identify any articles addressing the consequences of CSA. Daytime fatigue, insomnia, disrupted sleep, and effects of hypoxia are likely. Unlike OSA, there is no associated pleural pressure swing or sympathetic burst, which may avoid some of the cardiovascular problems seen with OSA.

Diagnosis: Like OSA, the gold standard of diagnosis is polysomnography. The typical patterns of Cheyne-Stokes respiration or bursts of respiration without intervening episodes of obstruction are, rather than ventilatory failure, easy to identify. Arterial blood gases will identify hypercapnia. Evaluation for congestive heart failure (echocardiography, etc.) may be indicated, and review of the patient's medications is appropriate.

Imaging: Use of imaging techniques is not an integral part of the evaluation of the patient of CSA, except to evaluate and treat related conditions.

Laboratory: Arterial blood gases and thyroid function studies may be helpful.

Treatment: Based primarily on etiology. Best therapy for heart failure–associated CSA is successful treatment of heart failure. Therapy such as resynchronization therapy has been shown to be helpful. Atrial overdrive pacing may be helpful in central apnea, but not in obstructive apnea (N Engl J Med 2002;346:404). Reduction in narcotics may be helpful if narcotic related. Persistent abnormalities are treated by restoring integrity to the feedback loop. Supplemental oxygen can reduce the tendency to oscillation caused by excessive sensitivity of chemoreceptors. Very small increases in CO_2 in inspired air can stimulate chemoreceptors, and this has been tested in several trials. Alteration of acid–base balance with acetazolamide can stimulate respiration. Direct respiratory stimulants such as progesterone can also be used, although men may be quite resistant to using the drug because of side effects. CPAP has been found to be effective in some patients; the mechanism is not known for certain. Bilevel PAP acts as a direct aid to ventilation, but incorrect settings may worsen oscillation if $PaCO_2$ is reduced excessively. In the United States, CMS and other insurers have strict guidelines for the use of NIPPV in CSA. Practitioners should familiarize themselves with local rules and policies (http://reimbursement.respironics.com/downloads/Helpful_Hints_RAD_2006.pdf 2006;2007).

11.3 Obstructive Sleep Apnea (OSA)

Epidemiology: Estimates are that 4% of US men and 2% of US women have OSA. Numbers will almost certainly grow as population ages and average BMI increases. Risk factors for illness include age, male sex, and obesity. OSA is associated with illnesses that have associated craniofacial abnormalities: trisomy 21, acromegaly, hypothyroidism (large tongue), and various congenital craniofacial disorders. Patients with bulbar palsies are also at greater risk. Consensus is that the condition is underdiagnosed and undertreated (only ~10% of patients with apnea are under treatment).

Pathophysiology: Sleep apnea is described as state dependent: it only occurs when sleeping. The primary pathophysiology is that of inadequate stimulation of dilator muscles of the upper airway during sleep, leading to a small airway caliber (Clin Chest Med 2003;24:179). This may occur in the context of an already anatomically abnormal airway, with a long, redundant soft palate, reduced AP diameter of the oropharynx, reduced lateral wall diameter of the oropharynx, large tongue, recessed jaw, or any combination thereof. Small airway caliber in turn increases airflow velocity, further reducing airway caliber by Bernoulli effect (pulls the airway walls inward). Poor muscle tone in the tongue and soft palate may be enhanced by supine position, where both structures fall backwards reducing AP diameter. Cessation of inspiration (apnea) or incomplete cessation of inspiration (hypopnea) triggers a response consisting of an arousal (short return to awake state and interruption of sleep), sympathetic surge, pleural pressure swing, temporary reduction in cardiac output, short period of hypertension, ±hypoxia, and a short period of bradycardia followed by tachycardia. The neural/behavioral consequence is that of sleep fragmentation and interference with normal sleep stage cycling (see **Polysomnography**). Long-term cardiovascular consequences of repetitive episodes of hypoxia, hypertension, sympathetic surge, and varying cardiac output are now recognized, and untreated sleep apnea confers significant increase in risk for MI, stroke, CHF, and hypertension (Clin Chest Med 2003;24:195). Obesity reduces airway caliber by fatty infiltration of the neck and throat structures. Severity of apnea is graded by RDI/AHI (interchangeable terms) indicating number of respiratory events per hour (<5, normal; 5–15, mild; 15–30, moderate; >30, severe). In the United States there are standardized definitions for apnea and hypopnea, and it is expected that interpretation and scoring of PSG will adhere to the definitions. Sleep specialists recognize that increased work of breathing against a partially obstructed airway may cause arousal and the cardiac response described, but without cessation of airflow. These are termed *RERAs* (REspiratory-Related Arousals) but are not counted as apneas or hypopneas for purposes of calculation of RDI. This may cause significant difficulty obtaining treatment for the patient from a third-party payor. A recent development is the formal identification of complex sleep apnea, a condition where the patient presents with obstructive sleep apnea and undergoes treatment with CPAP. While on CPAP, the patient's obstructive events are well controlled but the patient has central apneas as well. While long accepted as coexisting illnesses by clinicians, the entity has gained recognition by Medicare and other insurers, and is now an accepted indication for bilevel NIPPV, including a backup rate if necessary.

Symptoms: Patients with OSA classically present with excessive daytime somnolence. Sleepiness should be differentiated from fatigue; look for problems with staying awake driving, in conferences, and watching TV. The typical patient is obese and snores. A less typical patient may have insomnia. Often there are frequent reports of witnessed apnea from the bed partner and very restless sleep. Interruption of REM and delta sleep may also cause odd nocturnal behaviors such as sleep talking. These are symptoms of sleep deprivation and relate directly to number of arousals. Cardiovascular problems typically include hypertension; severe cases may present as respiratory failure with congestive heart failure or daytime CO_2 retention. Exam of the patient will often demonstrate a short, heavy neck. Oral and pharyngeal findings may include a recessed or small jaw (retrognathia, micrognathia), overbite, a long and redundant soft palate, large tongue, and a small inlet to the posterior oropharynx produced by adipose in lateral walls and/or the abnormal soft palate. Thinner patients with apnea often have an anatomic abnormality such as jaw problems and a high, arched palate. Nasal obstruction is contributory but not causative of apnea, helping make upper airway pressure more negative and prone to collapse.

Complications: Neurobehavioral consequences of apnea include motor vehicle and machinery accidents, depression, poor job performance, impaired sexual performance, poor decision making, and impaired interpersonal relationships. Some patients may experience a reduction in socioeconomic status. Cardiovascular consequences have been recognized more recently. Hypoxia, pleural pressure swings, abnormal sympathetic tone, activation of the inflammatory cascade, and abnormal cardiac loading increase the risk of hypertension, stroke, congestive heart failure, and myocardial infarction. Control of apnea appears to reduce cardiovascular risk (Clin Chest Med 2003;24:195, Clin Chest Med 2003;24:207). Caples (Ann Intern Med 2005;142:187) is a particularly good, succinct review of the abnormal physiology. Sleep apnea has been recognized as a significant surgical anesthetic risk. Preoperative cardiopulmonary dysfunction, difficult airway, rapid desaturation during apnea related to intubation (unfavorable body mass to FRC ratio), and exquisite sensitivity to sedatives, narcotics, and anesthetic agents increase the hazards of providing anesthesia and analgesia to this patient group (Anesthesiology 2006;104:1081).

Diagnosis: Differential diagnosis includes narcolepsy (apnea patients do not have cataplexy, but ~10% of narcolepsy patients have apnea), restless legs/PLMs, and sleep restriction (too little time in bed). Depression, chronic illness, and multiple medications can nonspecifically induce sleepiness. Some patients complain of fatigue and sleepiness but will have relatively normal or minimally abnormal studies. A small number of patients may complain of insomnia, particularly if they awaken repetitively at the beginning of the night. The standard for diagnosis is polysomnography (see **Polysomnography**). Because of the expense involved and lag time to testing, there is interest in identifying individuals who are at high risk for the condition and who can be tested and treated rapidly. One screening tool is the Berlin questionnaire, which has been validated (Ann Intern Med 1999;131:485), and if positive will yield a high percentage (85%) of patients with moderately severe to severe apnea. Other tools are in use as well (Am J Respir Crit Care Med 1994;150:1279). Interest has also been raised regarding a combination of screening, home testing, and home CPAP titration for rapid diagnosis and treatment (Ann Intern Med 2007;146:157). Implementation of this streamlined approach is limited in the United States by the insurers' requirement that full, attended polysomnography documents apnea. Other criteria apply to length of test and severity of disease before equipment is covered by insurance. Presumably, this is to prevent unnecessary testing and incorrect diagnosis. Patients with milder disease may have significant night-to-night variability, and if the test is inconsistent with pretest probability, retesting is warranted (Chest 2000;118:353). Many labs attempt split-night studies: the first half of the night is for diagnosis and severity classification, and the second half of the night is used for fitting and titration of NIPPV. In most labs, approximately 60–70% of patients who ultimately require NIPPV can be diagnosed and titrated in one night. CMS released a decision in March 2008 indicating that it will reimburse unattended home-based sleep studies. Implementation of this decision is under way, and it is likely that local carriers and CMS will pay for home-based sleep studies and accept results from these studies as adequate documentation for the prescription of NIPPV by the end of 2008 at the latest. It is probable that other third-party payors will also pay for this mode of testing and accept the results in the near future.

Imaging: Does not play a major role in initial diagnosis; CT scan of head and cephalometric X-rays for surgical/dental planning may play a role in treatment.

Laboratory: Evaluation of thyroid status is prudent. There are no specific lab abnormalities, but severe cases may have daytime hypercarbia on blood gases.

Treatment: Consists of surgery, dental appliances, and positive pressure airway management. *NIPPV,* either with CPAP or bi-level PAP, is unequivocally effective when tolerated and properly managed. A column of pressurized air is applied to the upper airway, acting as a pneumatic splint to maintain airway patency during inspiration and preventing collapse during expiration. Effective therapy requires coordinated management among the sleep laboratory, equipment provider, and clinician/specialist. Compliance is greatest in patients who experience relief of symptoms in a supportive atmosphere with comfortable, well-adjusted equipment. For this reason, global compliance statistics are misleading: local practice environment can foster very high or very poor compliance. During initiation of therapy, most patients are started on CPAP and may be switched to bi-level PAP for CPAP intolerance, central apnea episodes, or requirement for very high CPAP pressures that are intrinsically difficult to tolerate. Reimbursement plays a large role in management, with many third-party payors requiring evidence of "CPAP failure" prior to permitting the use of a bi-level unit. There are a variety of masks (nasal, full face, nasal pillows that connect directly to nostrils), head straps, connectors, and compressor units so that a patient should be able to be fitted comfortably. Humidification of the air flow improves compliance, and some patients require low-dose nasal steroids to reduce stuffiness and nasal obstruction. Some patients with chronic sinusitis cannot tolerate NIPPV. *Dental appliances* serve to advance the mandible with respect to the maxilla and in so doing move the tongue forward, increasing oropharyngeal caliber. Tolerance is variable, as is efficacy. In general, patients who are thinner, have more positional apnea, and lower AHI tend to do better with this therapy. A variety of mechanisms are available (Clin Chest Med 2003;24:355). *Operative management* is appealing, especially to younger, more mobile patients. However, there is almost universal opinion among pulmonary physicians and sleep specialists that surgical treatment of adult apnea is second-line therapy. Every effort should be made to obtain patient compliance with properly adjusted NIPPV. If this is not possible, a variety of interventions are available including uvulopharyngoplasty, genioglossus and hyoid advancement, and maxillomandibular advancement. The purpose of all of these operations is to reduce anatomic obstruction, either by reducing the size of the soft palate, bringing the tongue forward, or bringing both the maxilla and mandible forward. Surgical techniques include standard surgery, laser-assisted tissue destruction, and radiofrequency ablation. Because UPPP is technically easier and less invasive, it is often attempted first. However, most results indicate that ~50% of patients have an ~50% reduction in AHI (Clin Chest Med 2003;24:365). Sleep specialists will depart from the CPAP first rule when a severe, obvious upper airway abnormality is identified (e.g., kissing tonsils in an adult, severe craniofacial abnormality). Surgery may be a useful adjunct in patients with nasal obstruction (turbinate reduction) (Laryngoscope 2001;111:1783). Surgical planning and intervention are best undertaken by surgeons who have experience in apnea surgery. *Weight loss* is effective in overweight patients, but sustained reduction in BMI is difficult for most patients. Successful therapy of any sort will produce objective, quantifiable reductions in daytime sleepiness and ability to maintain vigilance, cognition, and coordination. Successful therapy is also associated with reduction in cardiovascular risk. While there are no effective medications for reversing the abnormal physiology, there is a subset of patients who, despite appropriate NIPPV therapy, have residual daytime sleepiness. These patients can benefit from the use of stimulants such as dextroamphetamine (10–20 mg/day, often controlled release), methylphenidate (5–40 mg/day as a combination of immediate and controlled release), or modafinil (200 mg/day). These medications should not be instituted until the practitioner is convinced that physiology has been rendered as close to normal as feasible. Management of patients with sleep disorders is challenging; these patients are often noncompliant, unhappy, irritable, and have difficulty comprehending explanations and instructions. There is often conflict with their spouse or partner. Patience, kindness, careful explanations, and a sense of humor can help a patient regain their equanimity and functionality as they undergo therapy.

Chapter 12

Pulmonary Vascular Disease

12.1 Pulmonary Arterial Hypertension and Pulmonary Hypertension (PAH and PH)

Epidemiology: Identification of elevated pulmonary artery pressures is
common, particularly given the widespread use of echocardiography with its ability to perform noninvasive assessment of pulmonary artery pressure by measuring the velocity of tricuspid
regurgitation. Changes in classification and nomenclature make
it difficult to provide precise incidence figures (Clin Chest Med
2007;28:1).

Pathogenesis: Pulmonary hypertension is defined as mean pulmonary
artery pressure greater than 25 mmHg at rest or 30 mmHg during
exercise. The WHO recently (2003) held a conference reclassi-
fying pulmonary hypertension (J Am Coll Cardiol 2004;43:5S).
Rather than primary and secondary PH, the system now defines
types 1 through 5. Type 1 is termed *pulmonary artery hypertension* and is used to describe elevated pulmonary artery pressures
that arise from anatomical abnormalities and dysregulation at
the pulmonary arteriole level. This includes PPH (primary
pulmonary hypertension). Types 2 through 5 are referred to as
pulmonary hypertension. In these groups, the primary defect
occurs outside the pulmonary arteriole and corresponds to what
previously was considered secondary PH. The main values of

this reclassification (to my mind, at least) are twofold: first, it addresses the ambiguous classification of PH produced by some collagen vascular diseases and toxins. Second, it provides a thorough etiologic classification of PAH and PH. Table 12.1 outlines the classification scheme and provides additional relevant information. Pulmonary hypertension places an increased load on the right ventricle, causing right ventricular dilation and a low output state. This in turn produces system venous hypertension with peripheral fluid retention. The low output state produces dyspnea and hypoxia. The mechanism of elevated pulmonary artery pressures varies among the etiologies. Plexogenic arteriopathy is a histologic picture of fibrosis, vessel narrowing, and proliferation that is seen in idiopathic PAH as well as portopulmonary hypertension. The mechanism of the initial medial intimal hypertrophy is unknown. In idiopathic PAH, there is evidence of abnormal bone morphogenetic protein receptor type II (BMPR2) function, and many of these conditions have defects of endothelial regulation and nitric oxide production. Collagen vascular disease injures vessels through fibrosis and medial proliferation. COPD causes pulmonary hypertension through reduction of the total cross-sectional area of the alveolar-capillary bed and by hypoxia. In COPD, pulmonary hypertension appears to correlate more with hypoxia than with structural lung damage. Congenital heart disease and acquired ventricular (and atrial) septal defects produce hypertension by volume overload of the right-sided circulation. Left-sided atrial disease, left-sided valvular disease, and left-sided congestive heart failure increase pulmonary venous back pressure, increase lung water, and produce hypoxia, all of which increase pulmonary artery pressures. Of particular interest is the role of diastolic dysfunction producing elevated pulmonary pressures in the face of seemingly mild left ventricular dysfunction (Int J Cardiol 2007;epub). Thrombotic disease is primarily mechanical obstruction of the vessels with increased back pressure on the right ventricle. Pulmonary veno-occlusive disease

Table 12.1 WHO Classification of Pulmonary Hypertension

Type 1 Pulmonary artery hypertension (add'l diagnostic requirements of mean pulmonary artery pressure >25 mmHg at rest or >30 mmHg with exercise, **AND** pulmonary capillary wedge pressure <15 mmHg, **AND** pulmonary vascular resistance (PVR) >120 dynes/sec/cm^5, **AND** transpulmonary gradient >10 mmHg, defined as the difference between the mean pulmonary arterial pressure and the pulmonary capillary wedge pressure)	Idiopathic	Preponderance in young women
	Familial	Similar molecular defect to idiopathic
	Collagen vascular	Scleroderma, lupus, RA
	Intracardiac shunt	VSD, ASD
	Anorexigens	Fenfluramine, dexfenfluramine, diethylpropion
	Stimulants	Cocaine, amphetamines
	HIV disease	HAART appears to help hemodynamics
	Portal hypertension	Rodriguez-Roisin, 2004, #510
Type 2 Pulmonary hypertension with left heart disease	Left atrial or ventricular disease	Left heart failure, left heart diastolic dysfunction, pericardial disease
	Left-sided valvular disease	Mitral stenosis, regurgitation
Type 3 Pulmonary hypertension associated with lung diseases and/or hypoxemia	COPD	PH correlates with hypoxia
	Interstitial lung disease	PH correlates with hypoxia
	Sleep-disordered breathing	OSA
	Alveolar hypoventilation	Obesity hypoventilation, chronic musculoskeletal disease
	Developmental abnormalities	Eisenmenger syndrome
Type 4 Pulmonary hypertension due to chronic thrombotic and/or embolic disease	Prox. thrombotic occlusion	Acute PE, chronic PE
	Distal thrombotic occl.	Chronic embolization
	Occl. w/ foreign material	Schistosomiasis
Type 5 Pulmonary veno-occlusive disease	Obstruction of large pulmonary veins by fibrosing diseases such as fibrosing mediastinitis, tumor, sarcoidosis, Langerhans histiocytosis	

Note: The far-right two columns describe recognized subgroups, example conditions, and further comments.
Data from Simonneau J Am Coll Cardiol 2004 43(125),55

PULMONARY VASCULAR DISEASE

produces hypertension by extrinsic compression of the pulmonary venous system. This is most easily envisioned with conditions such as fibrosing mediastinitis, where the fibrosis reduces vascular caliber. Irrespective of initial mechanism, the role of hypoxia is fundamental. In the presence of hypoxia, restoration of normal oxygen tensions is the most powerful pulmonary vasodilator available.

Symptoms: The majority of cases of elevated pulmonary artery pressure are in the context of preexisting cardiac or pulmonary illness. The manifestations of pulmonary hypertension may well be dispersed among those of the primary condition. Shortness of breath, peripheral edema, atypical chest pain, reduced exercise tolerance, and hypoxia are all reported. Examination may reveal accentuated pulmonary heart sounds with an enhanced P2 and right-sided heave.

Prognosis and Complications: Elevated pulmonary artery pressures carry a poor prognosis. Survival from sporadic IPAH is poor with 35% 5-year survival in the absence of therapy. Because these patients typically are young, years of potential life lost are great and the effect on young families is difficult. In patients with PH, the prognosis depends upon the underlying condition. Usually, PH is a marker of advanced coexisting disease and the additive effect of the PH may be difficult to isolate. Clinically, patients with PAH and PH have severe and progressive dyspnea, right heart failure, hypoxia, and edema. Their tendency to intrapulmonary thrombosis is considerable, and anticoagulation is recommended (Clin Chest Med 2007;28:1).

Imaging: Attenuated peripheral vascular markings may be seen on plain chest X-ray. CT scan is not recommended for diagnosis of PH or PAH, but on studies conducted for other purposes one may see a large right ventricular cavity or enlarged central pulmonary vessels. Most imaging abnormalities will reflect related pathologic processes such as filling defects in the pulmonary arteries in chronic thromboembolic disease, DPLD, or advanced emphysema.

Laboratory Testing: Pulmonary function testing will reflect a related underlying condition or may show mild restriction. Hypoxia will be present on blood gases, and erythrocytosis may be seen in the CBC. Serologic testing may be appropriate if collagen vascular diseases are suspected. Echocardiography (transthoracic or transesophageal) is the mainstay of noninvasive or minimally invasive diagnosis. The primary parameter studied is that of the tricuspid jet velocity. This investigation has significant limitations and overall is more sensitive than specific. Nonetheless, it is a useful tool for determining who may need more evaluation. Echocardiography may give information regarding the function of other valves, left ventricular function, and any structural abnormalities such as ASD or VSD (Clin Chest Med 2007;28:59). Right heart catheterization (and sometimes pulmonary angiography) may be the definitive procedure(s) used for the diagnosis of PH/PAH or to detect the presence of pulmonary thromboembolic disease.

Diagnosis: Pulmonary hypertension should be considered when patients with predisposing conditions as outlined in Table 12.1 have symptoms in excess of what their pulmonary function tests, cardiac function, or imaging would suggest. These patients should undergo echocardiography. Patients with a familial history should be investigated early in life and monitored to try and limit or delay damage. Sporadic PAH is sometimes difficult to detect but should be considered in a young person (typically but not exclusively female) who complains of atypical chest pain and exercise intolerance. Given the widespread availability and use of echocardiography, it is likely that there will be less delay now than in the past in establishing a diagnosis in these patients.

Treatment: Identification of pulmonary hypertension should elicit the following steps:
1. Identify the underlying cause.
2. Treat the underlying cause.
3. Characterize the severity of the hypertension.

4. Correct hypoxia.
5. Apply standard therapies such as diuresis and digoxin.
6. Consider institution of anticoagulation.
7. Consider the use of pulmonary vasodilators.
8. Consider the use of advanced techniques.

These steps are appropriate regardless of the patient. Table 12.1 should be reviewed and diagnostic/therapeutic steps taken as appropriate given the patient's presentation and known comorbidities. Vasodilator treatment of pulmonary hypertension is complex, and even many pulmonary physicians and cardiologists will defer to subspecialized colleagues. Current agents include calcium channel blockers, oral and parenteral prostanoids, endothelin 1 receptor antagonists, and phosphodiesterase inhibitors. None of these drugs should be initiated by a primary care clinician. Many authorities argue that a patient considered for vasodilator therapy should undergo right heart catheterization and have their response to an intravenous short-acting vasodilator assessed to evaluate for safety and efficacy. Patients who have progressive symptoms and are unresponsive to therapy may be candidates for heart-lung transplantation. Other surgical interventions include atrial septostomy to reduce right heart pressures (Clin Chest Med 2007;28:91, Clin Chest Med 2007;28:117, Clin Chest Med 2007;28:127, Clin Chest Med 2007;28:187). Portopulmonary hypertension requires aggressive therapy of the underlying liver disease. Pulmonary artery hypertension may contraindicate transplantation in patients with advanced liver disease.

12.2 Pulmonary Embolism (PE)

Thrombotic Embolism

Introduction: The prevention, diagnosis, and treatment of deep venous thrombosis and pulmonary embolism have been and remain one of the most vexing endeavors of modern clinical medicine. The condition is associated with significant morbidity and mortality, and missed diagnosis can have disastrous consequences but so can unnecessary treatment. Symptoms are nonspecific. Tests are expensive, have limited specificity and sensitivity, and occasionally are dangerous. Treatment is prolonged, expensive, and subject to complication. As technology has changed and improved, successive studies have provided increasingly accurate algorithms for diagnosis. Treatment and prophylaxis have benefitted from new means of anticoagulation, and there is an enhanced recognition of the dangers of heparin-induced thrombocytopenia (HIT).

Epidemiology: The true incidence of pulmonary embolism is unknown, but the condition is common, and particularly so in patients ill enough to require hospitalization. A large proportion of events are clinically inapparent and/or undiagnosed/misdiagnosed, probably on the order of 50%, and several hundred thousand episodes of PE are identified each year. The incidence of deep venous thrombosis is even higher. Risk is higher in the specific clinical conditions that are enumerated below.

Pathogenesis: Thrombotic pulmonary embolism is the consequence of an intravascular blood clot breaking off from its site of origin and depositing in the pulmonary circulation. The physiologic consequences of deposition in the pulmonary vasculature are complex. The total cross-sectional area of the pulmonary vasculature increases as the number of subdivisions of the arteries increases. This means that a clot with a cross-sectional area of 2 cm^2 lodging in the main pulmonary artery will have a different effect on pulmonary artery pressure and load placed on the right ventricle than the same clot lodging 3 or 4 generations more distal. There can be a direct loading effect on the right ventricle, causing acute pulmonary hypertension, acute right heart strain, and/or failure with a large proximal clot. Blockage of a pulmonary artery will create wasted ventilation, with no blood flow to areas of persistent ventilation. Patients who accumulate multiple small distal emboli may gradually develop pulmonary hypertension and chronic right heart failure. Acute obstruction of a pulmonary artery may lead to severe tissue hypoxia of the affected lung and produce pulmonary infarction. After thinking about this for a few minutes, the reader will identify a number of inconsistencies that imply that the embolism must have more than mechanical effects. First, the lung at rest has a great potential for recruitment: why should an embolism lodging in a segmental artery cause dyspnea and hypoxia? Why shouldn't the lung simply recruit inactive gas exchange units and take up the slack? Second, the lung has a dual circulation, with pulmonary and bronchial circulations. Why should lung infarction be possible? Third, why do patients wheeze and cough and complain of chest pain in the absence of tissue hypoxia? The answer to these questions lies in viewing the embolism as more of a chemical bomb thrown at the lungs rather than just an inert slug shot from the legs. The thrombus is rich in fibrin degradation products, by-products of the clotting cascade, and many mediators of inflammation. The effects of these substances may include bronchospasm, vasospasm, and other less definable consequences. Physiologic effects of embolism include hypoxemia, altered V/Q relationships, pulmonary tissue hypoxia, bronchospasm, pulmonary hypertension, right heart strain, and outright right heart failure.

Pulmonary emboli derive from thrombi. Most clinically significant emboli arise in either the thigh or pelvic veins; a smaller number can arise from more distal leg veins, the right heart, or the upper extremities. It should be noted, however, that most *thrombi* (as opposed to *emboli*) will arise in the distal legs, distal to the popliteal fossa. Propagation of clot into the proximal lower extremity increases the risk of embolization. Detection of extremity thrombi is achieved primarily with ultrasound and Doppler studies. Pelvic veins are more difficult to evaluate, but some information can be derived from ultrasound and Doppler imaging. The 1999 ATS statement on diagnosis of venous thromboembolism is dated with respect to the embolism workup, but quite useful in terms of detection and evaluation of thrombosis (Am J Respir Crit Care Med 1999;160:1043). Venous thrombosis is a result of Virchow's triad of venous stasis, tissue trauma, and hypercoagulable state. Risk factors for venous thrombosis are in Table 12.2.

Symptoms: Clinical manifestations of pulmonary embolism are non-specific. The most common symptoms are dyspnea, chest pain, cough, and hemoptysis. Signs often include tachycardia, tachypnea, and rales in the affected area. Hypotension or shock is uncommon; most patients who have an embolism large enough to cause shock die before they get to medical attention. However, when hypotension is present in the context of PE, it is a grave prognostic sign and requires immediate intervention. The accuracy of clinical examination to determine the presence or absence of lower-extremity deep venous thrombosis is that of a coin toss: 50%.

Table 12.2   Risk Factors for Deep Venous Thrombosis

Immobilization
Surgery within the last 3 months
Stroke
History of venous thromboembolism
Malignancy
Preexisting respiratory disease
Chronic heart disease
Factor V Leiden mutation
Antithrombin deficiency
Protein S deficiency
Protein C deficiency
Collagen vascular disease (e.g., lupus anticoagulant)
Additional risk factors identified in women:
   Obesity (BMI 29 kg/m)
   Heavy cigarette smoking (>25 cigarettes per day)
   Hypertension
   Pregnancy

PULMONARY VASCULAR DISEASE

Prognosis and Complications: The majority of patients who suffer PE and survive to reach medical attention recover without pulmonary sequelae. The number of patients who do not survive to reach medical attention is thought to be anywhere between 20% and 50% of patients with this diagnosis. Resolution of embolism often takes 2–3 months even with consistently therapeutic anticoagulation. A small percentage of patients go on to have nonresolution of clot leading to chronic pulmonary thromoboembolic disease and pulmonary hypertension. Patients who do not resolve their pulmonary symptoms after 2–3 months of therapy should undergo further imaging to determine if vascular filling defects are still present. Selected patients in this group may benefit from pulmonary endarterectomy, and all should be on indefinite anticoagulation (Eur Respir J 2004;23:637). This condition is one of the few causes of pulmonary hypertension that is curable. Deep venous thrombosis injures leg veins, causes venous incompetence, and predisposes to further thrombotic events. Chronic problems may warrant compression stockings and/or vascular surgical consultation.

Imaging: Chest X-ray may show a variety of findings. The classic description is that of atelectasis and elevation of a hemidiaphragm. Other findings may include an infiltrate in the area of infarction, and rarely it is possible to see an area of hypoperfusion manifesting as hyperlucency. Plain chest X-ray provides little diagnostic information in PE except to determine if another process is responsible for the patient's complaints or to identify a comorbid condition. Spiral CT scan of the chest with intravenous contrast bolus is the primary imaging modality for PE in many (if not most) centers in the United States. A good technical quality study permits identification of cutoff signs in the pulmonary arteries and visualizing filling defects. Originally, CT angiography was thought to approach conventional angiography in sensitivity and specificity. This is probably not the case. However, studies and meta-analyses should be interpreted with caution as to precise figures as scanner technology and interpreter/ operator skill have improved rapidly over the last 10 years. For many years, V/Q scanning was used as a means of evaluating for pulmonary embolism. The limitations of this test have been recognized for decades, and optimal use of a suboptimal test culminated in the PIOPED studies (JAMA 1990;263:2753). V/Q scan results are reported as normal, low probability, indeterminate, and high probability. A normal scan virtually excludes PE, irrespective of pretest probability. A high probability scan is also of significant value in the context of a high pretest probability. Low and intermediate probabilities do not have good predictive value and are dependent on pretest probability; many patients go on to have further testing with low or intermediate probability tests. Venous imaging with ultrasound can be used as an adjunct to the diagnosis of PE. Sensitivity and specificity are in the 95% range in patients who are not excessively obese. Attempts to optimize use of these tests are discussed in greater detail in the diagnosis section.

Laboratory: A variety of laboratory abnormalities may be seen in PE including elevations of the BNP and troponin, and elevated WBC. These are not useful and may be misleading. The test of greatest interest is the D-dimer, which is a by-product of fibrinogen to fibrin conversion. The test is intellectually appealing in that it should have elevated levels in the presence of clot formation. However, many inflammatory states, injury, infection, and recent surgery all may elevate the D-dimer, rendering its specificity close to useless (particularly given characteristics of the at-risk patients). However, a normal D-dimer titer assures that PE is not present. This high-quality negative predictive value will be employed in the diagnostic strategies outlined below.

Diagnosis: PE should be considered clinically in the context of sudden onset of pulmonary symptoms such as chest pain, dyspnea, or cough. The diagnosis should be considered seriously if the patient has predisposing factors. Wells et al. developed bedside criteria for estimating the likelihood of pulmonary embolism that have been validated repeatedly. These are outlined in Table 12.3. This ability to identify patients who have a high pretest probability and low pretest probability of having PE permits much more cost-effective and safe testing by following this general algorithm: If the pretest probability is low, and the test is conclusively negative, PE can be excluded. If the pretest probability is high, and testing is conclusively positive, it is safe to assume that the patient has PE and should be treated. If pretest probability is in the middle ground, a conclusively positive or negative group of test results is effective in making a final diagnosis. Discordant or persistently indeterminate test results dictate further testing and/or continued observation. A recent paper by Huisman et al., the Christopher Study group (JAMA 2006; 295:172), offers an elegant approach to diagnosis that couples the predictive power of two noninvasive evaluations, the application of the Wells criteria and the D-dimer, to exclude from further testing patients who do not require imaging or further testing. This algorithm is outlined in Figure 12.1. Although many hospitals

Table 12.3 Wells Criteria to Determine Probability of Pulmonary Embolism

Clinical Finding	Point Value
Sx and symptoms of deep vein thrombosis (min. of leg swelling, pain to palpation of deep veins)	3
Alternative diagnosis less likely than PE	3
HR >100/min	1.5
Immobilization >3 d or surgery in prev. 4 wks	1.5
Previous PE or DVT	1
Hemoptysis	1
Active malignancy (under Rx **OR** Rx in last 6 mo. **OR** undergoing palliation	1

Note: Add together point value for all true statements. If score ≤4, PE is unlikely. If score >4, PE is likely.
Data from Wells, Ann Int Med 1998 129(12);997

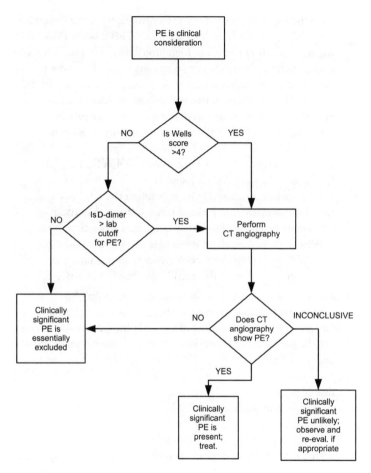

Figure 12.1 Decision algorithm for diagnosis of pulmonary embolism based on Well criteria, D-dimer, and CT angiography. Data from Huismann et al., 2006. (See text for citation.)

have the capability to perform CT angiography, many organizations still need to rely on V/Q scanning. This test has value when the result is either normal or high probability; a normal V/Q scan excludes clinically significant pulmonary embolism, and a high-probability scan with a high pretest probability confirms the presence of PE. The decision tree becomes more difficult within the extremes of range because V/Q scanning does not provide a yes/no answer, and the utility of the answer depends upon the pretest probability. A second decision tree, based upon V/Q scanning as the primary imaging test, is provided in Figure 12.2 (J Thromb Haemost 2007;5 Suppl 1:41). Sensitivity and specificity values are discussed in more detail in the reference materials. Occasionally, the question is not if the patient had a pulmonary embolism, but if they need anticoagulation. If the patient is physiologically stable and it is easier to make a diagnosis of deep venous thrombosis rather than pulmonary embolism, proof of venous thrombosis may be all that is necessary.

Treatment: Treatment of pulmonary embolism relies on physiologic support, prevention of further embolic events, and clot lysis. Depending upon the severity of the embolism, ICU level of care may be necessary including vasopressors, supplemental oxygen, and mechanical ventilation. Volume resuscitation may also be necessary to provide adequate right heart filling pressures in the face of pump failure and poor venous return. Prevention of further embolism depends on long-term anticoagulation and on lysis of existing clot.

Interruption of the clotting cascade initially with heparin or a similar drug followed by warfarin is the most common approach to treatment. By preventing coagulation, fibrinolytic mechanisms are permitted to work unopposed on an existing clot and promote clot lysis. Additionally, further thrombus formation is prevented. Unfractionated heparin is inexpensive and effective. However, continuous infusion, difficulty achieving goals of anticoagulation,

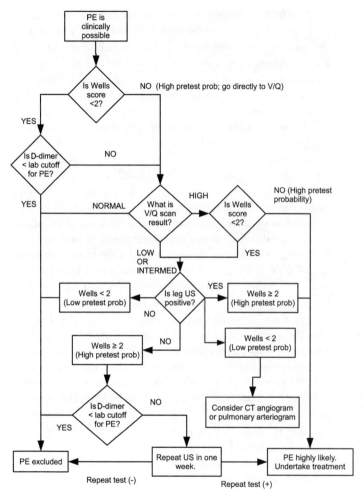

Figure 12.2 Algorithm for diagnosis of PE based on V/Q scanning. Data from Wells, 2007.

12.2 Pulmonary Embolism **451**

need for frequent laboratory testing to monitor the activated PTT, and heparin-induced thrombocytopenia (HIT) can make the use of heparin cumbersome and occasionally dangerous. For this reason, many authorities recommend the use of low-molecular-weight heparin (LMWH) for uncomplicated venous thrombosis and patients with pulmonary embolism who are physiologically stable. LMWH is very appealing in that dosing is simple, therapy consists of one or two subcutaneous injections per day, and in patients with normal renal function no laboratory monitoring is required. Unfractionated heparin continues to be recommended for patients with renal insufficiency (due to lack of widespread fast assays for Factor Xa inhibition needed for LMWH monitoring needed in renal disease) and patients who are hypotensive or otherwise compromised (absorption of SC injectate is unpredictable because of poor cutaneous blood flow). Unfractionated heparin also makes sense if interruption of anticoagulation for further invasive procedures is anticipated in the near term or there is concern that the patient is at high risk for bleeding complications. LMWH can be administered at home, and has the advantage of safety in pregnancy (as opposed to warfarin). Currently available LMWH products include enoxaparin, tinzaparin, nadroparin, and dalteparin. Fondaparinux is a synthetic heparin-like drug that has efficacy similar to that of LMWH preparations. The risk of HIT is diminished with fondaparinux. The FDA indications for individual LMWH preparations and fondaparinux is changing rapidly as new information becomes available. Current dosing guidelines and indications should be reviewed before prescribing.

HIT is a feared complication of heparin use. Type I HIT is a transient, modest drop in platelet count that often resolves spontaneously. Type II HIT is an immunologically mediated form of disseminated intravascular coagulation and requires immediate anticoagulation with a non-heparin agent such as argatroban or lepirudin. Warkentin provides an excellent overview (Chest 2004;126:311S). Warfarin (trade name Coumadin, so common it is subject to the "Kleenex" effect) is an oral or IV vitamin K antagonist used for long-term use. It is an effective agent but requires sustained monitoring. For this reason, many communities have instituted warfarin-management clinics. The major complications of warfarin use include bleeding (for the life of me I don't understand why the FDA has a black box warning on Coumadin that an anticoagulant can cause life-threatening bleeding) and skin necrosis. Despite these concerns, many patients on warfarin go on to have effective anticoagulation with few side effects and a low hassle factor. Most authorities recommend 3 months of anticoagulation for DVT/PE with a clearly defined etiology and where the risk factor has resolved (e.g., young otherwise healthy person with PE from a broken leg and casting). Six to 12 months of anticoagulation is recommended for the *first* event of DVT/PE where an etiology cannot be identified. Indefinite (i.e., permanent) anticoagulation is recommended where the patient has repeated episodes of DVT/PE without obvious etiology or where an irreducible risk (Factor V-Leiden deficiency, protein S, C deficiencies) has been identified. Anticoagulation should be initiated with a heparin-type product (or another acutely acting anticoagulant such as fondaparinux, lepirudin, or argatroban) and continued for 5–10 days. Coumadin should not be started for at least 3 days, and heparin should be continued until therapeutic levels of vitamin K inhibition (measured by prothrombin time and INR) are achieved and sustained (Chest 2004;126:401S).

Venal caval interruption with a filter mechanism (Greenfield filter) may be indicated in certain clinical situations. These filters do not prevent all clots, and if the filter is obstructed with a heavy clot burden, collateral circulation may carry clots through other vessels. However, it will be able to prevent a large, potentially clinically significant clot from reaching the pulmonary circulation. Filter deployment is recommended without controversy in patients who have an absolute contraindication to anticoagulation, who have further embolic events in the face of adequate anticoagulation, or patients who develop severe bleeding complications during anticoagulation. Many practitioners will also arrange for filter placement if there is a sense that the patient would suffer severe physiologic compromise or death if they were to sustain any further embolic events. Typically, this candidate is a patient with limited physiologic reserve at the outset and has a substantial clot burden. This indication is somewhat more controversial, but is generally accepted. Filters appear to reduce short-term risk of PE. Patients with and without vena caval filters have similar 2-year mortalities, and patients with filters may have a higher rate of IVC thrombosis (Br J Haematol 2006;134:590, J Vasc Interv Radiol 2003;14:425, N Engl J Med 1998;338:409).

The most controversial aspect of treatment concerns thrombolysis and the treatment of patients who sustain massive PE (defined as PE with systolic systemic BP <90 mmHg). Most patients with massive PE die before reaching medical care. A small number of patients will have varying forms of severe physiologic compromise but survive to receive care. Clot thrombolysis with either systemic or catheter-directed thrombolytics (tPA, streptokinase, etc.) has been studied. Potential indications include sustained hypotension (systolic <90 mmHg), refractory hypoxemia, very large perfusion defect, right ventricular dysfunction, and free-floating RV thrombus. Most authorities agree that persistent hypotension is an indication for therapy, but that the other indications should be invoked on a case-by-case basis. Unlike anticoagulation, which sometimes should be undertaken presumptively pending confirmatory testing, the risks associated with thrombolytic therapy are high enough to require confirmation of the diagnosis prior to treatment. Thrombolysis for DVT alone is actively discouraged with the exception of extensive clot burden producing severely impaired venous return from the limb(s) (phlegmasia cerulea dolens). Consideration of thrombolysis should prompt automatic consultation with someone experienced in ICU care and thrombolytic management. Thrombolysis does appear to offer short-term benefits, but group mortality was similar to that of patients treated with heparin alone. Systemic therapy rather than catheter-directed therapy is currently recommended (Chest 2004;126:401S, Circulation 2006;113:577). My own view is that subgroup analysis has not yet identified those individuals who will benefit.

Prevention of venous thrombosis so as to avoid the problem of PE altogether is an important component of therapy. Risk of DVT in hospitalized patients ranges anywhere from 10–80% depending upon risk factors and underlying conditions. Current agents include low-dose unfractionated heparin, LMWH, warfarin, fondaparinux, and venous compression devices applied to the lower extremities. The choice of agent/modality, duration of therapy, intensity of anticoagulation, observed risk reduction, and complication rates varies widely among risk groups, so much so that it is difficult to present this information succinctly. We strongly recommend DVT prophylaxis in patients with high-risk conditions such as prolonged critical illness, major trauma, acute spinal cord injury, and major orthopedic procedures. We strongly recommend DVT prophylaxis in virtually any patient who will be bedridden for more than 48 hours. We further recommend that if your hospital does not have individualized protocols in place for DVT prophylaxis in specific conditions, they should be created. This will permit the best application of an evidence-grounded, diagnosis-based approach to your entire patient population. Current comprehensive, evidence-based recommendations are available in Geerts (Chest 2004;126:338S).

Other Embolic Phenomena

Septic Embolism

Septic emboli are foci of metastatic infection in the lung. The nidus of infection may be infected thrombus or simply a bolus of bacteria or fungi. Typically, these patients will be physiologically unstable with fever and other manifestations of systemic infection. Chest X-ray may show single (usually multiple), round, poorly marginated fluffy infiltrates. Cavitation may be present. This X-ray appearance has a specific differential diagnosis (see **Cavity**). If embolism is a consideration, evaluation for an endovascular focus (right heart endocarditis, IV catheter infection, intravenous drug use) is appropriate. Other etiologies should be sought if an endovascular source is not identified immediately (Circ J 2007;71:772).

Amniotic Fluid Embolism

This is a life-threatening complication of pregnancy and delivery where amniotic fluid enters the maternal circulation. This event causes hypoxia, ARDS, and circulatory collapse. Stated mortality is as high as 90%, and there is no specific therapy except support. Amniotic fluid embolism typically occurs at or just after delivery, and should be in the differential diagnosis of a postpartum woman with hypoxia and circulatory collapse. Although much of the debris in the amniotic fluid is trapped by the lung, an immunologic response leads to catastrophic consequences. Thankfully, this is a rare condition (AANA J 2003;71:120).

Fat Embolism

Fat embolism syndrome occurs when marrow fat enters the circulation. This is often a consequence of long bone or pelvic fractures, occasionally associated with sickle cell crises as well. Overall incidence in long bone fractures is uncommon, probably 3% or less. The clinical syndrome includes hypoxia and diffuse pulmonary infiltrates. Because some fat enters the systemic circulation as well, neurologic abnormalities and a petechial rash may be seen. Treatment consists primarily of support, and early immobilization of a fracture will reduce the incidence of a fat embolism event. Some authors recommend prophylactic methylprednisolone in the context of a high-risk injury (Orthopedics 1996;19:41).

12.3 Sickle Cell Anemia and the Lung

Am J Respir Crit Care Med 2001;164:2016, Postgrad Med J 2003;79:384

Epidemiology: Sickle cell anemia (sickle cell disease, SCD) is a hemoglobinopathy seen (in the United States, at least) overwhelmingly in patients of African descent (of the five sickle hemoglobin haplotypes, four are African and one is Arab-Indian). Sickle trait is present in 30–40% of black Americans, and disease is present in ~1 in 600 African-Americans. SCD is a cause of morbidity and premature mortality.

Pathogenesis: A complete discussion of the sickle cell hemoglobinopathy, genetics, and mechanisms of sickling are beyond the scope of this book. (N Engl J Med 1999;340:1021 and N Engl J Med 1997;337:762 are two excellent reviews for further reading about SCD molecular biology.) SCD disease affects all organ systems. Pulmonary problems are common and are the greatest cause of fatality in this disease. The lungs are affected through a variety of mechanisms. Pulmonary vaso-occlusion gives rise to infarction and severe pain. Bony infarction may cause fat emboli when outside the chest, and rib infarction may lead to atelectasis and hypoventilation. Areas of poorly perfused and damaged tissue make the lung susceptible to infection, and chronic splenic infarction may lead to the equivalent of autosplenectomy, enhancing susceptibility to infection by encapsulated organisms such as *S. pneumoniae*. Long-term pulmonary injury from vaso-occlusive events may lead to pulmonary hypertension and pulmonary fibrosis. Although clinical manifestation of disease is uncommon in patients with sickle cell trait, sudden death has been reported in patients undergoing intense physical training such as that seen in the military or correctional "boot camps."

Symptoms: The most serious pulmonary manifestation of sickle cell disease is acute chest syndrome, defined as chest pain, fever, and a new pulmonary infiltrate on chest X-ray. Many times it is impossible to say whether the episode is infarction, infection, embolization, or some combination of all three. Most episodes are precipitated by infection, fat embolism, or infarction when an etiology can be identified. There are multiple triggers to vaso-occlusion and infarction, including dehydration, exercise, hypoxia, etc. Patients with acute chest syndrome can go on to become severely ill, with some series quoting an ~10–15% incidence of intubation and mechanical ventilation. Patients who have bony chest wall pain will complain of chest pain, but fever and infiltrate will be absent. Patients who suffer repetitive episodes of vascular and parenchymal injury will have obliteration of their alveolar-capillary bed with pulmonary hypertension and fibrosis. These patients will have a course typical of end-stage pulmonary hypertension and pulmonary fibrosis with progressive dyspnea, abnormal chest X-ray and CT scan, and evidence of right heart failure (Medicine (Baltimore) 1988;67:66). Some authors describe an increased incidence of reactive airway disease, and sleep apnea is noted with increased frequency in the pediatric population.

Course and Prognosis: Patients with SCD have many organs involved and many complications. Survival to the 5th or 6th decade is more common now than in the past with better understanding of pathophysiology and treatment (such as hydroxyurea). It is thought that ~4–5% of patients with SCD go on to have severe SCD chronic lung disease.

Imaging: Depending upon the acute problem and/or phase of disease, an X-ray picture may vary widely with infiltrates, atelectasis, and fibrosis dominating. Increased pulmonary vasculature and an enlarged cardiac silhouette is also possible.

Laboratory: Acute chest syndrome may demonstrate hypoxia. Laboratory assessment cannot be used to reliably distinguish between baseline sickling and acute chest syndrome and/or crisis. Reduced pulmonary function (low DLCO, reduced lung volumes) is common and can be progressive. As indicated above, obstructive lung disease and reactive airway disease is seen with increased frequency in this population.

Differential Diagnosis: Adult patients will present with an established diagnosis of SCD, so de novo diagnosis is not an issue. It is not possible to distinguish between infarction and infection. Although sickle cell disease does not provide immunity from other forms of pulmonary fibrosis or pulmonary hypertension, it is generally a safe assumption that an SCD patient with pulmonary fibrosis and/or hypertension can attribute those problems to his or her SCD.

Treatment: Treatment of an acute chest syndrome episode is supportive with prevention of hypoxia (critical to prevention of further sickling), judicious hydration (overhydration may cause pulmonary edema), and empiric antibiotics. Control of pain with opioid analgesia is also standard and critical. Patients with progressive respiratory failure may benefit from exchange transfusion. Hydroxyurea therapy has been shown to reduce the number and severity of crises. Other important prophylactic measures include appropriate vaccinations and penicillin prophylaxis. The treatment of pulmonary hypertension and pulmonary fibrosis is supportive; no specific therapies have been identified.

12.4 Pulmonary Arteriovenous Malformations (AVMs)

Am J Respir Crit Care Med 1998;158:643

Epidemiology: This is an uncommon condition, presented primarily for interest. Pulmonary AVMs are closely associated with hereditary hemorrhagic telangectasia (HHT, also referred to as Osler-Weber-Rendu disease). If there is an affected family in the community, local incidence may be high.

Pathogenesis: Pulmonary AVMs are low-resistance connections between the arterial and venous pulmonary circulations. No gas exchange occurs as blood travels through the AVM, creating an anatomic right to left shunt. Consequences of these connections include (in extreme situations) high-output cardiac failure, chronic hypoxia, cyanosis, polycythemia, and poor exercise tolerance. The AVM bypasses the filtering function of the capillary bed, and both stroke and brain abscess have been described in this condition. The cause of AVM is unknown. Approximately 70% of patients with pulmonary AVM have HHT. These patients have systemic manifestations of HHT including GI AVMs, mucosal and skin telangectasias, brain AVMs, and epistaxis (N Engl J Med 1995; 333:918). Most AVMs are macroscopic and discrete. A small number of patients have a syndrome of diffuse, small AVMs that are difficult to identify and almost impossible to treat.

Symptoms: Surprisingly, the most common symptom is not pulmonary, but epistaxis because this is the most common manifestation of HHT. Patients with pulmonary involvement may have cyanosis, high-output heart failure, hemoptysis, and exercise intolerance. Hemothorax has been reported but is not common. Other manifestations of HHT such as GI bleeds and oral bleeding may bring the patient to attention.

Prognosis and Complications: These patients have a poor prognosis and a high rate of complication. In untreated patients, mortality has been described as high as 15% in some series, and post-mortem examination has shown evidence of cerebral infarction as high as 30% or 40%. AVMs tend to enlarge with age, rendering insignificant lesions as potential sources of hazard (Mayo Clin Proc 1999;74:671). As indicated above, brain infarction, brain abscess, massive hemoptysis, and hemothorax are the most dangerous complications.

Imaging: The majority (90%+) of patients with pulmonary AVM have some form of imaging abnormality. The classic chest X-ray finding is that of a nodule with enlarged, abnormal vessels connecting it to the hilum. More typically, the patient will have a smooth-bordered nodule (or nodules). CT imaging may then show feeder vessels. Often there are more AVMs identified on CT scan than on X-ray. Perfusion scanning of the lung may be dramatic with high concentrations of radionuclide in the AVMs. Magnetic resonance imaging is still under study.

Laboratory: A number of other tests may be of use. Hypoxemia and erythrocytosis may be present. Contrast echocardiography will detect intrapulmonary shunting very effectively (Am Heart J 2001;141:243). Shunt may also be detected clinically by having the patient breath 100% oxygen with a tightly fitting mask for 15–20 minutes and then performing the following calculation (QS/QT is shunt fraction) (Thorax 1968;23:563):

$$QS/QT = ((Pa_{O_2} - Pa_{O_2}) \times 0.003) / (((Pa_{O_2} - Pa_{O_2}) \times 0.003) + 5)$$

Pa_{O_2} is measured by blood gas.
$Pa_{O_2} = F_{IO_2} \times (P_{ATM} - P_{H_2O}) - (Pa_{CO_2}/R) + (Pa_{CO_2} \times F_{IO_2} \times (1 - R)/R)$. However, when the patient is breathing 100% oxygen $R = 1$ and $F_{IO_2} = 1$. The equation simplifies to:
$Pa_{O_2} = (P_{ATM} - P_{H_2O}) - Pa_{CO_2}$
$P_{ATM} = 760 \text{ mmHg} \times e^{(-\text{altitude in meters}/7000)}$
$P_{H_2O} = 47 \text{ mmHg} \times e^{((\text{Pt. temp in celsius}-37)/18.4)}$

A shunt fraction of >5% is abnormal.

Diagnosis: Typically, patients with HHT are diagnosed early in life on the basis of their family history and bleeding episodes. Occasionally, the diagnosis will be missed until adulthood. Patients with pulmonary AVMs alone may be asymptomatic, and the AVM is discovered by chest X-ray for another purpose. The AVM is often fully characterized with CT scan. Other patients may require perfusion scanning or even angiography to identify the lesion. AVM is in the differential diagnosis of solitary pulmonary nodule, and an SPN that appears particularly vascular on CT should be treated with some respect before biopsy. Other patients may present with progressive signs and symptoms of respiratory distress from the large shunt fraction and high cardiac output; investigation then reveals the cause of the exercise intolerance.

Treatment: The treatment of these lesions is controversial. There is agreement among authorities that AVMs with large (>2–3 mm diameter) feeder vessels should be treated as these lesions are prone to complication. Some authorities recommend treatment of *all* identifiable lesions; this is a minority view. Current therapy consists of embolization with a detachable balloon catheter or deployment of steel coils; other materials are used as well (J Vasc Interv Radiol 2006;17:35). Surgery is possible for these lesions, but it would appear that it is currently not the preferred method of intervention. Hormonal therapy is useful in HHT but has not been studied extensively with respect to pulmonary results. Bilateral lung transplantation can be considered for severe disease that is unresponsive to therapy. The anatomic shunt produced by the AVM puts the patient at risk for air embolism during IV therapy and paradoxic embolism from venous thrombosis and/or embolism.

Bibliography

Textbooks

Zackon, H. *Pulmonary Differential Diagnosis*. WB Saunders, 2000. ISBN 0-7020-2577-1. This unrecognized gem is out of print. If you can get a copy, do so. Excellent for running the gamut of diseases and making sure that you've covered all bases. (I included the ISBN number to help you hunt for the book online)

Mason, Broaddus, Murray, and Nadel. *Murray and Nadel's Textbook of Respiratory Medicine*, 4th ed. Elsevier Saunders, 2005. There are several multiple volume texts of respiratory medicine. Murray and Nadel has a lot of pathophysiology and thus wins my nod.

Fraser, Muller, Colman, and Pare. *Fraser and Pare's Diagnosis of Diseases of the Chest*, 4th ed. Saunders, 1999. Most pulmonary physicians and radiologists consider this four-volume set the authoritative text for pulmonary differential diagnosis and imaging. If you can't find it described in Fraser and Pare, it likely doesn't happen. A new edition is imminent.

Webb, Muller, and Naiditch. *High-Resolution CT of the Lung*, 3rd ed. Lippincott Williams Wilkins, 2001. Specialized text devoted to high-resolution CT scanning of the lungs; very useful for diffuse parenchymal lung disease problems.

Kryger, Roth, and Dement. *Principles and Practice of Sleep Medicine*, 4th ed. Elsevier Saunders, 2005. Authoritative text on sleep medicine.

Electronic

UpToDate, www.uptodate.com. If you have the money to buy only one book or subscription, buy this. Far and away the most useful, practical source of information for self-education and care of patients. I use it almost daily.

PubMed, www.ncbi.nlm.nih.gov/sites/entrez. This is the portal to the National Library of Medicine. It has become increasingly easy to use and productive as the search engine has improved. Use the Limits function.

CDC, www.cdc.gov. Treasure trove of information regarding infectious disease and public health.

NHLBI, www.nhlbi.nih.gov. Home page of the National Heart, Lung, and Blood Institute of the NIH. Many asthma resources are available here in electronic format, as well as information about other cardiovascular and pulmonary conditions.

www.pneumotox.com. Resource for possible pulmonary toxicity from drugs.

www.clinicaltrials.gov. Worldwide directory of clinical trials, searchable by disease, organ systems. Links provided to eligibility criteria, enrollment mechanisms, etc.

Journals

Important Basic and Clinical Research

American Journal of Respiratory and Critical Care Medicine

Annals of Internal Medicine

Chest

European Respiratory Journal

New England Journal of Medicine

Thorax

Review-Oriented Publications

Clinics in Chest Medicine

Critical Care Clinics

Seminars in Respiratory and Critical Care Medicine

Index